6/98

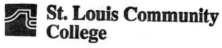

PHYSICIAN-ASSISTED SUICIDE

Medical Ethics Series
David H. Smith and Robert M. Veatch, Editors

Norman L. Cantor. *Advance Directives and the Pursuit of Death with Dignity*

Norman L. Cantor. *Legal Frontiers of Death and Dying*

Arthur L. Caplan. *If I Were a Rich Man Could I Buy a Pancreas? And Other Essays on the Ethics of Health Care*

James F. Childress. *Practical Reasoning in Bioethics: Principles, Metaphors, and Analogies*

Cynthia B. Cohen, ed. *Casebook on the Termination of Life-Sustaining Treatment and the Care of the Dying*

Cynthia B. Cohen, ed. *New Ways of Making Babies: The Case of Egg Donation*

Roger B. Dworkin. *Limits: The Role of the Law in Bioethical Decision Making*

Larry Gostin, ed. *Surrogate Motherhood: Politics and Privacy*

Christine Grady. *The Search for an AIDS Vaccine: Ethical Issues in the Development and Testing of a Preventive HIV Vaccine*

A Report by the Hastings Center. *Guidelines on the Termination of Life-Sustaining Treatment and the Care of the Dying*

Paul Lauritzen. *Pursuing Parenthood: Ethical Issues in Assisted Reproduction*

Joanne Lynn, M.D., ed. *By No Extraordinary Means: The Choice to Forgo Life-Sustaining Food and Water, Expanded Edition*

William F. May. *The Patient's Ordeal*

Richard W. Momeyer. *Confronting Death*

Thomas H. Murray, Mark A. Rothstein, and Robert F. Murray, Jr., eds. *The Human Genome Project and the Future of Health Care*

S. Kay Toombs, David Barnard, and Ronald Carson, eds. *Chronic Illness: From Experience to Policy*

Robert M. Veatch. *The Patient as Partner: A Theory of Human-Experimentation Ethics*

Robert M. Veatch. *The Patient-Physician Relation: The Patient as Partner, Part 2*

Robert F. Weir, ed. *Physician-Assisted Suicide*

PHYSICIAN-ASSISTED SUICIDE

ROBERT F. WEIR, EDITOR

INDIANA UNIVERSITY PRESS
Bloomington and Indianapolis

The paper used in this publication meets the minimum requirements of American National Standard for Information Sciences—Permanence of Paper for Printed Library Materials, ANSI Z39.48–1984.

Manufactured in the United States of America

Library of Congress Cataloging-in-Publication Data

Physician-assisted suicide / Robert F. Weir.
    p.   cm. — (Medical ethics series)
Includes index.
ISBN 0-253-33282-6 (cl : alk. paper)
1. Assisted suicide. 2. Assisted suicide—United States.
I. Weir, Robert F., date   II. Series.
R726.P49   1997
179'.7—dc21   96-49417

2   3   4   5   02   01   00   99   98

CONTENTS

PREFACE   *Robert F. Weir*   vii

Part I. Historical Interpretations

1. The Significance of Inaccurate History in Legal Considerations of Physician-Assisted Suicide   3
   Darrel W. Amundsen
2. Doctors and the Dying of Patients in American History   33
   Harold Y. Vanderpool

Part II. Ethical Assessments and Positions

3. Self-Extinction   69
   The Morality of the Helping Hand
   Daniel Callahan
4. Physician-Assisted Suicide Is Sometimes Morally Justified   86
   Dan W. Brock

Part III. Medical Practices and Perspectives

5. Physician-Assisted Suicide Is *Not* an Acceptable Practice for Physicians   107
   Ira R. Byock
6. Assisting in Patient Suicides *Is* an Acceptable Practice for Physicians   136
   Howard Brody

Part IV. Potentially Vulnerable Patients

7. Physician-Assisted Death in the Context of Disability   155
   Kristi L. Kirschner, Carol J. Gill, and Christine K. Cassel

8.   Physician-Assisted Suicide, Abortion, and Treatment   167
     Refusal
     Using Gender to Analyze the Difference
     Susan M. Wolf

     Part V. Public Policy Options and Recommendations

9.   Considerations of Safeguards Proposed in Laws and   205
     Guidelines to Legalize Assisted Suicide
     Steven Miles, Demetra M. Pappas, and Robert Koepp
10. Physician-Assisted Suicide   224
     Evolving Public Policies
     William J. Winslade

APPENDIXES
  People v. Kevorkian, Supreme Court of Michigan, 1994   243
  Compassion in Dying v. State of Washington, United States 246
     Court of Appeals, Ninth Circuit, 1996
  Quill v. Vacco, United States Court of Appeals, Second   253
     Circuit, 1996
CONTRIBUTORS   257
INDEX   259

PREFACE

Robert F. Weir, Ph.D.

Physician-assisted suicide (PAS) is one of the perennial ethical problems in medicine. A frequently quoted portion of the Hippocratic Oath is the sentence that declares, "I will neither give a deadly drug to anybody if asked for it, nor will I make a suggestion to this effect."[1] This statement, written in Greece sometime during the fifth to fourth centuries B.C.E., has had considerable influence in the history of Western medicine, with that influence increasing over the past two centuries as modern medical societies, both national and international, have again drafted professional codes of ethics. The oath set forth a normative view of physician conduct that came to transcend the time, place, and religious beliefs ("I swear by Apollo Physician and Asclepius and Hygieia and Panaceia and all the gods and goddesses . . .") of its author(s).[2] A central feature of that normative view was that physicians were neither to cause nor to help bring about the ultimate harm that could befall their patients, namely the patients' deaths.

This ancient code of medical ethics, frequently cited by modern physicians as though it represents universal truths, was actually a minority statement at the time of its origin. Physicians in ancient Greece, having a status similar to other itinerant craftsmen, were poorly equipped to relieve the suffering of persons who turned to them for help. Very often, it seems, such persons regarded suicide as a means of escaping painful illness and the suffering that accompanied dying. A widespread method of committing suicide was by taking poison, and a common practice involved getting a poisonous solution from someone identifying himself as a physician.[3–8] In this context, the Hippocratic Oath represented an effort by an apparently small group of physicians to build public trust and respectability by distancing themselves from other physicians who would sometimes assist seriously ill persons to commit suicide by giving "a deadly drug . . . if asked for it."

Now, once again, PAS is a major ethical issue in medicine, as well as an issue that involves law and public policy. With media attention being focused on medical and legal cases connected with Jack Kevorkian, M.D., a retired pathologist in Michigan, and Timothy Quill, M.D., an internist in New York, PAS has become an issue of substantial public interest.[9] It is also an issue that has become the subject of significant professional interest on the part of physicians, biomedical ethicists, and health-law attorneys.[10-19] The American Medical Association has developed a policy opposing PAS, as have the American Geriatrics Society and the National Hospice Organization.[20-22] The interdisciplinary Society for Health and Human Values has published a thoughtful, well-balanced document that addresses many of the factors that make PAS a complex issue that divides physicians, other health care professionals, and the general public.[23]

Six aspects of this debate over PAS are worth noting at the beginning of this book. First, considerable *conceptual confusion* clouds the debate about PAS. Some conceptual clarity can be gained by pointing out that an assisted suicide involves someone (a patient or other person outside a clinical setting, or a patient in a clinical setting) who has suicidal motives, intends to die, wants to do something to cause his or her death, and is noncoerced in deciding to kill himself or herself. In contrast to "normal" suicides, an assisted suicide requires aid from a relative or friend, a physician, or some other person who carries out the role of "enabler." The enabler can assist the suicidal person in any number of ways: by supplying information on the most effective ways of committing suicide, purchasing a weapon of self-destruction, providing a prescription for a lethal dose of pills, or helping the suicidal individual in the actual act of killing (e.g., by helping the person close the garage doors, turn on the gas, or take the pills). Nevertheless, the person who carries out the act of self-destruction is the person who wants to die. When a physician is in the role of enabler, he or she typically receives a request by a patient for assistance in committing suicide, assesses the patient's medical condition (including, one hopes, the possibility of depression), makes the difficult decision to help the suicidal individual, and then responds to the request for assistance by providing a potentially lethal prescription as well as information on how to use the prescription to achieve the patient's desired goal of death.[24]

Second, reasonable persons disagree about *whether acts of PAS,* at a conceptual level, *are different* from (a) acts of abating life-sustaining treatment and/or (b) acts of voluntary euthanasia. Several of the authors in this volume disagree on this point, especially as it pertains to suicidal persons with disabilities, as do some of the major court decisions on PAS. Lest this point of disagreement seem to be conceptual only, it is also important in terms of political strategy. Proponents of legalizing PAS in the states of Washington and California failed in statewide referenda earlier this decade at least in part because they lumped PAS with voluntary euthanasia under the category of "aid in dying," whereas proponents of legalizing PAS in Oregon succeeded in part because they did not include euthanasia as part of the referendum. In addition, it is also the case that however the acts of abating life-sustaining treatment, PAS, and voluntary euthanasia are framed conceptually, there continues to be a serious, ongoing debate about whether significant *moral differences* exist among these actions. On this question, as well, several of the authors in this volume disagree.

Third, as PAS is discussed in the multidisciplinary professional literature, at medical conferences, by the courts, in state legislatures, and in conversations among citizens, there is disagreement and uncertainty about the *kinds of medical conditions* that might convince some persons that death, whatever it may mean, is preferable to the agonizing suffering they currently experience. Three actual case descriptions may be helpful.

(a) The British Columbia Case of Sue Rodriguez:

> The facts of this case are straightforward and well known. Sue Rodriguez is a 42-year-old woman living in British Columbia. She is married and the mother of an 8-year-old son. Ms. Rodriguez suffers from amyotrophic lateral sclerosis (ALS), which is widely known as Lou Gehrig's disease; her life expectancy is between two and 14 months but her condition is rapidly deteriorating. Very soon she will lose the ability to swallow, speak, walk and move her body without assistance. Thereafter, she will lose the capacity to breathe without a respirator, to eat without a gastrostomy and will eventually become confined to a bed. Ms. Rodriguez knows of her condition, the trajectory of her illness and the inevitability of how her life will end; her wish is to control the circumstances, timing and manner of her death. She does not wish to die so long as she still has the capacity to enjoy life. However, by the time she no longer is able to enjoy life, she will be physically unable to terminate her life without assistance. Ms. Rodriguez seeks an order which will allow a qualified medical practitioner to set up technological means by which she might, by her own hand, at the time of her choosing, end her life.[25]

(b) The New York Case of "Jane Doe," according to her court declaration:

> I have a large cancerous tumor which is wrapped around the right carotid artery in my neck and is collapsing my esophagus and invading my voice box. The tumor has significantly reduced my ability to swallow and prevents me from eating anything but very thin liquids in extremely small amounts. The cancer has metastasized to my plural [sic] cavity and it is painful to yawn or cough. . . . In early July 1994 I had the [feeding] tube implanted and have suffered serious problems as a result. . . . I take

a variety of medications to manage the pain. . . . It is not possible for me to reduce my pain to an acceptable level of comfort and to retain an alert state. . . . At this time, it is clear to me, based on the advice of my doctors, that I am in the terminal phase of this disease. . . . At the point at which I can no longer endure the pain and suffering associated with my cancer, I want to have drugs available for the purpose of hastening my death in a humane and certain manner. I want to be able to discuss freely with my treating physician my intention of hastening my death through the consumption of drugs prescribed for that purpose.[26]

(c) The New York Case of William Barth, according to his court declaration:

In May 1992, I developed a Kaposi's sarcoma skin lesion. This was my first major illness associated with AIDS. I underwent radiation and chemotherapy to treat this cancer. . . . In September 1993, I was diagnosed with cytomegalovirus ('CMV') in my stomach and colon which caused severe diarrhea, fevers and wasting. . . . In February 1994, I was diagnosed with microsporidiosis, a parasitic infection for which there is effectively no treatment. . . . At approximately the same time, I contracted AIDS-related pneumonia. The pneumonia's infusion therapy treatment was so extremely toxic that I vomited with each infusion. . . . In March 1994, I was diagnosed with cryptosporidiosis, a parasitic infection which has caused severe diarrhea, sometimes producing 20 stools a day, extreme abdominal pain, nausea and additional significant wasting. I have begun to lose bowel control. . . . For each of these conditions I have undergone a variety of medical treatments, each of which has had significant adverse side effects. . . . While I have tolerated some [nightly intravenous] feedings, I am unwilling to accept this for an extended period of time. . . . I understand that there are no cures. . . . I can no longer endure the pain and suffering . . . and I want to have drugs available for the purpose of hastening my death.[27]

Fourth, considerable attention has been given in recent years to the *attitudes of physicians* toward PAS. What do physicians (especially family-practice doctors and internists) think about the morality of PAS, the possible legalization of such practices, and their own personal involvement in responding affirmatively to requests by their patients for assistance in committing suicide? Some surveys of physicians' attitudes have focused on physicians in medical specialties most likely to receive patient requests for PAS.[28–31] Other surveys have concentrated on physicians in particular states. For example, a survey of physicians in Washington State found that 50 percent of the respondents regard PAS as sometimes ethically justified and 40 percent would be willing to help a patient commit suicide, with a slightly smaller number (42 percent and 33 percent) expressing the same views toward euthanasia.[32] A subsequent survey of physicians in Washington State found that 12 percent of responding physicians (in family practice and internal medicine) had received one or more explicit requests for PAS, that they could provide 207 case descriptions (largely of patients with cancer, AIDS, or neurological diseases), that 24 percent of the patients (38 of 156 patients) requesting PAS had received prescriptions (21 patients died as a result), that 58 patients had requested euthanasia and 14 of them died after receiving parenteral medication, and that patients requesting PAS and euthanasia had a number of nonphysical concerns (e.g., losing control, being a burden, loss of dignity, and being dependent on others for personal care) in addition to their medical problems.[33]

Surveys of physicians in several other states have yielded similar results. A survey by the Massachusetts Medical Society found that 43 percent of the physicians favored legalizing PAS and 54 percent said that if the actions were legal, they would consider participating in cases of PAS; a survey of physicians in New Hampshire had similar results on the question of legalization, with 19 percent of the physicians indicating that they would consider participating in PAS even if such actions remain illegal.[34] Among Michigan physicians, 56 percent of the physicians surveyed indicated that they would prefer legalization of PAS to a legal ban of the practice, with 35 percent reporting that they would consider participating in PAS if it were legal.[35] Among Oregon physicians, 60 percent of the physicians stated that they thought PAS should be legalized, 21 percent of them said that they had previously received requests for PAS, and 7 percent indicated that they had complied with such a request.[36] By contrast, a survey of Iowa physicians found closely divided opinion, with 51 percent opposing PAS and 49 percent supporting it in some cases.[37] In Rhode Island, 88 percent of the physicians surveyed indicated that they would *not* engage in PAS, with most of them giving religious beliefs as the reason for their opposition to PAS.[38]

Fifth, surveys focusing on the *attitudes of the general public* show considerable support for PAS, for physicians who engage in assisted suicide, and for the legalization of PAS. For example, a compilation of the results from twenty-one national opinion surveys on end-of-life questions spanning forty years demonstrated that persons surveyed over the years increasingly have supported the legalization of treatment abatement, PAS, and voluntary euthanasia.[39] A survey of older adults in the United States found that 41 percent of the respondents support the legalization of PAS.[40] In Michigan, 66 percent of the public supports the legalization of PAS, and in Iowa, 51 percent of the public supports making PAS a legal option for patients and physicians.[41–42]

A study at the University of Iowa focused specifically on the attitudes of patients. When asked about the role of physicians in assisting some of their patients to commit suicide, 91 percent of the adult family-practice patients indicated that they think a physician who assists with suicide is a caring person, 85 percent said that such a physician would still be able to offer emotional support to surviving family members, and 90.5 percent stated that a physician who had engaged in PAS would be as trustworthy as any other physician in providing care for them in the event of critical illness. Only 5 percent indicated that they would probably change physicians if they discovered their physician had assisted in a patient's suicide.[43]

Sixth, *legal developments* are decidedly mixed. In Michigan, the controversial actions of Jack Kevorkian have resulted in an ongoing debate in the state legislature regarding the legality of Dr. Kevorkian's participation in the multiple cases (forty-six cases as of this writing) of persons who have sought his help in their deaths. In addition, the Michigan legislature passed a temporary statute banning PAS (the statute is now defunct), the Michigan Supreme Court ruled on the constitutionality of the statute (see an excerpt in the appendix), and three unsuccessful efforts have been made to convict Dr. Kevorkian of murder. In New York, the actions of Timothy Quill have resulted in grand jury hearings, a state medical society review, a trial court decision, and an influential decision on PAS by the U.S. Court of Appeals, Second Circuit (see the appendix). In Oregon, the citizens voted to legalize PAS in a 1994 referendum. The ensuing legislation, known as the "Oregon Death with Dignity Act," was subsequently challenged in court and held unconstitutional by the U.S. District Court of Oregon.[44] This decision was overturned by the U.S. Court of Appeals, Ninth Circuit, when the full panel of justices upheld a lower court decision in Washington (*Compassion in Dying v. State of Washington*) that found that state's ban of PAS unconstitutional. The Ninth Circuit specifically stated that the Oregon court's decision "is directly contrary to our holding" (see the appendix).[45] In the majority of states (thirty-two states at current count), PAS remains illegal based on either specific statutes or common law. Because of this mixed legal picture, the U.S. Supreme Court may decide to address the constitutional issues posed by PAS by taking one or more of these appellate-level cases on appeal.

The chapters in this book are intended to shed light and perspective on the issue of PAS. The authors were selected not only because of their experience and scholarship, but also because they would be able to provide readers with differing points of view on a complex subject. Writing from professional backgrounds in history, medicine, philosophy, religion, and law, the authors provide us with essays characterized by careful analysis, experienced insight, solid scholarship, and strong, sometimes passionate arguments.

Part I contains two historical interpretations that set the stage for the rest of the book. Darrel W. Amundsen, Ph.D., begins the volume by focusing on the views regarding the morality of suicide and assisted suicide that were dominant during the periods of classical antiquity and early Christianity, thereby demonstrating that some contemporary court decisions misinterpret those ancient views. Harold Y. Vanderpool, Ph.D., then describes a variety of traditional American views toward suffering and dying persons, including quite different views about the appropriate roles of physicians in relieving suffering and providing aid during the dying process.

Part II addresses the question of whether PAS is morally justifiable in individual cases. Daniel Callahan, Ph.D., argues that individual cases of PAS are frequently not morally justifiable and, further, that the acceptance of PAS will unfortunately lead to a general acceptance of voluntary euthanasia as well. For Dan W. Brock, Ph.D., individual cases of PAS are more easily justifiable, depending on the facts in such cases, because they promote individual self-determination and individual well-being; he is convinced, contrary to Callahan, that a general acceptance of PAS and voluntary euthanasia would be beneficial for our society.

Part III focuses specifically on the roles of physicians who have to decide, in at least some cases, whether they are morally obligated to take on the role of "enabler" when requested by one or more of their patients, or whether they are morally and legally obligated to turn down such requests. The chapters are written by two practicing physicians who have had leadership roles in several organizations (e.g., the Academy of Hospice and Palliative Medicine, the Michigan State Medical Society) that have wrestled with the issue of PAS in recent years. Ira R. Byock, M.D., argues that PAS is not an acceptable practice for physicians. In making his argument, Byock develops an alternative model for physicians who want to meet the needs of their suffering patients with appropriate end-of-life care. Howard Brody, M.D., Ph.D., agrees on the importance of palliative care at the end of life but argues that physicians are morally obligated to relieve their patients' suffering and to respect the autonomous choices of their patients even when, in a few cases, the patients choose to move beyond hospice care to request PAS.

Part IV focuses on persons with disabilities and women who may, at least in some cases, be inclined to request assistance in committing suicide because of serious problems connected with their disabilities or gender: their more limited options, their imposed roles and socialization, their feelings of dependency, or the quality-of-life judgments made about them by other people. Kristi L. Kirschner, M.D., Carol J. Gill, Ph.D., and Christine K. Cassel, M.D., argue that before physicians carry out requests for PAS from persons with disabilities, the physicians should carefully consider a number of factors related to those persons' perceived quality of life—not merely respond affirmatively to what seems like an autonomous choice for death. Susan M. Wolf, J.D., then addresses the issue of gender as it relates to decisions about PAS, arguing against the grounding of a right to PAS in rights to abortion (as the Ninth Circuit did) and the abatement of treatment (as the Second Circuit did).

Part V addresses PAS as an issue of law and public policy. Steven Miles, M.D., Demetra M. Pappas, J.D., and Robert Koepp, M.A., argue that current proposals to legalize PAS do not contain adequate safeguards and that once the medical profession is legally empowered to engage in an action whose central purpose is to cause death, substantial guidelines will be necessary to protect patients and minimize abuses. William J. Winslade, J.D., Ph.D., concludes the discussion of PAS by proposing that the laws that currently criminalize PAS be revised so that physicians willing to participate in PAS would have a legal excuse to engage in such actions in limited circumstances, thereby avoiding criminal liability.

Several persons need to be acknowledged for their help along the way to the completion of this book. Dan Brock, Richard Caplan, Diane Meier, and Steve Miles read an early proposal for the book and gave me instructive suggestions for improvement. Robert Sloan, my editor at Indiana University Press, and David Smith and Robert Veatch, the series editors, also made helpful suggestions that improved the book. Melanie DeVore did the word-processing of the manuscript—with patience, understanding, and an endlessly cooperative spirit. Jerry Weir, my wife, participated in numerous conversations on the subject of PAS, a subject that most of us would surely choose not to dwell on for very long, or very often. To each of these persons, my sincere thanks.

NOTES

1. Tom L. Beauchamp and James F. Childress, *Principles of Biomedical Ethics,* 2d ed. (New York: Oxford University Press, 1983), p. 329.

2. Stanley J. Reiser, Arthur J. Dyck, and William J. Curran, eds., *Ethics in Medicine: Historical Perspectives and Contemporary Concerns* (Cambridge, Mass.: MIT Press, 1977), p. 3.

3. L. T. Cowley, E. Young, and T. A. Raffin, "Care of the Dying: An Ethical and Historical Perspective," *Critical Care Medicine* 20 (1992): 1473–82.

4. Danielle Gourevitch, "Suicide among the Sick in Classical Antiquity," *Bulletin of the History of Medicine* 43 (1969): 501–18.

5. W. B. Fye, "Active Euthanasia: An Historical Survey of Its Conceptual Origins and Introduction into Medical Thought," *Bulletin of the History of Medicine* 52 (1978): 492–502.

6. Paul Carrick, *Medical Ethics in Antiquity* (Dordrecht: D. Reidel, 1985).

7. John M. Cooper, "Greek Philosophers on Euthanasia and Suicide," in Baruch A. Brody, ed., *Suicide and Euthanasia: Historical and Contemporary Themes* (Dordrecht: Kluwer, 1989), pp. 9–38.

8. Darrel W. Amundsen, "The Physician's Obligation to Prolong Life: A Medical Duty without Classical Roots," *Hastings Center Report* 8 (1978): 23–30.

9. David A. Kaplan, "Is It a Wonderful Life?" *Newsweek*, April 15, 1996, p. 62.

10. Sidney H. Wanzer et al., "The Physician's Responsibility toward Hopelessly Ill Patients: A Second Look," *New England Journal of Medicine* 320 (1989): 844–49.

11. Timothy E. Quill, "A Case of Individualized Decision Making," *New England Journal of Medicine* 324 (1991): 691–94.

12. Timothy E. Quill, "Doctor, I Want to Die. Will You Help Me?" *JAMA* 270 (1993): 870–73.

13. Edmund D. Pellegrino, "Compassion Needs Reason Too," *JAMA* 270 (1993): 874–75.

14. Christine K. Cassel and Diane E. Meier, "Morals and Moralism in the Debate over Euthanasia and Assisted Suicide," *New England Journal of Medicine* 323 (1990): 750–52.

15. David Orentlicher, "Physician Participation in Assisted Suicide," *JAMA* 262 (1989): 1844–45.

16. Yale Kamisar, "Are Laws against Assisted Suicide Unconstitutional?" *Hastings Center Report* 23 (1993): 32–41.

17. Howard Brody, "Assisted Death—A Compassionate Response to a Medical Failure," *New England Journal of Medicine* 327 (1992): 1384–88.

18. Ira R. Byock, "The Euthanasia/Assisted Suicide Debate Matures," *American Journal of Hospice and Palliative Care* (March–April 1993): 8–11.

19. Franklin G. Miller et al., "Regulating Physician-Assisted Death," *New England Journal of Medicine* 331 (1994): 119–23.

20. Council on Ethical and Judicial Affairs of the American Medical Association, *Code of Medical Ethics* (Chicago: American Medical Association, 1994–95 edition), p. 51.

21. Ethics Committee of the American Geriatrics Society, "Physician-Assisted Suicide and Voluntary Active Euthanasia," *Journal of the American Geriatrics Society* 43 (1995): 579–80.

22. Ethics Committee of the National Hospice Organization, *Proactive Responses to the Euthanasia/Assisted Suicide Debate* (Washington, D.C.: National Hospice Organization, in press).

23. Report of the Task Force on Physician-Assisted Suicide of the Society for Health and Human Values, "Physician-Assisted Suicide: Toward a Comprehensive Understanding," *Academic Medicine* 70 (1995): 583–90.

24. Robert F. Weir, "The Morality of Physician-Assisted Suicide," *Law, Medicine and Health Care* 20 (1992): 116–26.

25. Rodriguez v. British Columbia, 107 DLR4th 342, 349 (1993).

26. Quill v. Vaaco, 1996 WL 148605 (2nd Cir. [N.Y.]).

27. Ibid.

28. C. Crosby, "Internists Grapple with How They Should Respond to Requests for Aid in Dying," *Internist* 33 (1992): 10.

29. P. V. Caralis and J. S. Hammond, "Attitudes of Medical Students, Housestaff, and Faculty Physicians toward Euthanasia and Termination of Life-Sustaining Treatment," *Critical Care Medicine* 20 (1992): 683–90.

30. L. Slome et al., "Physicians' Attitudes toward Assisted Suicide in AIDS," *Journal of Acquired Immune Deficiency Syndrome* 5 (1992): 712–18.

31. David J. Doukas et al., "Attitudes and Behaviors on Physician-Assisted Death: A Study of Michigan Oncologists," *Journal of Clinical Oncology* 13 (1995): 1055–61.

32. J. S. Cohen et al., "Attitudes toward Assisted Suicide and Euthanasia among Physicians in Washington State," *New England Journal of Medicine* 331 (1994): 89–94.

33. Anthony L. Back et al., "Physician-Assisted Suicide and Euthanasia in Washington State," *JAMA* 275 (1996): 919–25.

34. Diane M. Gianelli, "Survey Yields Admissions of Doctor-Assisted Suicide," *American Medical News,* October 10, 1994, p. 6.

35. Jerald G. Bachman et al., "Attitudes of Michigan Physicians and the Public toward Legalizing Physician-Assisted Suicide and Voluntary Euthanasia," *New England Journal of Medicine* 334 (1996): 303–309.

36. Melinda A. Lee et al., "Legalizing Assisted Suicide—Views of Physicians in Oregon," *New England Journal of Medicine* 334 (1996): 310–15.

37. Tom Carney, "Assist Suicide? Doctors Narrowly Split," *Des Moines Register,* March 17, 1996, p. 1A.

38. T. R. Fried et al., "Limits of Patient Autonomy: Physician Attitudes and Practices Regarding Life-Sustaining Treatments and Euthanasia," *Archives of Internal Medicine* 153 (1993): 722–28.

39. Robert J. Blendon, Ulrike Szalay, and Richard Knox, "Should Physicians Aid Their Patients in Dying?" *JAMA* 267 (1992): 2658–62.

40. Larry Seidlitz et al., "Attitudes of Older People toward Suicide and Assisted Suicide: An Analysis of Gallup Poll Findings," *Journal of the American Geriatrics Society* 43 (1995): 993–98.

41. Bachman et al., "Attitudes of Michigan Physicians," pp. 303–309.

42. Thomas A. Fogarty, "Most Iowans Oppose Law Banning Assisted Suicide," *Des Moines Register,* April 6, 1996.

43. Mark A. Graber et al., "Patients' Views About Physician Participation in Assisted Suicide and Euthanasia," *Journal of General Internal Medicine* 11 (1996): 1–6.

44. Lee v. State of Oregon, 891 F.Supp. 1429 (D.Or. 1995).

45. Compassion in Dying v. State of Washington, 1996 WL 94848 (9th Cir. [Wash.]), p. 33.

Part I

Historical Interpretations

1

THE SIGNIFICANCE OF INACCURATE HISTORY IN LEGAL CONSIDERATIONS OF PHYSICIAN-ASSISTED SUICIDE

Darrel W. Amundsen, Ph.D.

History and the Courts

Justice Blackmun, writing in 1973 for the majority in Roe v. Wade, says, "we have inquired into, and in this opinion place some emphasis upon, medical and medical-legal history and what that history reveals about man's attitudes toward the abortion procedure over the centuries."[1] In his dissent, Justice Rehnquist compliments the majority's bringing "to the decision of this troubling question both extensive historical fact and a wealth of legal scholarship."[2] More recently, in his 1993 "Opinion and Order concerning the Constitutionality of the Michigan Statute Proscribing Assisted Suicide" in the ongoing legal saga of retired pathologist Jack Kevorkian, Michigan Circuit Court Judge Richard C. Kaufman writes, "Most strikingly, in Roe v. Wade . . . the Court justified its result, in part, by an appeal to history. . . ."[3] Kevorkian had insisted that a right to commit suicide is fundamental to those liberty interests protected by the Fourteenth Amendment. Judge Kaufman writes, "The prosecutor argues that a right cannot be deemed fundamental, and thus entitled to protection through the 'liberty' provision of the Fourteenth Amendment, unless it is based upon our Nation's history and tradition. In contrast, the defendant insists that history and tradition can be completely ignored in distilling the existence of a fundamental liberty interest. This Court rejects both approaches."[4]

In order to arrive at this decision, Judge Kaufman felt it incumbent

3

"to analyze whether the claimed right is 'deeply rooted in this Nation's history and traditions.'"[5] After mentioning that "Many commentators . . . have disputed the Roe Court's historical analysis," he asseverates: "To the extent that Roe's historical analysis is not totally accurate, the decision is grounded more in a contemporary view of what is 'implicit in the concept of ordered liberty.'"[6] Hence, it is reasonable to assume that in formulating his own legal opinion Judge Kaufman would (1) be very cautious in accepting as "totally accurate" the Roe Court's historical analysis; and (2) be extremely thorough in his own historical research so as to ensure that his own historical analysis be "totally accurate." He concludes his historical analysis with the exclamation, "It is striking that so much of the historical analysis of the Roe Court with respect to abortion mirrors historical traditions with respect to suicide."[7]

Greece and Rome

Judge Kaufman writes, "Just as the Roe Court found some support for abortion being freely practiced in Greek and Roman times, there is significant support that historical attitudes toward suicide were not in line with a blanket proscription. The idea that one's honor or one's quality of life would allow society to recognize the act of suicide as not contrary to societal norms has great historical support."[8] The "great historical support," which Judge Kaufman marshals in reference to ancient attitudes toward suicide, is a popularized account written by a poet, literary critic, and writer of fiction and screenplays, Alfred Alvarez.[9]

Judge Kaufman asserts, "Much of what we know about Greek society supports the conclusion that suicide in many circumstances was acceptable." In support of this statement he quotes Alvarez:

> Plato . . . suggested that if life itself became immoderate, then suicide became a rational, justifiable act. Painful disease or intolerable constraint were sufficient reasons to depart. . . . Within a hundred years of Socrates' death, the Stoics had made suicide into the most reasonable and desirable of all ways out.[10]

"These attitudes toward suicide," Judge Kaufman writes, "continued during Roman times." He again quotes Alvarez:

> The evidence is, then, that the Romans looked on suicide with neither fear nor revulsion, but as a carefully considered and chosen validation of the way they had lived and the principles they had lived by. . . . According to Justinian's *Digest,* suicide of a private citizen was not punishable if it was caused by "impatience of pain or sickness, or by

another cause," or by "weariness of life . . . lunacy, or fear of dishonor." Since this covered every rational cause, all that was left was the utterly irrational suicide "without cause," and that was punishable. . . .[11]

After summarizing and quoting from Alvarez's assessment of the effect of Christianity on Western attitudes toward suicide, Judge Kaufman quotes from Roe v. Wade: ". . . only the Pythagorean school of philosophers frowned upon the related act of suicide." He then says:

> The Roe Court goes on to determine that the Pythagorean school was a minority view, and "'[i]n no other stratum of Greek opinion were such views held or proposed in the same spirit of uncompromising austerity.'[12] . . . Edelstein then concludes that the Oath originated in a group representing only a small segment of Greek opinion and that it certainly was not accepted by all ancient physicians. He points out that medical writings down to Galen (A.D. 130–200) 'give evidence of the violation of almost every one of its injunctions.' But with the end of antiquity a decided change took place. Resistance against suicide and against abortion became common. The Oath came to be popular. The emerging teachings of Christianity were in agreement with the Pythagorean ethic. The Oath 'became the nucleus of all medical ethics' and 'was applauded as the embodiment of truth.' Thus, suggests Dr. Edelstein, it is 'a Pythagorean manifesto and not the expression of an absolute standard of medical conduct.'"[13]

The Roe Court's dependence on Edelstein is unfortunate, for Edelstein was somewhat of an iconoclast. While his analysis of the so-called Hippocratic Oath is the fruit of exquisitely competent classical scholarship, his support of his thesis of the Pythagorean authorship of the oath, which is now accepted by few, if any, specialists in ancient medical history,[14] suffers from the inevitably debilitating effects of special pleading. Alvarez's amateurish survey is rife with minor errors of fact. Nevertheless, what Judge Kaufman provides from Alvarez and from Justice Blackmun is accurate insofar as it conveys the fact that throughout classical antiquity there was *no blanket prohibition of either abortion or suicide*. It should be stressed, however, that in classical antiquity there also was a strong, though minority, view that would sanction abortion and suicide *only under the most circumscribed conditions*. Much evidence for that position can be found outside the oath.[15]

Early Christianity

While Justice Blackmun's and Judge Kaufman's assessments of suicide in classical antiquity are merely simplistic, the latter's analysis of suicide in early Christianity is blatantly inaccurate.[16] He maintains:

> Presently, the teachings of mainstream Christian and Judaic faith find
> suicide anathema. Yet, Alvarez points out that this was not always the
> case: "The idea of suicide as a crime comes late in Christian doctrine, and
> as an afterthought. It was not until the sixth century that the Church
> finally legislated against it, and then the only Biblical authority was a
> special interpretation of the Sixth Commandment: 'Thou shalt not kill.'
> The bishops were urged into action by St. Augustine; but he, as Rousseau
> remarked, took his arguments from Plato's *Phaedo,* not from the
> Bible."[17]

Judge Kaufman next observes:

> Alvarez indicates that when the Christian Church decided to adopt a
> prohibition on suicide it had a difficult time in supporting this new
> position on the basis of the Scriptures: "They also reflect the difficulty
> the Church had in rationalizing its ban on suicide, since neither the Old
> nor the New Testament directly prohibits it. There are four suicides
> recorded in the Old Testament—Samson, Saul, Abimelech and
> Achitephel—and none of them earns adverse comment. In fact, they are
> scarcely commented on at all. In the New Testament, the suicide of even
> the greatest criminal, Judas Iscariot, is recorded as perfunctorily; instead
> of being added to his crimes, it seems a measure of his repentance. Only
> much later did the theologians reverse the implicit judgment of St.
> Matthew and suggest that Judas was more damned by his suicide than
> by his betrayal of Christ. In the first years of the Church, suicide was such
> a neutral subject that even the death of Jesus was regarded by Tertullian,
> one of the most fiery of early Fathers, as a kind of suicide."[18]

Judge Kaufman then asserts:

> Although theologically rooted in the concept of the sanctity of life, the
> change in Christianity's attitude toward suicide was, as Alvarez persua-
> sively argues, primarily motivated by practicalities. He explains that the
> cult of martyrdom led to a rapid increase of actual suicide in the name
> of religion. In order to preserve its numbers the early Church needed to
> stop this practice: "Viewed from the Christian Heaven, life itself was at
> best unimportant; at worst, evil: the fuller the life, the greater the
> temptation to sin. Death, therefore, was a release awaited or sought out
> with impatience. In other words, the more powerfully the Church
> instilled in believers the idea that this world was a vale of tears and sin
> and temptation, where they waited uneasily until death released them
> into eternal glory, the more irresistible the temptation to suicide became.
> Even the most stoical Romans committed suicide only as a last resort;

they at least waited until their lives had become intolerable whatever its conditions. Why, then, live unredeemed when heavenly bliss is only a knife stroke away? Christian teaching was at first a powerful incitement to suicide."[19]

If Judge Kaufman had not relied exclusively on Alvarez but had consulted others who speak with authority regarding the place of suicide in early Christianity, he would have had little difficulty finding the works of scholars from various fields whose perspectives are similar to Alvarez's. In *The Sanctity of Life and the Criminal Law,* the noted philosopher Glanville Williams writes:

> There is no condemnation of suicide in the New Testament, and little to be found among the early Christians, who were, indeed, morbidly obsessed with death. . . . The Christian belief was that life on earth was important only as a preparation for the hereafter; the supreme duty was to avoid sin, which would result in perpetual punishment. Since all natural desires tended toward sin, the risk of failure was great. Many Christians, therefore, committed suicide for fear of falling before temptation. It was especially good if the believer could commit suicide by provoking infidels to martyr him, or by austerities so severe that they undermined the constitution, but in the last resort he might do away with himself directly.[20]

Likewise the philosopher Margaret Pabst Battin, in her *Ethical Issues in Suicide,* writes:

> Christianity *invites* suicide in a way in which other major religions do not. . . . The lure exerted by the promise of reunion with the deceased, release of the soul, the rewards of martyrdom, and the attainment of the highest spiritual states, including union with God, all occur in Christianity. . . . Thus the question of the permissibility of suicide arises, though often only inchoately, for any sincere believer in a religious tradition of this sort, whether that individual's present life is a happy one or filled with suffering. Religious suicide is not always a matter of despair; it is often a matter of zeal. The general problem presented by the promise of a better afterlife may be strongest in Christianity, since the afterlife of spiritual bliss depicted by Christianity is a particularly powerful attraction. . . . The early Christian community appeared to be on the verge of complete self-decimation in voluntary martyrdom and suicide until Augustine took a firm position against such practices. . . . Although there is little reason to think that Augustine's position is authentically Christian . . . it nevertheless rapidly took hold and within an extremely short time had become universally accepted as fundamental Christian law.[21]

The historical and theological presuppositions and conclusions of Alvarez and of these two (and other) philosophers, as well those of many sociologists, anthropologists, psychologists, and popular authors who have written, even incidentally, on suicide in early Christianity during the last several decades are typically as follows:

1. So eager were many early Christians to realize their fullness of joy in heaven that they committed suicide if they were unable to provoke pagans to put them to death as martyrs.

2. So depressing was the burden of sin and guilt of many early Christians that they killed themselves in despair.

3. So intensely did many early Christians despise their sinful flesh that they killed themselves, often through severe asceticism.

4. So low a regard did early Christians have for their lives that they were willing to die for their faith, some even volunteering for or provoking martyrdom. And martyrdom, of course, is suicide.

5. Augustine was the first Christian to denounce suicide as a sin. His negative influence has subsequently tempered the Christian attitude to suicide, including both active and passive euthanasia.

Such views of suicide in early Christianity suggest not only an ignorance of early Christian theology and history but also the conceptual influence of Emile Durkheim, the father of academic sociology in France. In *Le suicide: Etude sociologique,* published in 1897 but not translated into English until 1951,[22] Durkheim created three categories of suicide that he viewed as etiologically explicable with reference to social structures: (1) egoistic (resulting from a lack of social integration); (2) anomic (precipitated by the destabilizing effects of sudden negative or positive social change); and (3) altruistic (resulting from overintegration, especially when the individual is completely controlled by religious or political groups).

Durkheim's definition of suicide is very well known to students of the social sciences: "All cases of death resulting directly or indirectly from a positive or negative act of the victim himself, which he knows will produce this result."[23] Durkheim was determined to avoid the question of motivation or even whether the individual actually desired to die. It is suicide if one believes that one's actions or passivity will eventuate in one's own death. Hence he classifies the death of Christian martyrs as (altruistic) suicide, since they,

> without killing themselves, voluntarily allowed their own slaughter.
> ... Though they did not kill themselves, they sought death with all their
> power and behaved so as to make it inevitable. To be suicide, the act
> from which death must necessarily result need only have been performed

by the victim with full knowledge of the facts. Besides, the passionate enthusiasm with which the believers in the new religion faced final torture shows that at this moment they had completely discarded their personalities for the idea of which they had become the servants.[24]

According to Durkheim, dying for one's beliefs is suicide. Since those who commit suicide are, in Durkheim's construct, victims of pathological social phenomena, martyrs are victims not of the people who kill them but of their own religious group's demand for excessive integration, control, and regimentation.

It is not surprising that when scholars who appear to be as ignorant of historic Christianity as they likely are of Buddhism apply Durkheim's grid to the history of early Christianity the results are as distorted as those quoted and summarized above. Consequently, when two theologians, Arthur J. Droge and James D. Tabor, both trained in history and in patristics, recently wrote *A Noble Death: Suicide and Martyrdom among Christians and Jews in Antiquity*,[25] one could reasonably have anticipated a more perspicacious historical analysis. But they have added confusion to inaccuracy. Rejecting for their purposes the word *suicide* as "a recent innovation and pejorative term," they prefer the designation *voluntary death*. "By this term we mean to describe the act resulting from an individual's intentional decision to die, either by his own agency, by another's, or by contriving the circumstances in which death is the known, ineluctable result." They concede that their definition of voluntary death is quite similar to Durkheim's definition of suicide and assert that theirs is "intended to be morally neutral, since our enterprise is not one of moral (or clinical) judgment but an attempt to understand the ways in which voluntary death was evaluated in antiquity."[26]

Emphasizing that both "suicide" and "martyrdom" are semantically and conceptually ambiguous, Droge and Tabor think that they have reduced the ambiguity and confusion by providing the concept of "voluntary death" as a much more objective grid for the historian. They dislike the word suicide especially because of its typically pejorative connotations. They, of course, convey a positive view of voluntary death; after all, a voluntary death is a noble death, as the title of their book declares. They acknowledge in their conclusion that their purpose had been "to deconstruct the 'linguistics of suicide' by examining the precise terms and formulations employed in antiquity to denote the act of voluntary death."[27]

"It is a profound irony of Western history," they maintain, that Christian theologians, beginning with Augustine, "condemned the act of voluntary death as a sin for which Christ's similar act could not atone. . . .[28] Despite the claim of Augustine and later theologians, the New Testament expresses no condemnation of voluntary death. . . . Yet, to say only that the writers of the New Testament did not condemn voluntary death is to miss the positive significance they attached to the act. The authors of the Gospel created [sic] a Jesus who died by his own choice, if not by his own hand."[29] They ask regarding Jesus' death, "Was it the legal execution of a criminal, an example of heroic martyrdom, or a case of suicide?"[30] Judas' death was similar to Jesus' in that both were voluntary: "In the *Umwelt* of early Christianity the act of taking one's life was judged to be acceptable and, in certain circumstances, noble. . . . this was Matthew's implicit judgment on Judas' death. Judas was condemned for betraying the Messiah, not for killing himself. According to Matthew, Judas' act of self-destruction was the measure of his remorse and repentance."[31]

Droge and Tabor are especially interested in the apostle Paul's supposed "fascination with death and his desire to escape from life"[32] and suggest that "for Paul, an individual could kill himself and be 'glorifying God with his body' by doing so. . . . In a world-negating system like the apostle Paul's, the question became how to justify continued existence in the world rather than voluntary death."[33] "Voluntary death," as they conclude their book, "was one of the ideals on which the church was founded."[34]

These authors begin and end their book with reference to the current debate regarding physician-assisted suicide (PAS). While insisting that "when the conventional distinction between 'suicide' and 'martyrdom' is read back into antiquity, it conceals rather than reveals the issues,"[35] it is their own faddish linguistic deconstructionism and historical revisionism that are blatantly anachronistic and do violence to the texts that they "deconstruct." So effectively have they blurred even the most commonsensical distinctions between different categories of so-called voluntary death and created such a conceptually amorphous and morally ambiguous realm in which to include PAS that Derek Humphry, founder of the Hemlock Society, enthusiastically exclaims on their book's dust jacket, "This book will upset traditional Christian views about the right to choose to die."

Droge and Tabor's determination to label such a diverse variety of motives and actions "voluntary death" is so conspicuously special pleading and hence so entangles them in contradictions and inconsistencies that it becomes laughable. Two of a plethora of examples: (1) When dealing with the Old Testament, Droge and Tabor discuss the suicides of Abimelech, Saul and his armor-bearer, Samson, Ahithophel, and Zimri, then say of Elijah's request that God take his life (1 Kings 19:4–5): "Though no act of self-destruction is involved, we might term this a 'voluntary departure' or perhaps even a 'voluntary death.'"[36] Aaron's "death is voluntary in the sense that he submitted to God's decision" that it was time for him to die.[37] They speculate that "whether Moses himself took a hand in his own death or not is left unclear, though it might well be implied," then say, "The point we want to emphasize here is that the distinctions tend to be blurred between a request that God take one's life, God's determining the time of death, and one's taking a hand to carry out such a choice or decision."[38] Indeed. (2) A recurring theme in their book is that Augustine condemned "voluntary death." Nevertheless, they maintain that he "attempted to draw a distinction between two kinds of voluntary death: 'self-homicide' and 'martyrdom.' The former was condemned as reprehensible; the latter was praised as noble and ennobling."[39] It appears, then, that although Augustine ostensibly condemned "voluntary death," nevertheless, since he made a distinction between "self-homicide" (i.e., "suicide"), which he condemned, and "martyrdom," which he praised, he did not actually condemn Droge and Tabor's meaningless category of "voluntary death" per se. After all, who could? Only Durkheim and his followers who insist that any willingness to die, even to sacrifice one's life to save others or forfeit it rather than go against conscience is suicide. Labeling as "voluntary death" everything that Durkheim calls "suicide" proves nothing other than that it is, at best, as meaningless, or, at worst, as tragically a misleading grid to apply to any period of history (not to speak of the present) as is Durkheim's. Both have in common, as their Achilles' heel, their inclusion of martyrdom and self-sacrificial death as suicide or voluntary death.

Martyrdom as Suicide

Christians reacted to persecution in four ways: (1) apostatizing; (2) fleeing; (3) accepting whatever penalties that were inflicted, including death; and (4) volunteering for or provoking martyrdom.[40] The first of these was always condemned and the third always approved during the patristic period.[41] The second and the fourth were much more problematic and evoked considerable disagreement within the Christian community especially between rigorists and moderates.

Martyrdom in the early church is a rich field from which Droge and Tabor harvest examples of "voluntary death": "The martyrs are portrayed as going to their death in one of three ways: either as a result of being sought out, by deliberately volunteering, or by actually taking their own lives. On the basis of the evidence that has survived, it would appear that the majority of Christian martyrs chose death by the second and third means."[42] Only a statistical breakdown of all recorded cases of martyrdom during the patristic era could irrefutably disprove this assertion. The preponderance of known cases of martyrdom that occurred before the legalization of Christianity in 313 are of those who did not actively seek martyrdom but, when arrested, were martyred rather than apostatize, or who, as spectators of others' being interrogated, tortured, or executed, identified themselves as Christians and suffered the consequences. These varied from the theatrically eager to the resigned. This is not to say that there were not some who actively sought to provoke pagans to martyr them. *Indisputable* examples of such, however, are extremely rare. Droge and Tabor are hard pressed to provide many except by the most contorted hermeneutical gymnastics.

There is an even greater scarcity of recorded instances of their third category, i.e., those who "actively [took] their own lives" as a means of martyrdom. The extremely small number of Christians who are recorded as "actively taking their own lives" before the legalization of Christianity in 313 did so only under extreme duress. There are three categories:

1. Those who killed themselves to avoid being arrested and subjected to extreme suffering. I have found only one instance. It is recorded by Eusebius (ca. 265–339) and occurred during the "Great Persecution" (303–312):

> Need I rekindle the memory of the martyrs at Antioch, who were roasted over lighted braziers, not roasted to death but subjected to prolonged torture? Or of others who plunged their hands right into the fire sooner than touch the abominable sacrifice? Some of them were unable to face such a trial, and before they were caught and came into the hands of their would-be destroyers, threw themselves down from the roofs of tall houses, regarding death as a prize snatched from the scheming hands of God's enemies.[43]

Eusebius records this incident with neither approval nor disapproval. As we shall see below, Ambrose (ca. 339–97) implicitly and Jerome (ca. 345–ca. 419) explicitly condemn suicide to avoid the tortures that typically attended martyrdom.[44] Both, however, were born decades after the legalization of Christianity, but Eusebius lived through the "Great Persecution." This may suggest why the latter does not condemn the act. Augustine (354–430) was extremely thorough in his various analyses of suicide. Yet he makes no reference to this category of self-killing, although he appears to have scoured both pagan and Christian literature for references to suicide. Hence it is reasonable to conclude that such types of suicide by Christians had occurred very rarely while Christians were still a persecuted minority.

2. Those who had already been arrested but dramatically ended their lives before being executed. I know of only two examples, both recorded by Eusebius: The first occurred in Alexandria in 249 under Decius:

> Next they seized the wonderful old lady Apollonia, battered her till they knocked out all her teeth, built a pyre in front of the city, and threatened to burn her alive unless she repeated after them their heathen incantations. She asked for a breathing-space, and when they released her, jumped without hesitation into the fire and was burnt to ashes.[45]

The second was during the "Great Persecution":

> [T]here was a conflagration in the palace at Nicomedia, and through a groundless suspicion word went round that our people were responsible. By imperial command God's worshippers there perished wholesale and in heaps, some butchered with the sword, others fulfilled [*teleioō* = perfected, made perfect or complete] by fire; it is on record that with an inspired and mystical fervour men and women alike leapt on to the pyre.[46]

3. Virgins and married women who committed suicide to avoid defilement. The earliest examples appear to be from the "Great Persecution." Nearly a century after the legalization of Christianity, Rome was captured and ravaged by Alaric and his Goths, who raped pagan and Christian women alike. Some Christian women committed suicide to preserve their chastity. It is a consideration of such suicides that prompted Augustine to write a lengthy but diversionary discussion of suicide in book one of his *City of God*.

Leaving aside these three categories of suicide that arise in the context of persecution/martyrdom or, in the case of those women who committed suicide to preserve their chastity, in the face of immanent ravishing by barbarians, let us return to the subject of martyrdom. I have already mentioned that there was considerable disagreement within the Christian community, especially between rigorists and moderates, regarding the two extremes of fleeing in the face of persecution and volunteering for or provoking martyrdom. All Christians held that martyrdom was the most perfect display of love toward God and was to be desired above any other form of death. Never could any other form of death provide the spiritual glory and rewards that martyrdom guaranteed. Accordingly, for moderates (a strong majority in our sources), who condemned seeking or provoking martyrdom, the very basis for their condemnation of actively contriving that one most coveted form of death would *eo ipso* preclude (1) their approving of one's intentionally ending one's own life through some lesser means, much less (2) their formulating a theological justification for taking one's own life by one's own hand. For rigorists (a minority in our sources), who approved of volunteering for martyrdom, any form of death, including suicide, would be an obstacle to that one most cherished form of death, martyrdom. Hence it is not surprising that in the entirety of extant patristic literature written before the legalization of Christianity, there is not even one recorded instance of Christians' committing suicide after having failed to provoke pagans to martyr them.

Suicide

Suicide is never discussed, much less condemned, in the New Testament. The only suicide recorded there is that of Judas (hardly a model of Christian virtue), and his self-destruction is reported without comment (Mt. 25:5; Acts 1:18). Suicide arises incidentally on some other occasions. When Jesus said, "'Where I go, you cannot come,' this made the Jews ask, 'Will he kill himself?'" (Jn. 8:21–22). One suicide is prevented in the New Testament. Paul and Silas had been freed from prison in Philippi by an earthquake. When the jailer was about to kill himself in despair, Paul intervened by offering him salvation, which he joyfully accepted (Acts 16:25–34). In some cases of demon possession, self-destructive tendencies are manifested, e.g., in Mark's accounts of the Gerasene demoniac (Mk. 5:5) and of the mute boy (Mk. 9:14–29). In the latter, the boy's father told Jesus that the demon had "often thrown him into the fire or water to kill him" (Mk. 9:22). The New Testament contains no other reference to potential or realized suicide.

Although suicide is a topic that excited little comment by church fathers before Augustine, one encounters passing references. An anonymous author of the *Shepherd of Hermas,* a work that was composed in stages between 90 and 150, contends that one who is harassed by distress (*incommoda*) should be assisted, for "many bring death on themselves by reason of such calamities when they cannot bear them. Whoever therefore knows the distress of such a man, and does not rescue him, incurs great sin and becomes guilty of his blood."[47] This suggests that the author held the suicide of one who resorted to such a deed because of distress as so serious a matter that whoever could have helped but failed to do so was guilty not only of a serious sin but of the suicide's blood.

Justin Martyr (ca. 100–165) envisages a pagan exclaiming, "All of you, go kill yourselves and thus go immediately to God and save us the trouble." Justin responds, "If . . . we should kill ourselves we would be the cause, as far as it is up to us, why no one would be born and be instructed in the divine doctrines, or even why the human race might cease to exist; if we do act thus, we ourselves will be opposing the will of God."[48] This passage occurs in juxtaposition to Justin's assertion of Christians' willingness to die for their faith. Although the passage is an unequivocal condemnation of suicide for Christians, it is only an explanation provided to pagans of why Christians do not kill themselves. Justin appears not to have felt it incumbent upon himself to provide any moral explanation or scriptural defense of his position. Although his argument is sufficiently Platonic to be familiar to educated pagans, it contains ingredients that even Platonists would find unpalatable: Christians must not kill themselves because God wants them in the world and humanity needs them, for if there were no Christians not only would there be no one to instruct pagans in the truth, but also, since God sustains the world for his people's sake, the human race would cease to exist if all Christians were removed from the face of the earth.

A similar message is contained in the late second-century, anonymous *Epistle to Diognetus:*

> The soul is locked up in the body, yet is the very thing that holds the body together; so, too, Christians are shut up in the world as in a prison, yet are the very ones that hold the world together. Immortal, the soul is lodged in a mortal tenement; so, too, Christians, though residing as strangers among corruptible things, look forward to the incorruptibility that awaits them in heaven. The soul, when stinting itself in food and drink, is the better for it; so, too, Christians, when penalized, increase daily more and more. Such is the important post to which God has assigned them, and it is not lawful for them to desert it.[49]

The similarity of the reasoning of Justin and of the author of the *Epistle to Diognetus* is striking. The presence, in such early Christian sources, of a Christianized form of the Platonic argument that God has assigned people to a post that they must not abandon renders the assertion of Rousseau and others that Augustine took his arguments from Plato's *Phaedo* less than compelling. Clearly Augustine inherited a Christian argument that was already more than two centuries old.

In the so-called Clementine *Homilies,* probably redacted to their present form in the mid–fourth century but based on a late second- or early third-century original, the apostle Peter encounters a pagan woman who is considering killing herself because of various afflictions. He says to her, "Do you suppose, O woman, that those who destroy themselves are freed from punishment? Are not the souls of those who thus die punished with a worse punishment in Hades for their suicide?"[50] It is uncertain whether the conviction that suicide will compound one's future punishment was in the original or added by a fourth-century redactor.

Clement of Alexandria (ca. 155–ca. 220) viewed as a *praeparatio evangelica* those features of Greek philosophy that he regarded as consonant with divine revelation. He especially admired the Stoic concept of *apatheia* (insensibility to suffering). But in his thought the Stoic concept is so thoroughly informed by scriptural principles that the *apatheia* that he lauds as a Christian ideal could never reasonably lead to, much less justify, suicide:

> [By] going away to the Lord [the Christian] does not withdraw himself from life. For that is not permitted to him. But he has withdrawn his soul from the passions. For that is granted to him. And on the other hand he lives, having put to death his lusts, and no longer makes use of the body, but allows it the use of necessaries, that he may not give cause for dissolution [of the body].[51]

Clement's was a Stoicism that had been Christianized to such a degree that suicide was permitted neither in the active sense (i.e., "withdrawing from life," a popular Stoic expression for suicide) nor in the passive sense (i.e., allowing the dissolution of the body by failing to provide it with necessities).

Tertullian (ca. 160–ca. 220), commenting on Christ's having commanded his followers "to give to the one who asks," says that "if you take His command generally, you would be giving not only wine to a man with a fever, but also poison or a sword to one who wanted to die."[52] It was regarded as exceedingly harmful for the febrile to consume wine. Tertullian includes in the same category assisting one to commit suicide. A Christian simply will not supply the means if asked. In another work, Tertullian classifies as demented or insane (possibly demon possessed) anyone who "cuts his own throat."[53]

There is no suggestion in the sources thus far surveyed that for contemporary Christians suicide either posed a theoretical, much less a practical, problem or was an attraction to them. Such will continue to be the case through the end of the patristic era.

Lactantius (ca. 240–320), appointed professor of oratory in Nicomedia by the emperor Diocletian and later converted to Christianity, resigned his position when the "Great Persecution" began in 303. He intended his major apologetic work, the *Divine Institutes,* to persuade educated pagans of the truth of Christianity and to edify and encourage Christians who were troubled by philosophical attacks against their faith. Discussing various pagan philosophers, he says that many of them, "because they suspected that the soul is immortal, laid violent hands upon themselves, as though they were about to depart to heaven." He then asserts that

> nothing can be more wicked than this. For if a homicide is guilty because he is a destroyer of man, he who puts himself to death is under the same guilt, because he puts to death a man. Yea, that crime may be considered to be greater, the punishment of which belongs to God alone. For as we did not come into this life of our own accord; so, on the other hand, we can only withdraw from this habitation of the body which has been appointed for us to keep, by the command of Him who placed us in this body that we may inhabit it, until He orders us to depart from it. . . . All these philosophers, therefore, were homicides.[54]

Some years later Lactantius yielded to requests to write an abridgment of the *Divine Institutes*. In his *Epitome* he asks whether we should approve those

> who, that they might be said to have despised death, died by their own hands? Zeno, Empedocles, Chrysippus, Cleanthes, Democritus, and Cato, imitating these, did not know that he who put himself to death is guilty of murder, according to the divine right and law. For it was God who placed us in this abode of flesh: it was He who gave us the temporary habitation of the body, that we should inhabit it as long as He pleased. Therefore it is to be considered impious, to wish to depart from it without the command of God. Therefore violence must not be applied to nature. He knows how to destroy His own work. And if any one shall apply impious hands to that work, and shall tear asunder the bonds of the divine workmanship, he endeavours to flee from God, whose sentence no one will be able to escape, whether alive or dead. Therefore they are accursed and impious, whom I have mentioned above, who even taught what are the befitting reasons for voluntary death; so that it was not enough of guilt that they were self-murderers, unless they instructed others also to this wickedness.[55]

In his *Divine Institutes* Lactantius condemns suicides as worse than homicides on the Christianized Platonic grounds that suicides desert the place to which God has appointed them. In his *Epitome* he adds the offenses of attempting to flee from God by committing violence against nature and encouraging others to do likewise. In his second work his tone is even more vitriolic and outraged than in the first: suicides are not only homicides but are impious as well.

Lactantius's contemporary, Eusebius, whom we have already considered in our discussion of martyrdom, writes:

It is worthy of note that, as the records show, in the reign of Gaius . . .
Pilate himself, the governor of our Saviour's day, was involved in such
calamities that he was forced to become his own executioner and to
punish himself with his own hand: divine justice, it seems, was not slow
to overtake him. The facts are recorded by those Greeks who have
chronicled the Olympiads together with the events occurring in each.[56]

Eusebius clearly regarded Pilate's suicide from despair as God's just
penalty, a condemnation for his sin of sentencing Jesus to death by
crucifixion.

Eusebius quotes from the anti-Montanist work of Bishop Apolinar-
ius of Hierapolis, written during the reign of Marcus Aurelius, the
following account of the deaths of Montanus (the founder, in the late
second century, of the charismatic and prophetic sect that bears his
name) and one of his prophetesses, Maximilla:

[I]t is thought that both of these were driven out of their minds by a
spirit, and hanged themselves, at different times; and on the occasion of
the death of each, it was said on all sides that this was how they died,
putting an end to themselves just like the traitor Judas. . . . But we must
not imagine that without seeing them we know the truth about such
things, my friend: it may have been in this way, it may have been in some
other way, that death came to Montanus . . . and [his] female associate.[57]

Neither Eusebius nor his source would vouch for the accuracy of this
account. Including it, however, they suggest death by suicide as
appropriate for two whom they regarded as notorious heretics.

John Chrysostom (349–407), writing on Galatians 1:4 (Jesus "gave
himself for our sins to rescue us from the present evil world, according
to the will of our God and Father"), castigates those dualistic heretics
who viewed the material world as evil. He takes the words "evil world"
to mean

evil actions, and a depraved moral principle. . . . Christ came not to put
us to death and deliver us from the present life in that sense, but to leave
us in the world, and prepare us for a worthy participation of our
heavenly abode. Wherefore He saith to the Father, "And these are in the
world, and I come to Thee; I pray not that Thou shouldest take them
from the world, but that Thou shouldest keep them from the evil," i.e.,
from sin. Further, those who will not allow this, but insist that the
present life is evil, should not blame those who destroy themselves; for
as he who withdraws himself from evil is not blamed, but deemed
worthy of a crown, so he who by a violent death, by hanging or
otherwise, puts an end to his life, ought not to be condemned. Whereas
God punishes such men more than murderers, and we all regard them

with horror, and justly; for if it is base to destroy others, much more is it to destroy one's self.[58]

Chrysostom thus asserts that dualistic heresy encourages suicide. True Christians—"we all" would be the orthodox community—according to Chrysostom justly regard suicide with horror. Such a statement would be preposterous if there had been any sympathy within the orthodox community with suicide to escape "the present evil world."

Augustine's erstwhile mentor Ambrose (ca. 339–97) says of Paul's statement "For to me, to live is Christ and to die is gain" (Phil. 1:21):

> For Christ is our king; therefore we cannot abandon and disregard His royal command. How many men the emperor of this earth orders to live abroad in the splendor of office or perform some function! Do they abandon their posts without the emperor's consent? Yet what a greater thing it is to please the divine than the human! Thus for the saint "to live is Christ and to die is gain." He does not flee the servitude of life like a slave, and yet like a wise man he does embrace the gain of death.[59]

Once again we see a Christianized form of the Platonic argument against suicide. Elsewhere Ambrose writes to his sister Marcellina:

> You make a good suggestion that I should touch upon what we ought to think of the merits of those who have cast themselves down from a height, or have drowned themselves in a river, lest they should fall in the hands of persecutors, seeing that holy Scripture forbids a Christian to lay hands on himself.[60]

He gives the example of a virgin's committing suicide to preserve her chastity and then of a woman's enduring torture that resulted in her death. The implied answer to Marcellina's question is that suicide to avoid persecution is wrong but to preserve chastity is right. It is very significant that Ambrose simply states that Scripture forbids suicide and does not seem to feel compelled to defend that contention. He speaks with the same degree of confidence that his audience will agree as does Chrysostom when he says, "we all regard suicides with horror, and justly."

In a letter to the lady Paula, who was distraught over the death of her daughter Blaesilla, Jerome (ca. 345–ca. 419) asks:

> Have you no fear, then lest the Savior may say to you: "Are you angry, Paula, that your daughter has become my daughter? Are you vexed at my decree, and do you, with rebellious tears, grudge me the possession of Blaesilla? You ought to know what my purpose is both for you and for yours. You deny yourself food, not to fast but to gratify your grief,

and such abstinence is displeasing to me. Such fasts are my enemies. I receive no soul which forsakes the body against my will. A foolish philosophy may boast of martyrs of this kind; it may boast of a Zeno, a Cleombrotus, or a Cato. My spirit rests only upon him 'that is poor and of a contrite spirit and that trembleth at my word' [Is. 66:2]."[61]

Jerome qualifies this apparently unlimited condemnation of suicide elsewhere: "It is not ours to lay hold of death, but we freely accept it when it is inflicted by others. Hence, even in persecutions it is not right for us to die by our own hands, except when chastity is threatened, but to submit our necks to the one who threatens."[62]

Both Ambrose and Jerome make one exception to their otherwise inclusive condemnation of suicide: if it is done for the preservation of chastity. Only a small minority of patristic sources prior to Augustine mention this category of suicide; those that do approve it.[63]

Augustine

Augustine's rejection of the probity of suicide to preserve chastity led him to engage in a thorough analysis of suicide in book one of the *City of God*. The first installment of this massive work was published in 414, four years after the Goths' sack of Rome.

In sections 16–28 Augustine condemns the following motivations for suicide: (1) to avoid or escape from temporal problems; (2) to avoid or escape from another's sinful actions (including doing so to preserve chastity); (3) because of guilt over past sins; (4) because of a desire for heaven; and (5) to avoid sinning. If there were any conceivably justifiable cause for suicide, Augustine says, it would be the last, but yet even the sin of such a well-motivated suicide would be greater than any sin that one might avoid by killing oneself. The basis of his condemnation of suicide is fourfold:

1. Scripture does not expressly permit, much less command, suicide as a means of achieving heaven or as a way to escape or avoid evil.
2. A prohibition of suicide is explicit in the sixth commandment.
3. Since no private party has the authority to kill a criminal who deserves capital punishment, those who kill themselves are homicides.
4. Suicide allows no opportunity for repentance.

His only reference to martyrdom in this digression on suicide is his refutation of pagan approval of suicide to avoid captivity. He argues that the patriarchs, prophets, and apostles did not commit suicide to escape persecution or martyrdom.

About a decade before he published the first installment of the *City of God*, Augustine had devoted some attention to martyrdom, not to that of Catholics persecuted by pagans but rather to the courting of martyrdom by and, when unsuccessful, the theatrically spectacular suicides of members of a schismatic, heretical group, the Donatists.[64] The Donatist movement (named after its earliest leader, Donatus) had been formed in the early fourth century by rigorists who condemned the church's accepting back into fellowship those who had apostatized during the "Great Persecution." Donatists viewed themselves as upholders of the purity of discipline in the face of Catholic "compromise with the world" that they viewed as having worsened since the legalization of Christianity. From its very beginning, the movement was a thorn in the flesh for the Catholic leadership. Persecution of the Donatists by the Catholic Church and by the imperial government began in 317. Finally, in 415, the death penalty was enacted for those Donatists who continued to assemble. It was especially then that some Donatists, primarily a fringe group known as the Circumcellions, increased their indiscriminate as well as systematic acts of violence against Catholics (even once attempting to ambush and kill Augustine) and their provoking the authorities to put them to death. Some Donatists staged sensationalistic suicides as well.

Intermittently, for nearly twenty years, Augustine composed anti-Donatist treatises. A frequent focus of these tracts was the Donatists' attitude toward and practice of suicide. Space permits only a brief summary of the major themes in his anti-Donatist writings that do not occur in his digression on suicide in book one of the *City of God*:

1. Provoking martyrdom is a form of suicide and hence a sin.
2. "Heroic" suicide by those who are unable to provoke others to martyr them is a sin.
3. The Donatists' suicides violate the foundational Christian principle of patient endurance. This argument is presented in one of his last anti-Donatist writings (*Letters* 204, composed in 420).

An Augustinian Reversal?

In 415 Augustine had written a treatise entitled *De patientia,* in which, without specifically naming the Donatists, he chided them with the example of Job's endurance:

> At him let those men look who bring death upon themselves when they are being sought out to be given life, and who, by taking away their present life, reject also the life to come. For, if they were being forced to deny Christ or to do anything contrary to justice, they ought, as true martyrs, to bear all things patiently rather than to inflict death upon themselves in their impatience. If he could have done it righteously to escape evil, holy Job would have destroyed himself so that he might have

escaped such diabolic cruelty in his own possessions, in his own sons, in his own limbs.[65]

Patient endurance proved to be the climax of Augustine's final statement on the subject of suicide, in book 19 of the *City of God,* published in 426 or 427.

The theme of patient endurance was, of course, not unique to Augustine. Even a casual reading of the church fathers shows that they saw suffering as an essential component of God's sanctifying work. This conviction, coupled with a firm belief in divine sovereignty and an equally firm confidence that God does all things for the ultimate good of his people, engendered in them a sense of responsibility to preach and practice endurance in the face of all afflictions. An outstanding but not atypical example is Cyprian (ca. 200–258). Writing to his fellow Christians while the city was being ravaged by plague, he comments on the phenomenon that some of them were troubled because this

disease carries off our people equally with the pagans, as if a Christian believes to this end, that, free from contact with evils, he may happily enjoy the world and this life, and, without having endured all adversities here, may be preserved for future happiness. . . . But what in this world do we not have in common with others as long as this flesh . . . still remains common to us?

As examples he gives famine, the devastation of war, drought, shipwreck, "and eye trouble and attacks of fever and every ailment of the members we have in common with others as long as this common flesh is borne in the world."[66] He reminds his readers that this

endurance the just have always had; this discipline the apostles maintained from the law of the Lord, not to murmur in adversity, but to accept bravely and patiently whatever happens in the world. . . . We must not murmur in adversity, beloved brethren, but must patiently and bravely bear with whatever happens.[67]

Hence, "the fear of God and faith ought to make you ready for all things," such as loss of possessions, sickness, loss of loved ones. So

let not such things be stumbling blocks for you but battles; nor let them weaken or crush the faith of the Christian, but rather let them reveal his valor in the contest, since every injury arising from present evils should be made light of through confidence in the blessings to come. . . . [C]onflict in adversity is the trial of truth.[68]

Cyprian consistently emphasizes the activity of God and the passivity of Christians in death. He asserts that Christians who died of the current plague "have been freed from the world by the summons of the Lord."[69] Later he avers that "those who please God are taken from here earlier and more quickly set free, lest, while they are tarrying too long in this world, they be defiled by contacts with the world." He then advises that "when the day of our own summons comes, without hesitation but with gladness we may come to the Lord at His call." For "rescued by an earlier departure, you are being freed from ruin and shipwrecks and threatening disasters!" Hence, "Let us embrace the day which assigns each of us to his dwelling, which on our being rescued from here and released from the snares of the world, restores us to paradise and the kingdom." He encourages them to consider their loved ones already in heaven and the joys that await them there. "To these, beloved brethren, let us hasten with eager longing! Let us pray that it may befall us speedily to be with them, speedily to come to Christ."[70]

It is God who calls; it is he who issues the summons. God takes Christians from the world; God frees them; God rescues them; God releases them; God restores them to heaven. Christians are passive— they *are being* freed; they *are being* rescued; they *are being* released; they *are being* restored. It is God who is the active party. Christians are to yearn for heaven and to pray for an early departure from life. Yearning for death and praying to die are categorically different from taking one's own life. There is *no room here for suicide.* Patient endurance of all afflictions, perseverance to the end, final resignation to God's will in the midst of those very circumstances that God is using to test and refine the Christian: such thought is antithetical to the taking of one's own life. And such thought permeates patristic literature.

The first paragraph of Droge and Tabor's conclusion reads:

> Why did the Augustinian condemnation of voluntary death succeed in reversing the perspective of an entire period of history, a period that Augustine himself is often thought to have brought to a close? We confess not to have a satisfying answer to that question, save for the obvious one of the enormous influence of Augustine's legacy in the West. But this does not explain why a similar attitude toward voluntary death came to be held in Eastern Christianity, where Augustine was little read. Have we then misinterpreted the evidence by making too much of the Augustinian "reversal"?[71]

They should have answered this last question "yes" and then repudiated their thesis and scrapped their manuscript. Even though they cannot account for the fact that the same position that Augustine articulates also prevails in Eastern Christianity,[72] they continue to defend the conceptually nebulous haze that they have generated in their attempt "to deconstruct the 'linguistics of suicide'"[73] in support of the "right-to-die" movement.

Did Augustine formulate the Christian position on suicide? The answer must be an unequivocal "no." He based his condemnation of suicide most fundamentally on the same presuppositions and values that had caused the earlier church fathers to condemn the act. Recall the terms with which they had condemned it: it is opposed to the will of God (Justin); it is not lawful (*Epistle to Diognetus*); suicides are punished more severely than others (Clementine *Homilies*); it is not permitted (Clement); God punishes suicides more than homicides and we all justly regard them with horror (John Chrysostom); nothing can be more wicked than suicide (Lactantius); Christ will not receive the soul of a suicide (Jerome); Scripture forbids Christians to lay hands on themselves (Ambrose). Augustine was simply the first Christian on record to discuss the issue thoroughly, although a century earlier Lactantius had already devoted several pages of his *Divine Institutes* to suicide and then amplified his treatment of the subject in his *Epitome*.

Did Augustine contribute anything new to the Christian position? Here the answer must be a qualified "yes," for three reasons.

First, although it is unlikely that any of the earlier sources that I have cited would have disagreed with any of his arguments except regarding suicide to preserve chastity, nevertheless, this is a significant disagreement. It is both ironic and intriguing that in this one area of dispute Augustine did not carry the day.

Second, in his unequivocal and absolute condemnation of suicide, Augustine painted himself into a corner. If committing suicide to preserve chastity is a sin, what is one to think of those women who had killed themselves during times of persecution and were then venerated as martyrs? Augustine's only explanations are that either divine authority instructed the church that they should be thus honored or these martyrs had followed a divine command that was personally revealed to them. The latter is the only explanation that he can imagine for the one "justifiable" suicide in Scripture, that of Samson. Hence, one may commit suicide only when one is the recipient of an unmistakable and entirely unambiguous command from God to do so. Augustine is noticeably uncomfortable with this apparently unavoidable conclusion.[74]

Third, the thoroughness with which he discusses suicide—in books 1 and 19 of the *City of God* and in his various anti-Donatist writings—results in his marshaling a much larger array of arguments against suicide than any of his predecessors. His appeal to the sixth commandment is interesting as the earliest example in the history of moral considerations of suicide. But it would be significant only if earlier church fathers had attempted to justify their condemnations of suicide by recourse to specific injunctions in Scripture, which they did not.

There is no evidence that before Augustine's time suicide was a debated issue in the Christian community. Martyrdom, however, was. The probity of provoking or volunteering for martyrdom was hotly disputed before the legalization of Christianity. Furthermore, those few "approved" suicides that we encounter in early Christian literature occurred under the extreme duress of persecution or imminent sexual violation. It was the questionable probity of the latter that stimulated Augustine to deal with suicide per se, bolstered by the antics of Donatist Circumcellions. Why was suicide not a debated issue within the Christian community? Surely not because the church fathers were reluctant to condemn sin and to confront their fellow Christians for their moral failings. Nevertheless, there does not appear to be even one exhortation to refrain from suicide even in the writings of those authors who condemn the act unequivocally. The absence of a debate over suicide should not suggest that Christians were indifferent to suicide as an ethical issue. It simply appears not to have been a sufficiently attractive and viable option for them to have regarded it as a threat to the moral integrity of the Christian community.

The condemnations of suicide that we encounter prior to Augustine's time are comparatively rare because they are not part of the broad moral indignation voiced by church fathers against pagan depravity. Their outrage, especially against abortion and infanticide, was greatly stimulated by the perceived helplessness of the victim, whether a fetus or an infant. So also with gladiatorial combat and viciously cruel forms of torture and execution. Even acts of sexual immorality were more severely condemned when there were victims such as slaves who were forced to be the objects of their owners' lusts or of their greed when they were compelled to act as prostitutes for their owners' profit. The moral indignation of Christian authors was especially animated by the helplessness of the victims of others' sins. Suicide, as practiced by pagans, simply did not evoke passionate denunciation, for it is not an act in which an innocent party is victimized but an act in which one harms only oneself.

Christian Morality, the Care of the Sick, and Suicide

Christianity not only condemned pagan immorality, but it also introduced moral obligations that were altogether foreign to the Greek and Roman ethos. One of these was a duty to care—not a duty to cure,[75] but a duty to care—an obligation to extend practical compassion to the destitute, the widow, the orphan, and the sick. This introduced a truly radical transformation in attitudes toward the sick. Henry Sigerist has observed that Christianity inaugurated

> the most revolutionary and decisive change in the attitude of society toward the sick. Christianity came into the world . . . as the joyful Gospel of the Redeemer and of Redemption. It addressed itself to the disinherited, to the sick and the afflicted. . . . It became the duty of the Christian to attend to the sick and poor of the community. . . . The social position of the sick man thus became fundamentally different from what it had been before. He assumed a preferential position which has been his ever since.[76]

Although early Christians lived in a secular milieu in which suicide by the ill was frequently practiced and its probity seldom questioned,[77] I am confident not only that there is no discussion of the issue in patristic literature but that there is also not a single example of Christians committing suicide, asking others' assistance in doing so, or requesting others to kill them directly, in order to escape from the grinding tedium of chronic or the severe suffering of terminal illness. The only ethical issues raised by illness in patristic literature are (1) the tendency of some Christians to seek medical care without first pondering the spiritual dimensions of their suffering; (2) their having recourse to pagan or magical healing alternatives; and (3) their occasionally frantic struggles to find and cling to any even meager hope of recovery. Not only is suicide by the ill never raised as an ethical issue in the literature of early Christianity but also there is not a scintilla of evidence that the preferential position that Christianity gave to the sick included an expedited "final exit." So foundational are the goodness of God and his sovereignty in patristic theology and patient endurance of affliction so regularly and consistently stressed as an essential Christian virtue that it is not in the least surprising that *patristic texts are void of any reference to suicide by the ill.*[78]

The Significance of Inaccurate History

We now return to the court decision regarding PAS in Michigan. As we have seen, Judge Kaufman adopts without reservations the Roe Court's acceptance of Edelstein's thesis that the Hippocratic Oath was a Pythagorean manifesto and that its condemnation of abortion therefore represented a minority view. "But with the end of antiquity," Judge Kaufman quotes Justice Blackmun, "a decided change took place. Resistance against suicide and against abortion became common. The Oath came to be popular. The emerging teachings of Christianity were in agreement with the Pythagorean ethic."[79] This is extremely ambiguous. An adequate discussion of the variety of possible alternative interpretations of these four sentences would take several pages. Very briefly, by "the end of antiquity" does Justice Blackmun mean the period that began with the legalization of Christianity (313) and closed with the "fall" of the western Roman Empire (476)? The "decided change" that he maintains took place then is that "resistance against suicide and against abortion became common." Justice Blackmun appears to be saying that there are two related causes for this change: (1) "The Oath came to be popular" and (2) "The emerging teachings of Christianity were in agreement with the Pythagorean ethic." Who were then resisting suicide and abortion? Apparently Christians. With whom did the oath come to be popular? Apparently Christians.

Just when were the teachings of Christianity, which ostensibly were consonant with the ethics of the oath (i.e., for Justice Blackmun, "with the Pythagorean ethic"), *emerging?* Is Justice Blackmun's suggestion that Christian teachings did not "emerge" until the "end of antiquity" an indication that he accepts the contention of some historians and theologians that it is inaccurate to speak of an orthodox or even a normative Christianity before late antiquity? That is quite unlikely. Even if he did work from that premise, he most certainly does not give the slightest intimation that he questioned the very well known and easily demonstrable fact that even the earliest post–New Testament Christian literature fervently and uncompromisingly condemned abortion.

I would hesitate to suggest that Justice Blackmun was so ignorant of the history of the issue that he was addressing that he could think that Christians had not begun to condemn abortion until several centuries after the advent of their religion. Judge Kaufman, however, either had no qualms about attributing such a view to Justice Blackmun or he was unaware that he was doing so. This is shown by (1) his exclaiming, "It is striking that so much of the historical analysis of the Roe Court with respect to abortion mirrors historical traditions with respect to suicide," and (2) his unquestioning endorsement of Alvarez's thesis that suicide was both approved and widely practiced by Christians before the "end of antiquity" (i.e., the time of the Augustinian "reversal").

Although he may well be a competent legal scholar, Judge Kaufman has proved to be singularly inept and careless in his historical analysis. In great part, his dismissing of "history and tradition" as irrelevant to the case[80] appears to have stemmed from his misunderstanding of history. This raises an obvious question. If Judge Kaufman's understanding of the history of the issue had not been distorted by the glaring inaccuracies of his one "authority," would he have been more inclined to see greater merit to the prosecutor's argument regarding the relevance of "history and tradition"? If the answer is affirmative, then inaccurate history has played and may continue to play a significant role in legal considerations of PAS.

NOTES

Abbreviations

AF   *Apostolic Fathers,* K. Lake, trans. (Cambridge: Harvard University
            Press, 1912–13)
ANF   *Ante-Nicene Fathers,* various translators, various dates (reprint,
            Grand Rapids: Eerdmans, 1951)
FC   *Fathers of the Church,* various translators (Washington, D.C.:
            Catholic University of America, 1948–)
NPNF-1   *Select Library of Nicene and Post-Nicene Fathers of the Christian
            Church,* various translators, 1st ser., various dates (reprint,
            Grand Rapids: Eerdmans, 1976–79)
NPNF-2   *Select Library of Nicene and Post-Nicene Fathers of the Christian
            Church,* various translators, 2d ser., various dates (reprint,
            Grand Rapids: Eerdmans, 1976–79)

1. *United States Reports: Cases Adjudged in the Supreme Court at October Term, 1972* (Washington, D.C.: United States Government Printing Office, 1974), vol. 410, pp. 116–17.

2. Ibid., p. 171.

3. 1993 WL 603212 (Mich. Cir. Ct.), p. 7.

4. Ibid., p. 6.

5. Ibid., p. 7.

6. Ibid., pp. 7–8.

7. Ibid., p. 10.

8. Ibid., p. 9.

9. Judge Kaufman's quotations are from Alfred Alvarez, "The Background," in *Suicide: The Philosophical Issues,* ed. M. P. Battin and D. J. May (New York: St. Martin's, 1980), pp. 7–32, which is chap. 1 of Alvarez's very influential book, *The Savage God: A Study of Suicide* (New York: Random House, 1970).

10. WL 603212 (Mich. Cir. Ct.), p. 9.

11. Ibid.

12. Justice Blackmun is here quoting Ludwig Edelstein, "The Hippocratic Oath." Originally published as a monograph in 1943, it is more readily available in *Ancient Medicine: Selected Papers of Ludwig Edelstein,* ed. Owsei Temkin and C. Lilian Temkin (Baltimore: Johns Hopkins University Press, 1967), pp. 3–63.

13. 1993 WL 603212, p. 10.

14. E.g., Karl Deichgräber, *Der hippokratische Eid* (Stuttgart: Hippokrates-Verlag, 1955); Fridolf Kudlien, "Medical Ethics and Popular Ethics in Greece and Rome," *Clio Medica* 5 (1970): 91–121; Charles Lichtenthaeler, *Der Eid des Hippokrates: Ursprung and Bedeutung* (Cologne: Deutscher Ärzte-Verlag, 1984); and Vivian Nutton, "Beyond the Hippocratic Oath," in *Doctors and Ethics: The Earlier Historical Setting of Professional Ethics,* ed. Roger K. French, Andrew Wear, and Johanna Geyer-Kordesch (Amsterdam: Rodopi, 1993), pp. 10–37.

15. For traditions of "respect for life" in classical antiquity, see Owsei Temkin, "The Idea of Respect for Life in the History of Medicine," in Owsei Temkin, William K. Frankena, and Sanford H. Kadish, *Respect for Life in Medicine, Philosophy, and the Law* (Baltimore: Johns Hopkins University Press, 1976), pp. 1–23. An extensive secondary literature continues to accumulate that assesses the practice of and attitudes toward suicide in classical antiquity. Still basic is R. Hirzel, "Der Selbsmord," *Archiv für Religionswissenschaft* 11 (1908): 75–104, 243–84, 417–76. A few examples in English: J. M. Rist, chap. 13, "Suicide," in his *Stoic Philosophy* (Cambridge: Cambridge University Press, 1969), pp. 233–55; Miriam Griffin, "Philosophy, Cato, and Roman Suicide," *Greece and Rome* 33 (1986): 64–77, 192–202; John M. Cooper, "Greek Philosophers on Euthanasia and Suicide," in Baruch A. Brody, ed., *Suicide and Euthanasia: Historical and Contemporary Themes* (Dordrecht: Kluwer, 1989), pp. 9–38; Anton J. L. van Hooff, *From Autothanasia to Suicide: Self-killing in Classical Antiquity* (London: Routledge, 1990); Elise P. Garrison, "Attitudes toward Suicide in Ancient Greece," *Transactions of the American Philological Association* 121 (1991): 1–34.

16. Although I shall include some new material, in the remainder of this chapter I shall draw extensively from my "Suicide and Early Christianity," which is chap. 4 of my *Medicine, Society, and Faith in the Ancient and Medieval Worlds* (Baltimore: Johns Hopkins University Press, 1996), pp. 70–126. This paper originally appeared in *Suicide and Euthanasia: Historical and Contemporary Themes,* Baruch A. Brody, ed. (Dordrecht: Kluwer, 1989), pp. 77–153, and is reprinted in a slightly abridged and revised form in *Medicine, Society, and Faith.*

17. WL 603212 (Mich. Cir. Ct.), p. 9.

18. Ibid.

19. Ibid., pp. 9–10.

20. Glanville Williams, *The Sanctity of Life and the Criminal Law* (1957; reprint, New York: Knopf, 1970), pp. 254–55. See also his article "Suicide" in *The Encyclopedia of Philosophy* (New York: Macmillan, 1967).

21. Margaret Pabst Battin, *Ethical Issues in Suicide* (Englewood Cliffs, N.J.: Prentice Hall, 1982), pp. 29, 71–73, 89.

22. Emile Durkheim, *Suicide: A Study in Sociology,* trans. J. A. Spaulding and G. Simpson (Glencoe, Ill.: Free Press, 1951).

23. Ibid., p. 44.

24. Ibid., p. 227; cf. p. 67.

25. Arthur J. Droge and James D. Tabor, *A Noble Death: Suicide and Martyrdom among Christians and Jews in Antiquity* (San Francisco: Harper, 1992).

26. Ibid., p. 4.

27. Ibid., p. 187.

28. Ibid., p. 5.

29. Ibid., p. 125.

30. Ibid., p. 114.

31. Ibid., p. 125.

32. Ibid., p. 119.

33. Ibid., pp. 124, 187.

34. Ibid., p. 189.

35. Ibid., p. 187.

36. Ibid., pp. 61–62.

37. Ibid., p. 62.

38. Ibid., p. 63.

39. Ibid., p. 179.

40. The numerous issues that make the subject of martyrdom in early Christianity complex are only tangential to our present concerns and, hence, must not detain us here. There is a continually expanding literature on martyrdom and persecution in early Christianity. Still the most authoritative and reliable treatment is W. H. C. Frend, *Martyrdom and Persecution in the Early Church* (Oxford: Blackwell, 1965).

41. Some groups that were peripheral to the orthodox community, e.g., the Gnostics, maintained that apostasy—even a cavalier denial of one's beliefs—was acceptable if death were the alternative, since what one said under duress was irrelevant to the condition of one's heart. The reaction of the orthodox community to such a perspective was unequivocally condemnatory.

42. Droge and Tabor, *A Noble Death*, p. 156.

43. *The History of the Church from Christ to Constantine,* trans. G. A. Williamson (New York: Penguin, 1965), 8.12.2 (p. 342).

44. Ambrose, *Concerning Virgins* 3.7.32; Jerome, *Commentarius in Ionam prophetam* 1.6.

45. Eusebius, *History of the Church* 6.41.7, p. 276 in Williamson's translation.

46. Ibid., 8.6.6, p. 334.

47. "Similitude" 10.4.3, in *Shepherd of Hermas,* in *AF* 2:305.

48. Justin Martyr, *2 Apology* 4, in *FC* 6:123.

49. *Epistle to Diognetus,* in J. Quasten, *Patrology,* vol. 1, *The Beginnings of Patristic Literature* (1950; reprint, Westminster: Christian Classics, 1983), p. 251.

50. *Clementine Homilies* 12.14, in *ANF* 8:295.

51. Clement, *Stromateis* 6.9, in *ANF* 2:497.

52. Tertullian, *Flight in Time of Persecution* 13.2, in *FC* 40:304.

53. Tertullian, *Apology* 23.3, in *FC* 10:71–72. See also ibid., 46.14, 50.4–11; *To the Martyrs* 4.9; and Timothy D. Barnes, *Tertullian: A Historical and Literary Study* (Oxford: Clarendon, 1971), pp. 218–19.

54. Lactantius, *Divine Institutes* 3.18, in *ANF* 7:88–89.

55. Lactantius, *Epitome* 39, in *ANF* 7:237.

56. Eusebius, *History of the Church* 2.7.1, p. 81 in Williamson's translation.

57. Ibid., 5.16.13 and 15, p. 220.

58. John Chrysostom, *Commentary on Galatians* 1:4, in *NPNF-1*, 13:5.

59. Ambrose, *Death as a Good* 3.7, in *FC* 65:73–74.

60. Ambrose, *Concerning Virgins* 3.7.32, in *NPNF-2*, 10:386.

61. Jerome, *Letters* 39.3, in *NPNF-2*, 6:51.

62. Jerome, *Commentarius in Ionam prophetam* 1.6, in *Patrologia cursus completus, Series Latina,* Jacques Paul Migne, ed. (Paris: J. P. Migne, 1844–65) 1.12:390–91 (my translation).

63. See also Eusebius, *History of the Church* 8.12.3–4, 8.14.14 and 17, and Chrysostom, *Homilia encomastica,* in *Patrologia cursus completus, Series Graeco-Latina,* Jacques Paul Migne, ed. (Paris: J. P. Migne, 1857–66), 49:579–84.

64. On the Donatist movement see W.H.C. Frend, *The Donatist Church* (Oxford: Clarendon, 1952).

65. Augustine, *Letters* 13.10, in *FC* 16:246.

66. Cyprian, *Mortality* 8, in *FC* 36:204–5.

67. Ibid., 11, p. 207.

68. Ibid., 12, p. 208.

69. Ibid., 20, p. 215.

70. Ibid., 26, pp. 220–21.

71. Droge and Tabor, *A Noble Death*, p. 185.

72. Not only was Augustine's influence minimal in Eastern Christianity, but it also became fashionable in some quarters of Eastern Orthodoxy virtually to excoriate Augustine, as is graphically illustrated by the mean-spirited tone of the Eastern Orthodox lay theologian and philosopher Christos Yanaras, who calls Augustine "the fount of every distortion and alteration in the Church's truth in the West"; see his *Freedom of Morality* (Crestwood, N.Y.: St. Vladimir's Seminary Press, 1984), p. 151 n. 10.

73. Ibid., p. 187.

74. See his *City of God* 1.26.

75. See the compelling study by Gary B. Ferngren, "Early Christianity as a Religion of Healing," *Bulletin of the History of Medicine* 66 (1992): 1–15.

76. Henry Sigerist, *Civilization and Disease* (Chicago: University of Chicago Press, 1943), pp. 69–70. That Sigerist, an avowed Marxist, was no apologist for Christianity is graphically demonstrated by an entry in his diary on June 8, 1935: "I firmly believe in the fundamental goodness and honesty of man. Give him a social security, a chance to work and his share in the goods of life and he has no reason to be wicked. Christianity came into the world as the religion of love, and failed. It was adopted because man was afraid of life. If you are not afraid of this life you need not wait for a hypothetical hereafter. Christianity failed to create satisfactory economic conditions. It did not prevent man from exploiting his fellow-men and therefore sowed hatred instead of love." *Henry E. Sigerist: Autobiographical Writings,* selected and translated by Nora Sigerist Beeson (Montreal: McGill University Press, 1966), p. 110.

77. See Danielle Gourevitch, "Suicide among the Sick in Classical Antiquity," *Bulletin of the History of Medicine* 43 (1969): 501–18, and van Hooff, *From Autothanasia to Suicide,* especially pp. 122–26.

78. Margaret Pabst Battin, one of the philosophers whom I quoted earlier, was as dogmatic as Alvarez in her conviction that Christians before Augustine were very favorably inclined toward suicide and that Augustine imposed a new perspective which, as she said, "there is little reason to think . . . is authentically Christian." She has apparently modified her views somewhat. It is interesting to note that she has recently written, "While Christian values clearly include patience, endurance, hope, and submission to the sovereignty of God, values that militate against suicide, they also stress willingness to sacrifice one's life, especially in martyrdom, and absence of the fear of death. Some early Christians (e.g., the Circumcellions, a subsect of the rigorist Donatist) apparently practiced suicide as an act of religious zeal. Suicide committed immediately after confession and absolution, they believed, permitted earlier entrance to heaven. Augustine (354–430) asserted that suicide violates the commandment 'Thou shalt not kill,' and is a greater sin than any that could be avoided by suicide. Whether he was simply clarifying earlier elements of Christian faith or articulating a new position remains a matter of contemporary dispute." Margaret Pabst Battin, "Suicide," in *Encyclopedia of Bioethics: Revised Edition* (New York: Simon and Schuster Macmillan, 1995), p. 2446.

79. 1993 WL 603212 (Mich. Cir. Ct.), p. 10.

80. Ibid., pp. 10–11.

2

DOCTORS AND THE DYING OF PATIENTS IN AMERICAN HISTORY

Harold Y. Vanderpool, Ph.D., Th.M.

This story of doctors and the dying of adult patients in colonial American and U.S. history is both new and seemingly familiar. It is new because it has not yet been fully told. It may seem familiar because several of its subplots deal with widely discussed contemporary issues that have been, in fact, subjects of discussion and divisiveness for generations.

The "traditions" narrated here consist of patterns of thought, advocacy, and practice on the part of colonial and U.S. physicians vis-à-vis how their patients died—for example, the tradition of soothing the physical and mental sufferings of persons until death ensued or the tradition of fighting death against all odds of recovery. Over the centuries new traditions of thinking and acting emerged, forged change, sometimes became submerged, but never vanished.

Because these traditions encompass professional, moral, religious, institutional, social, and technological dimensions of life, their history must be interdisciplinary. This story is informed by all of these dimensions, as well as by historical discussions concerning this topic,[1] some of which focus on professional-technological, intellectual,[2] institutional,[3] and socioeconomic[4] developments.

Doctors, Home Dying, and Assuaging Death

Before and after the American Revolution physicians apparently attended the beds of many dying persons, but they did not define such attendance as a professional duty until the 1840s. Criticizing the extravagance of funerals in New York, William Livingston in 1753 decried the "ridiculous" burden of families' giving scarves and rings to the rich, but was not opposed to "sending a genteel present in a private manner" to a deserving clergyman or physician for service to the deceased.[5] The life and letters of the notable American physician Nathan Smith (1762–1829) tell of his service during the "dying hours" of patients, and how, in turn, some of his medical colleagues attended to his dying "with kind ministrations."[6]

Smith and others were doing all they could to save the lives of their patients, which included the use of surgery and the "heroic" remedies of the time—copious bloodletting and huge doses of poisonous drugs to induce vomiting and defecating.[7] While the extent of their "kind ministrations" is not altogether clear, without question it included prolific use of the drug without which the practice of "physic . . . would be lame and deficient," opium.[8] Nathaniel Chapman, the author of the first (1817) systematic treatise on pharmacology in the U.S., called opium the most useful drug in the *materia medica*. Regarded as a stimulant and unmatchable analgesic, opium in liquid form as laudanum was used throughout the eighteenth and much of the nineteenth centuries to dull pain, induce sleep, alleviate coughs and headaches, and treat a wide range of communicable diseases.[9]

At the same time, Americans of all walks of life could procure laudanum or any number of patent (actually unpatented) medicines filled with opium or its active alkaloid, morphine (first isolated in 1817) without relying on doctors.[10] Readily available from druggists, published recipes, and traveling salesmen, opium- and morphine-laden concoctions were often self-prescribed for aches, pains, and the pangs of dying family members. Indeed, the widespread and liberal lay use of such medicinals led physicians to write about how to treat those who had overdosed. This literature continued during the many decades prior to the passage of U.S. federal legislation in 1906 that began to control the use of narcotics.[11]

With or without the aid of physicians, the drama of human death was enacted in the home. Surrounded by loved ones, friends, and neighbors, dying persons were observed with almost clinical detail, were given calculated doses of laudanum, and, most of all, were expected to inspire others with noble dying. Lest they be considered "very stupid," they were expected to know when they were dying, so that they could resign themselves to the hands of Providence, commission those around them to useful and righteous living, and think upon heavenly things until they expired naturally, peacefully, and, on occasion, triumphantly.[12] To die away from one's family was terrible. To die unaware or afraid was worse. Writing to his mother for details about the death of his "dear old pappy," a Missouri farmer drew together these themes:

> Mother i should have liked to have node whether he was resined to gow. . . . rite to me and let me now all about that gives me eas if he was perfectly risined to gow mother in that triing ower if he was prepared to gow what sweet thoughts to himself and all of his children.[13]

No wonder books and countless articles in religious periodicals recounted the final days, testimonies, and deaths of Americans of all walks of life with hardly a mention of physicians—unless the physician's own life displayed a notable aspect of the expected drama, such as returning home from travels so the dying doctor "might be among his friends before the closing scene."[14]

Narratives of the deaths of Americans in the nineteenth century often appeared in magazines under the title "Biography" or "Memoirs" rather than "Obituaries." Accounts of the decedents' afflictions, how they bore up under the afflictions, and detailed descriptions of their actions and quotations of their utterances constituted core features of their lives, their biographies.[15] To be present at a friend's, neighbor's, or family member's death was looked upon as a "great" or "very great privilege."[16]

By the end of the 1840s, U.S. physicians agreed that they should assume special responsibilities in the care of grievously sick and incurable patients. Their duties were set forth in the rules unanimously adopted by the newly formed American Medical Association in 1847. Regarded virtually as scripture by American physicians for the next sixty years, the text of this Code of Ethics is historic:

> . . . the physician should be the minister of hope and comfort to the sick; that, by such cordials to the drooping spirit, he may sooth the bed of death, revive expiring life, and counteract the depressing influence of those maladies which often disturb the tranquillity of the most resigned in their last moments. . . . A physician ought not to abandon a patient because the case is deemed incurable; for his attendance may continue to be highly useful to the patient, and comforting to the relatives around him, even in the last period of a fatal malady, by alleviating pain and other symptoms, and by soothing mental anguish. To decline attendance, under such circumstances would be to sacrifice . . . that moral duty, which is independent of, and far superior to, all pecuniary consideration.[17]

These responsibilities accord with the Continental and British medical literature on "euthanasia," the term denoting what doctors could and should do to ease and assuage the physical and mental trials of dying persons without ever shortening or ending life.[18] In keeping with centuries of Jewish, Catholic, and Protestant tradition,[19] U.S. physicians sought to "revive expiring life" and, in cases "deemed incurable," to alleviate "pain and other symptoms" and soothe mental anguish.

Why did American doctors begin to assume these duties? In part this practice developed as a result of the medical profession's increasing organization and influence throughout the first half of the nineteenth century.[20] Surely also notable physicians became aware of and actively opposed some of the ignorance and abuses of home dying. Highly influential through teaching and publications, Worthington Hooker (1806–1867) expressly addressed abuses associated with noble and holy dying. He described how a physician (probably himself) "found the family and the friends assembled around the bed of the patient weeping over him as a dying man," and how, in turn, by administering a cordial of medicine (likely laudanum) and his own "cordial" of prognostic hope, "The patient not only revived but recovered."[21] Hooker critiqued "erroneous" views and actions associated with the "perfect resignation" so "exceedingly desired" by his contemporaries—its monotony, its "semi-fatalism," the ways it was being falsely equated with "charity and fondness of friendship," and, most of all, the times in which it ran counter to the physician's highest duty, "the prolongation of life."[22] Hooker's views precisely paralleled the contents of the AMA's 1847 code, which held, as noted, that by administering "cordials to the drooping spirit," physicians would "sooth the bed of death, revive expiring life, and counteract the depressing influence of those maladies which often disturb the tranquillity of the most resigned in their last moments."

Hooker's passionate concern to "revive expiring life" fueled his criticisms of popular rituals of home dying. "To cure the patient," he said, is the doctor's "*vocation,* and nothing should be permitted to interfere with it."[23] For the sake of this calling, patients' surroundings should be "kept quiet," and doctors should let everyone know that it is "wrong to excite the mind of the patient on any subject." Revealing that the "subject" he had in mind was religion, Hooker added that clergy should "consult with the physician," rather than presume to act independently.[24]

We may be inclined to regard these formerly center-stage issues as antique curiosities. In fact, they display how Hooker and his American peers wrestled with a question that continues to plague modern medicine: By what means and to what extent should the physician try to prolong life? Hooker and his peers employed their knowledge, experience, and influence to the extent that they transformed ingrained patterns of home dying. Recognizing the limits of their craft, they believed that one of the most effective means of prolonging life emanated from the doctor's insistence on quiet, composed, and hope-imbued surroundings. Ever hopeful that most patients would recover, they nevertheless believed that once the doctor could determine that health could not be restored, they should, as reflected in the AMA code, comfort relatives, alleviate pain and other symptoms, and soothe mental anguish.[25] Holding to the same ideals, but less concerned about how they clashed with popular rituals surrounding home dying, European physicians decried the use of excessive and futile *medical* interventions. Their opposition to "dangerous and dubious therapeutic measures" for patients whose health could not be restored would soon be discovered in America.[26]

Like the 1847 AMA code and virtually all his contemporaries, Hooker did not discuss shortening or ending human life.[27] In one place he commented that when patients are dying, physicians "can generally give relief to suffering . . . and thus at least smooth the passage to the tomb"; and he adds that the number of those "whose diseases [the physician] can neither palliate nor cure is exceedingly small."[28] Given this silence, Worthington Hooker and other U.S. physicians of the time likely would have agreed with the pioneer educator Horace Mann: "The suicide, who eats poison and dies, strikes us with a just horror, for we feel it a heinous sin to spurn God's blessing of life."[29]

Seven Physician Responses over Euthanasia: 1870–1950s

Many factors contributed to the post-1870 turmoil over the morality of doctors' inducing the deaths of incurable and suffering patients. These factors include the development of the hypodermic syringe (brought to America in 1856), by which morphine could be injected with quick and powerful results;[30] the discovery of anesthesia in 1846 and the ensuing controversies over and refinements of its uses;[31] the emphasis on palliation of disease in the face of a discrediting of the heroic remedies of the eighteenth and nineteenth centuries;[32] the advance of pluralism and secularism in the face of cogent challenges to religious orthodoxy beginning in the last decades of the nineteenth century;[33] and the public's increasing appetite for painkillers and for physician assistance in relieving their aches and pains.[34]

In this chapter, and in keeping with modern usage, *physician-induced* or *physician-administered death* will be used synonymously with the term *euthanasia*. In spite of its historic meaning from the seventeenth into the nineteenth century, in America *euthanasia* began to denote physician-administered death beginning in 1873, even though the term was occasionally used in its historic sense into the 1920s.[35]

The turmoil over the morality of euthanasia began in the U.S. in 1873 with the published review of a debate that had been going on in England for three years. While the stories of doctors and the dying of patients in England and America are decidedly different, English opinion did, on occasion, influence the thinking and actions of American physicians.

The 1873 review was published in the then widely read *Popular Science Monthly*. The pros and cons of euthanasia set forth in this review are to this day regularly aired by defenders and opponents of mercy killing. The review centered on an essay by a schoolmaster and essayist, Samuel D. Williams, who defended the proposition

> that in all cases of hopeless and painful illness it should be the recognized duty of the medical attendant, whenever so desired by the patient, to administer chloroform, or such other anesthetic as may by-and-by supersede chloroform, so as to destroy consciousness at once, and put the sufferer at once to a quick and painless death.[36]

After outlining how to prevent abuses to such a duty—firmly establishing prognosis, assuring that the patient's wishes are clear, and so on, Williams described "the tortures of lingering disease," then marshaled his case: that instances of such suffering "abound on every hand"; that the patient desires to die because his life is "an intolerable burden to himself and others"; that the doctor possesses the medical means and skill to bring "his patient immediate and permanent relief"; that while we greatly value life, its "sacredness" under "grinding pain" is negated; and, reflecting the arguments of the philosopher David Hume (1711–76), that if Providence wills that humans should not seek to escape from pain, it must also will the absurd notion that humans should never strive to better the conditions of their lives and communities.[37]

Noting how Williams's article was being widely circulated and discussed in the English press and how most of the replies to it were "decidedly" opposed, the *Popular Science* reviewer outlined the positions of those opposed. Euthanasia could and would be abused. Overdoses of readily accessible laudanum, for example, could "do the business" of death without leaving a trace of evidence. Euthanasia would give rise to a "sea-change" of lessened care and concern for invalids. It would release social "instincts" of "selfishness and cruelty" toward helpless and vulnerable persons. It would undermine the care of the grievously sick and dying. While all of these arguments were well stated, none was more powerfully expressed than how euthanasia, if widely accepted, would undermine dying persons' sense of worth:

> A deathbed, instead of being the scene for calling forth the tenderest emotions and the noblest self-sacrifice, will be haunted by a horrid suspicion; the sick man fearing that his departure is earnestly desired.[38]

These pro and con arguments became and remain fixtures in the story of the U.S. struggle over the morality of euthanasia. Debates over its possible abuses and whether they could be controlled became the subject of unending discussion and controversy.[39] While physicians disproved Williams's assertions about the frequency of torturous dying,[40] all could relate agonizing cases of persons pleading for relief, but whose physical and mental sufferings could not be eased short of death.[41] Both sides of the debate appealed to the value and sacredness of life. Euthanasia's opponents claimed that reverence for life serves as the foundation for Western religion and the practice of medicine.[42] Its proponents held that life's sacredness was being confused with the ruthlessness of nature and the far greater worth of the many dimensions of life accompanying personal awareness.[43] A. A. Brill's opposition to euthanasia in 1936 on Freudian grounds—that "incalculable harm" would result from releasing humankind's cruelty and aggressiveness via authorized killing—represents an elaboration of the 1873 theme about euthanasia's giving rise to cruelty and selfishness.[44] Arthur J. Dyck's and Albert R. Jonsen's opposition to physician-assisted suicide (PAS) on the grounds that easily accessible doctor-aided death undercuts the need of expertise in terminal care expands on the 1873 theme of euthanasia's undermining the care of the dying.[45] Robert N. Wennberg's concern that legalized euthanasia will lead dying persons to feel guilty about their burdensomeness on the family precisely accords with the 1873 quotation already given.[46]

The replaying of themes during the first fifty years of controversy led a *JAMA* editorialist to remark that "like a recurring decimal, euthanasia becomes a subject of controversy periodically in the press."[47] In actuality, the controversy that began in 1873 became all the more heated, and new patterns of thought and practice were developed during the ensuing years.

The historical record between 1873 and the 1950s reveals that U.S. physicians responded to the questions posed by euthanasia in a variety of ways. Seven types and levels of response will be delineated here. Unlike the discreet categories of ethics and some historical accounts, these responses are many-faceted, often interrelated, and forecast a number of contemporary concerns that are often assumed to have arisen only recently.

The first response arose from the American Medical Association and contains a "no" and "yes": a no to euthanasia because it undermines the physician's duty to prolong human life, and a yes to the AMA's nineteenth-century tradition of continuing to care for terminally ill persons.

First the no. Expressly responding to the proeuthanasia arguments of Samuel Williams, an editorial in *JAMA* in 1885 called Williams's proposal "ghastly." Any doctor who would adopt such views displays "moral laxity" and might as well "don the robes of an executioner" or carry out the act of "a scientific assassin."[48] Other editorialists and authors voiced similar but less accusatory stances in the years to follow. In 1901, Louis J. Rosenberg and N. E. Aronstam presented a graphic case in which "euthanasia would be a godsend," but then argued that for "the welfare of society," it is better "to let a few suffer" than to "run the risk of creating crime and criminals."[49] In 1926 an editorialist opined that his opponents were advocating "the right to die," which cut against the grain of the doctor's duties to prolong life and never "bring life to a close."[50] Doctors continued to say no during the mid-1930s when debates over euthanasia intensified over its possible legalization in the House of Lords (1936) and in response to the activities of the British Voluntary Euthanasia Legislation Society (founded in 1935) and the Euthanasia Society of America (founded in 1938). During the heat of the controversies over the passage of legislation to permit euthanasia in the state of New York (1947), Willard L. Sperry, dean of the Harvard Divinity School, asserted in the *New England Journal of Medicine* that "the legal validation of euthanasia seems to cut against the whole basis and practice of medicine." If we forfeit reverence for life, the dean added, "we have slipped our moorings."[51] This tradition continued through the 1960s, 1970s, 1980s, and to the present time.[52]

The yes to the medical profession's duty to assuage the physical and mental anguish of dying persons was upheld from the 1870s through the 1950s by a few increasingly isolated physicians. The lack of concern over terminal care during these years is mirrored in the revisions of the AMA Code of Ethics. The two paragraphs from the 1847 code were reduced to four lines in 1903, then to this part of a sentence in 1912: ". . . a physician should not abandon or neglect the patient because the disease is deemed incurable. . . ." The widely separated publications of advocates of medicine's nineteenth-century legacy are readily identifiable, publications by Frank E. Hitchcock in 1889, Arthur MacDonald in 1921 and 1928, Alfred Worcester in

1935, and Walter C. Alvarez in 1952.[53] The authors indicate how their deeply held concerns were being neglected. All mention that "making death easy, gentle and placid" is not being taught in medical schools; and three of four say in effect that "there is little found in the medical literature on the management of the dying."[54] Alvarez expressed the concerns of all: "the handling of the slowly dying and their families is so important, it is unfortunate that so rarely does anyone ever discuss the subject in medical schools, at medical meetings, or in the journals." His best source of information was, he said, the "excellent little book" by Worcester, which "every physician in the land should read and re-read."[55] Each doctor had much to say about terminal care in the setting of his time—the life-prolonging and life-sustaining effects of candor, communication, and the physician's steadfast attention; what analgesics to use; differences between age groups; physician-family relationships; and the personal rewards of bringing comfort to dying persons and their families.

A second type of physician response to euthanasia followed in the footsteps of many nineteenth-century practitioners: the prolongation of life takes absolute priority over the easing of suffering.[56] In 1896, for example, Isaac N. Quimby was asked, "Is it right to prolong the agony of a patient if the physician knows positively that death is inevitable in a short time?" "To the bitter end," Quimby asserted. "A physician has no right to terminate the life of a patient, even when to prolong that life is to cause the most agonizing tortures." Pleased rather than alarmed by Quimby's position, other physicians agreed with him at the time.[57] Years later, but prior to the campaign that championed the patient's right to forego aggressive treatment, David A. Karnofsky reasserted Quimby's point of view. Before a large medical audience Karnofsky insisted on the necessity of "aggressive or extraordinary means of treatment" to prolong life. He then asked, "When should the physician stop treating [the] patient?" His answer: "I believe he must carry on until the issue is taken out of his hands."[58] The pervasiveness of this tradition in U.S. medicine will soon become evident.

Responding in the opposite direction, but seeking to uphold the basic premises of the AMA's stance, a third response recognized prolonging life as a priority that could, on occasion, sanction the shortening of life in order to ease pain and assuage suffering. This was the position taken by perhaps the first American doctor to admit publicly that he had "practiced" euthanasia—T. T. Robertson. Expecting that he would "shock some and antagonize the theologians," Robertson, at a meeting of the South Carolina Medical Association in 1879, said that he had administered narcotics to two patients dying with "loathsome and torturing disease," so "as to shorten life a few hours and secure [their] easy deaths."[59] Similar views and stories are found in the 1920s and 1930s. In 1950, having received numerous letters from doctors and nurses in response to his article in the *New England Journal of Medicine,* William Sperry recounted specific instances when doctors and nurses gave drugs that they knew would shorten life.[60] However frequent this practice may have been, it was not advocated as a policy until the 1980s. Given the frequency of doctors insisting that the time of death could not be accurately determined, those who shortened life could be accused of performing euthanasia.[61]

The fourth response is that which the AMA staunchly opposed: physician-administered death. Those advocating this view held that the physician's duty to assuage suffering should, on occasion, take priority over the duty to prolong life. During the ferment over the legalization of euthanasia in Ohio (1906), a physician wrote to the *New York Times* saying that "some means ought to be devised to provide an 'easy death' for those who desire it, who are a burden to themselves, a millstone to a struggling family, and a shuttlecock for the hospitals." He then related a case in which euthanasia would have been "of immeasurable benefit for everyone concerned," and added, "Physicians know it would be a benefit, but humanity will never legally allow it."[62] By 1917 at the annual meeting of the American Association of Progressive Medicine, 87 of the 111 delegates voted to have a committee draw up legislation supportive of euthanasia in "every State."[63] By 1945 the Euthanasia Society of America secured a symbolic 1,776 physician signatures in favor of legislation to permit euthanasia in New York. In 1972, a poll of physicians in two West Coast hospitals revealed that 27 percent were willing to end the lives of patients who were suffering and incurably ill.[64]

A fifth response was registered by physicians who wanted to extend euthanasia to populations of undesirable or unwanted human beings. While this response centered on the social desirability of ending the lives of "newborn monsters," on occasion doctors held that legalizing euthanasia "should include in its provisions such members of the community as are suffering from incurable diseases, lunatics, and idiots."[65] This view was backed by notable Americans between 1900 and 1939. In 1935 the Rockefeller Institute's famed Nobel Prize winner, Alexis Carrel, declared that "sentimental prejudice should not obstruct the quiet and painless disposition of incurables, criminals, hopeless lunatics."[66]

The sixth and seventh responses deserve much more exploration. The sixth held that while it is the "bounden duty" of doctors not to terminate life, physicians should be allowed to end the "living death" of persons "dying at the top"—those who are "past consciousness, past even suffering."[67] To use contemporary language, this approves of ending the lives of humans who are persistently unaware of their surroundings, which would include patients in comas.

The seventh response held that physicians should never end the lives of persons suffering from incurable diseases, but that suicide and suicide assistance should not be condemned. In the midst of restating *JAMA*'s opposition to euthanasia in 1904, one of its editors commented, "We may excuse the person who commits suicide to avoid inevitable torture or dishonor."[68] Speaking to the medical staff of the Massachusetts General Hospital in 1948, William Sperry opposed euthanasia but countenanced this case of physician-aided suicide/euthanasia:

> I have a friend who, with the connivance of her doctor, gave her husband, who was suffering from a cruelly painful and fatal disease, a heavy overdose of morphine. She said she had no scruples about doing so and had never had a single regret. You must know many more such examples than I.[69]

New Responses to the Dreadfulness of Hospitalized Dying, 1952–70

Walter C. Alvarez's article "Care of the Dying" in 1952 identified an emerging problem that would soon take center-stage—the problem of physician-controlled dying in the hospital. The article signals the difference between the expert and humane care Alvarez was giving in the homes of his patients and his sense of dread over what was occurring in hospitals. "When I myself lie dying," he wrote,

> I hope that I will have by me some wise and kindly physician who will keep interns from pulling me up to examine my chest, or constantly puncturing my veins, or putting a tube down my nose, or giving me enemas and drastic medicines. I am sure that at the end I will very much want to be let alone.[70]

Two factors account for the momentous changes that were occurring in the 1950s. First, ever-increasing numbers of Americans were dying in hospitals and institutions for the aged and infirm. Equated with social progress and the triumphs of scientific medicine, the number of general hospitals expanded exponentially—from fewer than 200 in 1873, to 4,438 in 1928, 5,237 in 1955, and 5,736 in 1965.[71] In theory and fact, hospitals became the locus of modern medical care. They became and remain the organized meeting place of medical professionals, patients, and developing technology. Hospitals and long-term care institutions thus replaced the home as the place in which increasing numbers of Americans spent the last months, weeks, and days of their lives. By 1949, these institutions were the sites of 50 percent of American deaths; by 1977, over 70 percent, and by 1983, perhaps 80 percent.[72]

Second, within hospitals—especially teaching hospitals that modeled first-class medicine for each generation of medical trainees—the priority of prolonging life against the background of ever-new forms of technological intervention emerged triumphant. In the first decades of the twentieth century, nasal tubes, masks, and positive pressure ventilation apparatuses were developed for resuscitation and anesthesia. Compressed air and oxygen were used to inflate the lungs, and injections of epinephrine (adrenaline) via long hypodermic needles directly into the heart were used to counteract cardiac arrest. With the advent of thoracic surgery in the early 1930s, surgeons discovered that direct hand massaging of the heart could restore its functioning; and by 1953, 28 percent success rates of surgically opened chest procedures were reported.[73] Penicillin and other antibiotics were employed to control infections after 1945; and in the early 1950s ventilators as "complete substitutes to spontaneous breathing" had been developed, the refinements of which continued to the present day. The newer respirators were designed to overcome chronic and progressive respiratory insufficiency of seriously sick, dying, and comatose patients.[74] The report of successful closed-chest or external heart massage/defibrillation in 1960 led to the rapid employment of portable, battery-powered defibrillators that became and remain standard equipment for cardiopulmonary resuscitation (CPR).

The practices and complex patterns of interaction between doctors, nurses, patients, and families within hospitals during the early 1960s were explored in depth by Barney G. Glaser and Anselm L. Strauss, who identified the following as the hospitals' overarching goal:

> Doctors, particularly the younger ones, often cannot bear the thought of losing a patient, which comes with recognizing that there is nothing more to do. Fired with the ideal of saving, they put patients on life-prolonging equipment, in the vain hope that they can achieve recovery after all. They search the literature for clues to new treatments.[75]

Glaser and Strauss indicate that several conditions in hospitals "encourage unduly extending the life of patients" even in "the 'nothing more to do' phase": uncertainty of the time of death; on occasion, a family's insistence on doing everything possible; the "favorite rationale" that prolonging life is the society's mandate to medical professionals; doctors' sense of helplessness and defeat when life could not be prolonged; and, most of all, the sheer "inertia of intense heroics" that "sometimes lead a doctor to continue an all-out effort to save a lost patient even though he is dimly aware that there is no hope."[76] Regardless of the reasons, the hospital's personnel believed that "once you come to the hospital," you ought to know that "everyone is concerned to preserve your life." "The person has no choice" in the matter.[77]

Beyond the tradition of giving absolute priority to prolonging life, several of the other responses charted earlier continued in the hospital. The tradition of assuaging physical and emotional suffering continued, but was revised as "comfort care," care that centered on the ideal of pain-free dying. Given the overriding belief at the time (a story in itself) that patients would be emotionally devastated if they discovered that their lives could not be prolonged, medical personnel and patients alike were "characteristically unwilling to talk openly about the *process* of dying" in the hospital.[78] Having surrendered the benefits of candor and openessness advocated by Worchester, Alvarez, and others earlier, elaborate measures were taken to *control* what patients and families knew and to keep ward-upsetting emotional outbursts from occurring.[79] Dying must be painless and peaceful.

Other responses continued, but in secretive fashion. Patients whose pain could not be controlled were at times euthanized. Lethal doses of narcotics were given "in the hope of achieving painless comfort." Both euthanasia and the practice of shortening life to relieve pain were designated "invisible acts" by hospital personnel.[80]

The countenancing of suicide continued. Called "auto-euthanasia," suffering patients were at times relegated to a separate "dying room," where with or without a "nurse's surreptitious assistance" (via providing pills at the bedside and leaving the patient "unwatched for comparatively long periods of time") the patient could and would "manage his own death." Sympathy for those suffering and dying fostered this tacit permission of suicide, whereby the patient could "arrange a painless, easy departure," forestall life prolongation, and mitigate the ordeals of both the family and the medical staff.[81]

Through it all, a "collective mood" developed—the desire not to be present at death.[82] All, or at least nearly all, of the expectations and meanings of death that had sustained nineteenth-century Americans' belief that to witness a person's passage from life was a "great privilege" had been lost. "General hospitals are unhappy places" for dying persons, a physician remarked in 1961; in them the dying "'crock' is a second class citizen."[83]

The ideal of "prolonging life" became and remains more replete with meaning than might be assumed. While the meaning of "prolonging" is now clear, the strange meaning of "life" requires explication. Within the beliefs and practices of the modern hospital, "life" referred and refers to a numinous, supremely valued substance that physicians, beyond all others, know about—when and how it resides within the inner working of the human body, and when it threatens to vacate that habitation. Physicians, therefore, became life's appointed guardians. When humans who still possess life but stand to lose it are rushed to the hospital, they consign themselves to the life-prolonging efforts of physicians. In American hospitals between the 1950s and 1970, life's prolongation had taken precedence over the lives, the biographies, experiences, wishes, and relationships of persons who possessed life.

The pre-1970 protests of the small number of doctors and others who decried the overuse of life-sustaining technology occurred against the backdrop of the technological, institutional, and conceptual changes just sketched. No voice, other than that of the Pope, quite matched that of an anonymous woman from the pages of the *Atlantic Monthly* in 1957. This is the way her essay began:

> There is a new way of dying today. It is the slow passage via modern medicine. If you are very ill modern medicine can save you. If you are going to die it can prevent you from so doing for a very long time.[84]

Only gleamings of the power of her article shine through selective quotations. Her husband had gone through "an ordeal which has somehow deprived death of its dignity." "Every new formula, all the latest wonder drugs, the tricks and artificial wizardry, are now prescribed and brought to bear. The dreary dreadful days and nights proceed." "Your husband went into a coma at eleven o'clock. We are doing all we can." "When the first doctor came on duty I accosted him and begged that they cease this torture. He explained that except under the most unusual circumstances they had to maintain life."[85]

The woman's anguish was heard by like-spirited physicians in the late 1950s and the 1960s. Quoting from her in 1962, Frank J. Ayd remarked that her article "should be read by all physicians. What a contrast there is between what this distressed widow portrayed" and what Alfred Worcester advocated "in his edifying lecture on 'The Care of the Dying'!"[86] Ayd opposed those who gave absolute priority to the prolongation of life by employing all possible therapeutic measures. Believing that this represents "the prolongation of agony," Ayd voiced a point of view that many might assume was never articulated before 1970. He maintained that every competent adult "has the right" to "not only refuse extraordinary means of prolonging life," but also to "reject means which are ordinary but artificial and which offer no hope of a cure." Ayd illustrated his second point by saying that the patient with terminal illness has the right to refuse antibiotics if she or he develops pneumonia.[87]

The primary "moralist" Ayd quoted as substantiating his views was Pope Pius XII (1876–1958), who in 1957 addressed the morality of using or ceasing to use extraordinary measures to prolong conscious life or, via artificial respirators, to maintain the lives of permanently comatose patients. The Pope held that in these instances the doctor "has no separate or independent right where the patient is concerned . . . he can take action only if the patient explicitly or implicitly, directly or indirectly, gives him permission."[88] Ayd was also taking cues from Edward H. Rynearson, who had referred to the teachings of the Pope and asserted that "the physician himself" is the one who causes "these extraordinary measures to be continued indefinitely."[89]

The position of Worchester, Alvarez, Rynearson, Ayd, and others[90] constitutes an eighth response to questions posed in the name of mercy by advocates of euthanasia. This response says "Yes!" to the tradition of gentle and natural dying stemming from the nineteenth century in the form of a "No!" to those who viewed life prolongation as an absolute priority. Those from the 1930s, 1950s, and 1960s who, against the tenor of their time, proclaimed that the acclaimed advances of scientific medicine were becoming instruments of oppression for dying persons were the prophets of an imminent revolution.

The Right to Refuse and the Duty to Care, 1970–

The revolution began in 1970 when a Protestant ethicist, Paul Ramsey, published *The Patient as Person,* a book that was in its fifth printing by 1975. Ramsey wrote *Patient as Person* after experiencing the "cultural shock" of two semesters of biweekly conferences over the moral aspects of medicine with faculty members at the Georgetown University Medical School.[91] He underscored an agenda of critical issues: (1) "Should a patient suffering from terminal illness be given life-sustaining procedures?" (2) Should "fragmented creatures in deep and prolonged coma from severe brain damage . . . be maintained 'alive' for years by a combination of artificial activators and by nourishment?" (3) Must patients suffering from incurable diseases be given "routine" measures, such as antibiotics for pneumonia? And (4) beyond these moral quandaries, is there not a positive "medical duty to (only) care for the dying" when they can no longer be cured?[92]

While the problems Ramsey addressed were precisely those Ayd and others had previously identified, Ramsey's approach was new. He both heralded these issues into the public domain and wrestled with them in light of Western philosophical and religious heritages. Physicians and other responsible professionals must, he said, "enter the thicket" of ethical discourse, the distinctions and import of which would test and reform existing "medical imperatives" according to clearly articulated "moral imperatives." The doctor must "make room for the primacy of human moral judgment on the part of [those] who are his patients, the relatives of his patients, and their spiritual counselors."[93]

Drawing upon a long tradition of Roman Catholic medical ethics and employing his own "canons of loyalty" derived from a "steadfast *faithfulness*" to God-human and human-human "covenants," Ramsey argued that the employment of all medical procedures is morally permissible only if they are perceived as beneficial from the patient's point of view. For example, on the matter of intravenous feeding Ramsey wrote that this "ordinary means may be out of place because of the condition of a patient—as out of place as unusual or heroic procedures" in other circumstances:

> All these procedures, some "natural," others "artificial," are appropriate means . . . of only caring for the dying, of physically companying with the dying. They are the embodied and effective gestures of soul to soul.[94]

"The patient," Ramsey added, "has entered a covenant with the physician for his complete *care,* not for continuing useless efforts to *cure.*"[95]

Paul Ramsey's voice was accompanied by a chorus of others. The year before *Patient as Person* appeared, a psychiatrist, Elisabeth Kubler-Ross, published *On Death and Dying,* which began with a graphic depiction of the dreadful circumstances of terminally ill persons in hospitals. Foreshadowing the title of Ramsey's book, Kubler-Ross held that the dying person is

> treated like a thing. He is no longer a person. Decisions are made often without his opinion. If he tries to rebel he will be sedated. . . . He may cry for rest, peace, and dignity, but he will get infusions, transfusions, a heart machine, or tracheostomy if necessary . . . he will get a dozen people around the clock, all busily preoccupied with his heart rate, pulse, electrocardiogram . . . his secretions or excretions but not with him as a human being.[96]

Kubler-Ross's book added fuel to the fire of an emerging "death and dying" movement that focused on the meanings of death, better communication with dying persons, their psychological responses to impeding death, and the need of palliative and hospice care. Within four years, half a million copies of her book had been sold.[97]

In 1969, the Hastings-on-Hudson Institute was organized to bring together leading scholars in medicine, philosophy, law, and the social sciences to collaborate on ethical problems associated with what it called "the biological revolution." It became "immediately evident" to the Institute's participants that questions related to human death would "occupy a special place" in its deliberations.[98] The Hastings Institute became a catalyst in the burgeoning "medical ethics movement" that began in the late 1960s, developed journals, published textbooks, and soon made the movement's presence known in ethics and humanities courses in medical schools, colleges, and seminaries across the nation.

Leading figures in this movement included Robert M. Veatch, who, while working with the Hastings Institute, proposed in 1972 that legislation regarding the right of patients to refuse medical treatment "is worthy of consideration as a public policy."[99] By 1976 Veatch published a book that explored in detail the ethical issues Ramsey had raised and assessed the pros and cons of various legislative options, several of which were under consideration in state legislatures. The emerging "right to refuse" laws enabled patients to fill out "living wills" that would hopefully keep them from having to endure unwanted life-sustaining interventions should they become terminally ill.[100] Veatch's bibliography displayed a virtual "who's who" of the many physician and nonphysician ethicists and humanists who had become engaged in the ever-broadening discussion.

What began as books soon made its way into magazines, newsweeklies, daily papers, and "right to die" television programs. By 1973, polls showed that some 62 percent of Americans believed that they ought to be able to tell their doctors to let them die rather than to extend life with no cure in sight. In 1970 and 1973, polls of doctors revealed that 59 percent and 80 percent, respectively, favored withdrawal of treatment under similar conditions.[101]

In 1973 Norman L. Cantor addressed worrisome legal issues surrounding patients' desires to decline lifesaving medical treatment. Noting that the issue was far from settled and that one professor of law had argued that compulsory lifesaving treatment by doctors was both permissible and desirable,[102] Cantor set forth a point of view that would soon become normative—that "an independent adult who genuinely objects to treatment . . . must be respected by the judiciary." Respect for the patient's bodily integrity and constitutional rights of privacy support the patient's right to decline treatment in spite of the "emotional strain" it would entail "both for physicians and judges."[103]

The Karen Ann Quinlan case in New Jersey (1976) extended this right of refusal (through patients' proxies or surrogates) to persons in persisting comas—the "fragmented creatures" Ramsey spoke about in

1970, who had also been subjects of concern as early as 1896. By 1991, thirty-one states had enacted durable power-of-attorney laws as mechanisms for the exercise of incompetent persons' rights to refuse medical care.[104]

In spite of all the ethical, legal, and popular ferment over the right to refuse life-prolonging medical procedures, the members of the President's Commission for the Study of Ethical Problems in Medicine and Biomedical and Behavioral Research thought that the complex issues that remained required attention. The Commission's report (1983) held that ethical principles and U.S. law (1) allow medical professionals to provide pain relief to dying patients, even if that treatment "entails substantial risks" of shortening life; (2) permit patients to refuse even "'ordinary' hospital interventions" such as tube-conveyed nutrition, hydration, and antibiotics; but (3) do not warrant any withdrawal of comforting and respectful patient care.[105]

The Commission also critically evaluated the strengths and weaknesses of "living wills" and other advance directives and reviewed the "natural death acts" that had been passed in fourteen states (beginning with California in 1976) to enable patients to forego life-sustaining treatment.[106] It furthermore addressed the morality of cardiopulmonary resuscitation (CPR) and concluded that a "presumption favoring" the use of CPR was justified when patients undergo "unexpected cardiac arrest in the hospital," that do-*not*-resuscitate (DNR) orders are also justified as long as the patient requests or consents to such orders, and that all medical institutions should establish "explicit policies and procedures" governing CPR and DNR procedures.[107]

Yet the issuance of the President's Commission report did not settle all the issues surrounding a person's right to refuse medical interventions. Worries continued over the degree to which the honoring of patients' choices was more illusory than real in hospitals.[108] And the case of Claire C. Conroy (1985), a woman who was mentally and physically impaired but neither brain dead nor in a chronic vegetative state and not even terminally ill, initiated controversy over the right of such patients and their proxies to refuse and remove nasogastric feeding. While ethical and legal discussion over the Quinlan case centered on discontinuing the use of respirators for patients in persisting comas and the uncertainty of death after respiratory therapy was withdrawn (Karen Ann Quinlan survived for ten years after she was taken off the respirator), the Conroy and other cases centered on the right of both mentally impaired and competent persons to refuse being fed through intravenous lines and stomach tubes, which would result in death within days.[109] Case law now upholds the right of refusal by mentally impaired and competent patients on grounds that their rights of free choice, self-determination, and privacy outweigh medicine's and the state's interests in prolonging life, preventing suicide or manslaughter, and protecting the goals and practices of modern medicine. Ethicists opposed to or cautious about such refusals point to their possible abuses, harmful consequences, and conflicts with certain religious traditions.[110] Those who favor this right point to the inhumanity of forcing treatment on persons whose quality of life is deemed intolerable; to the degree to which competent adults who refuse hydration and nutrition do not manifest suicidal behavior predicated on mental illness, self-hate, or feelings of worthlessness; to the right of free choice in societies with diverse understandings of the nature of life and the good life; and to its conformity with other religious traditions.[111]

The protests over the reign of technology in the 1930s through the 1960s became transformed during the ensuing decades into struggles over the extent to which both "high tech" and "low tech" medical procedures should be delimited for the benefit of persons.

Euthanasia, 1950s–

The literature on euthanasia from the 1950s to the present is far more limited than meets the eye. While it appears that this literature is vast, most of the books and articles that dealt with "euthanasia" were, in fact, wrestling over the issues just explored—the right to refuse medical treatment for various groups of patients. In spite of well-voiced criticisms at the time over the confusing uses of the term *euthanasia*,[112] the word was constantly associated with a wide range of practices. To forego or refuse medical treatment was often designated "passive euthanasia" or, at times, "negative" or "indirect" euthanasia. To end the lives of patients in persistent comas was called "direct involuntary" or "active involuntary" euthanasia. And the now common meaning of the term (physician-administered death out of mercy) was called "voluntary" or "direct voluntary" or "active" euthanasia. No wonder the literature seemed vast. Books that focused on the ethics and legality of terminating life-sustaining medical interventions were identified as works on euthanasia; and the ever-increasing number of medical ethics texts that contained sections on "euthanasia" were dealing with many issues other than mercy killing, if indeed that subject was covered at all in such sections.[113]

Although the literature on euthanasia (in its common sense) was limited, the issue itself had and has staying power because of its great moral import for individuals, the medical profession, and the public. We have seen how "mercy killing" became the subject of controversy in 1873 and never ceased to attract and alarm thereafter. The controversy continued both before and after World War II. While it is true that advocacy of euthanasia for undesirable or unwanted human beings—the fifth response identified previously—by and large ceased in the U.S. after the horrors of the Nazi holocaust became known, the widely held notion that proeuthanasia sentiment for incurable sufferers of disease was for many years sharply curtailed because of these horrors appears to rest more on fiction than fact.[114] In actuality, the Euthanasia Society of America began a new campaign to legalize euthanasia in New York—a campaign that kindled controversy throughout the 1950s and beyond—the very year World War II ended with the defeat of Germany and Japan (1945).

No single individual championed the cause of physician-administered death more than Joseph Fletcher, whose several books and articles from 1954 through the 1970s were widely reprinted in medical ethics texts and became staple items in college and medical school courses. In his book on medical ethics in 1954, Fletcher tackled the problem head on and at length. Drawing upon the ideas that empowered the proeuthanasia initiative in New York, he defended the morality of euthanasia as an act of mercy for patients who have no "reasonable hope of recovery" and for whom narcotics cannot relieve pain.[115] He had in mind horrible deaths experienced by persons such as the satirist and Irish clergyman Jonathan Swift, whose "mind crumbled to pieces" over the course of eight years of demoralization and degradation. Viewing Roman Catholic opposition to euthanasia as a form of fatalism that renders physiological life sacrosanct, Fletcher predicated his defense on the worth and sacredness of personal uniqueness, pleasure, freedom, and rational control and on the Christian beatitude, "Blessed are the merciful, for they shall obtain mercy."[116] After he offered his refutation of the ten "most common and most important" objections to the morality of doctor-induced death, he briefly mentioned three others. Fletcher dismissed the third of these—that to legalize mercy deaths might lead to the killing of persons with nonfatal illnesses and disabilities—as an "alarmist . . . old red herring."[117] Certain physicians at the time approved of euthanasia on grounds that precisely parallel those of Fletcher.[118]

In 1968 Fletcher gave his still ardently held views a new cast—that euthanasia offers an escape from modern medicine's propensity "to prolong life (or, perhaps, to prolong death)." "Nowadays," he said, persons die "sedated . . . betubed nasally, abdominally, and intravenously . . . more like manipulated objects than like moral subjects." Fletcher then asserted that medicine had succumbed to the errors he formerly attributed to Catholicism. Medicine had turned the "bare sentience" of biological life into an idol. Compared to the terrors and the "dehumanization" of "protracted terminal treatment," euthanasia offered escape, peace, and person-centered control.[119]

Fletcher's new emphasis on euthanasia as the means by which persons could control their own ends rather than be enslaved to the traditional sanctity-of-life ethics of religion and medicine, found full expression in 1973. "It is harder," he said,

> morally to justify letting somebody die a slow and ugly death, dehuman-ized, than it is to justify helping him to escape from such misery. This is the case at least in any code of ethics which is humanistic or personal-istic, i.e., in any code of ethics which has a value system that puts humanness and personal integrity above biological life and function.[120]

While he still spoke of compassion, the "exigent and tragic circum-stances" Fletcher now emphasized were conditions "that biomedical progress is forcing [on] us." Instead of the *sanctity of life*, ethical imper-atives should be derived from *"quality of life"* considerations. For Fletcher, quality-of-life concerns morally justify our "taking it into our own hands to hasten death for ourselves (suicide) or for others (mercy killing)."[121]

Joseph Fletcher's conceptual transformation illustrates why con-cerns over euthanasia and, almost two decades later, physician-assist-ed suicide continued to be the subjects of intense scholarly, legislative, and public controversy. In 1873 and for many decades to follow, debates over euthanasia centered on whether merciful, physician-induced death for persons with intractable pain could be permitted without undermining the fundamental goals of and trust in the pro-fession of medicine, the sense of worth of severely ill and debilitated persons who did *not* want to be painlessly killed, and abuses that might result from further compromising legal, moral, and religious prohibi-tions against killing. While it might appear that medicine's advances in pain control should have ended, or at least moderated, the debate, it did not. It did not because of the post-1960 horrors over "dehumanizing" technology-controlled dying.

An article in 1977 by a neurology resident, Thomas W. Furlow, Jr., exemplifies this change. Furlow decried how doctors and patients alike are "victim[s] to the tyranny of technology, whereby artificial life-support systems create and sustain the semblance of life, though the patient is devoid of any modicum of actual living." Furlow pointed out that "surreptitiously . . . euthanasia in its various forms is practiced by many physicians and the support for it is even greater." At the same time, most doctors believe that euthanasia "runs counter to the tenets of medical ethics." So why was Furlow one of the doctors who signed

"A Plea for Beneficent Euthanasia" that would grant patients "the right to live and die with dignity"?[122] Because, he answered, euthanasia could engender "magnificent comfort" in the place of "the agonizing dread of impending death felt by both patient and his family . . . when the healing arts and the patient alike had reached their limits."[123]

The highwater mark of controversy and consternation over euthanasia in the medical literature occurred with the "It's Over, Debbie" case published in *JAMA* in 1988. Within an acute care hospital, a resident physician was called to the bedside of a twenty-year-old woman named Debbie who was experiencing "unrelenting vomiting . . . receiving nasal oxygen, had an IV . . . suffering . . . severe air hunger . . . had not eaten or slept in two days . . . had not responded to chemotherapy." "It was a gallows scene," the resident said, "a cruel mockery of her youth and unfulfilled potential." Her circumstances and single utterance, "Let's get this over with," led the doctor to end her life with twenty milligrams of morphine sulfate. "She seemed peaceful at last."[124]

The case itself and the numerous, mostly negative, responses to it did not argue over what then and now (and in keeping with the changes just sketched) constitutes the quintessential horrors of human dying—life-sustaining measures to the point of prolonged, controlled, and emaciated death. Well-known physician ethicists who decried the resident's action appealed to historic arguments—its constituting premeditated murder, its undermining trust in and respect for physicians as healers, not killers, and its failure to give the patient relief and comfort rather than death.[125] Those who agreed with the resident's action spoke of his courage to do what they could not bring themselves to do, or they recounted graphic stories of loved ones who, for example, had their arms tied down as they were forced to exist "for sustained periods of time in a living hell."[126]

Debbie's case illustrates how appeals to mercy and compassion could be and were being used both to approve of euthanasia[127] and oppose it in the name of medicine's longstanding duty to comfort and care for dying persons.[128] To break past this standoff in light of the public's post-1970 fears over technology-dominated dying, proponents of euthanasia had to—and did—find a stronger appeal: patient autonomy. We have noted how that appeal empowered the right of patients to refuse life-prolonging interventions. The turmoil surrounding "It's Over, Debbie" demonstrates how this appeal had become a bedrock principle for proeuthanasia advocates, several of whom condemned the morality of the resident's actions because he failed to secure Debbie's clearly expressed and legally documented informed consent.[129]

Albert R. Jonsen has rightly argued that appeals to autonomy, not "intractable pain," became the ethical principle, the main "justifying argument," for euthanasia after the late 1970s, and that fears over the loss of personal autonomy due to mental deterioration—in particular, "the threat of Alzheimer's disease and other similar dementing disorders—empowered this change.[130] Beyond these fears, indeed fueling them, lay the two decades of repulsion over the loss of control, freedom, and selfhood due to technologized dying.

This accounts for the debates and turmoil that continue. Hotly contested and narrowly defeated (46 percent for, 54 percent opposed) voter-based referenda in Washington State (1991) and California (1992) sought to legalize or decriminalize euthanasia for terminally ill patients whose written requests would have to be witnessed by two nonrelatives who did not stand to gain from the patient's death.[131] Commenting on the defeat of California's Proposition 161, Alexander Capron noted that its defeat "should not obscure the remarkable fact that millions of people are so fearful of how they think they'll be treated by the health care system when they're very ill that they'd rather be dead."[132] This message has not been lost on doctors and others who plead up to the present time that physicians and nurses must recover the meaning of "the naturalness of dying" in the face of decades of "medicalized" overtreatment.[133]

The pro and con arguments first articulated in 1873 still infuse modern controversies over the morality of euthanasia, but the contention that continues is fed by new-found and more widespread concerns. Mercy found new forms—mercy not just for the few faced with intractable pain, but for the many, for any and all faced with agonizing medicalized dying. Mercy forged new linkages—sorrow, repulsion, and fear over technologized dying and the deterioration of acquaintances and loved ones in nursing homes. Linked to and empowered by the law, autonomy became the predominant moral means by which the proponents of euthanasia sought to ease these anxieties.

Physician-Assisted Suicide (PAS), 1990–

As indicated in the seventh response discussed above, by the late 1940s U.S. physicians and nurses were surreptitiously allowing and aiding incurably sick and suffering patients to take their own lives, and decades earlier, doctors expressly stated that they could not condemn patients for doing so. Throughout the 1970s and 1980s the tradition of secretively, or not so secretively, aiding persons with terminal or degenerative illnesses to die continued.[134] Doctor-aided suicide was also advocated by a few ethicists in the 1970s.[135] Prophetic of future developments, Sisella Bok commented in 1977 that the sufferings of terminally ill patients could be mitigated not only by offering them more "humane care" but also through the development of "more permissive attitudes toward the suicide of those in distress and terminally ill."[136] On the popular front, Derek Humphry, then a newspaper reporter for the *Los Angeles Times,* published *Jean's Way* in 1978, "the true story of one woman's plans to end her own life toward the end of a terminal [bone cancer] illness." Deluged with inquiries, Humphry refused to reveal the name of the doctor who had given him the drugs to induce his wife's "peaceful death."[137]

Prosuicide sentiment for persons suffering unto death gathered greater force in the 1980s. Formed as "a pressure group" in 1980 under the leadership of Humphry and his new wife, the Hemlock Society championed "self-deliverance for the dying." Humphry soon published *Let Me Die before I Wake,* a regularly revised book that included a number of personal narratives that explicitly revealed how persons with advanced illnesses or with serious incurable diseases could, with the assistance of physicians or friends, carry out "rational suicide." The motivations behind Humphry's and the Hemlock Society's work were overtly stated: "leaders of the medical profession . . . have only themselves to blame" for the appalling number of requests they are getting for assisted suicide. "The fearsome machinery . . . they have brought to their healing arts invokes a feeling of horror in many people . . . the thought of remaining hooked up to machines via tubes to our orifices, is, for many, the abnegation of human dignity."[138]

Even though the medical ethics literature had not yet passionately seized the topic of PAS, the *Bouvia v. Superior Court* case (1986), which was advanced as a "right to refuse" case, contained many of the ingredients of physician-managed suicide.[139] The case itself was pressed by Richard Scott, a physician, attorney, and founding member of the Hemlock Society.[140] In 1988 the Unitarian Universalist Association became the first U.S. religious group to "advocate the right to self-determination in dying, and the release from civil or criminal penalties of those who, under proper safeguards, act to honor the right of terminally ill patients to select the time of their own deaths."[141]

These traditions and developments formed the backdrop for the explosion of interest that greeted the 1990s: Dr. Jack Kevorkian's highly publicized assistance of Janet Adkins's death in 1990 and his supervision of the deaths of others thereafter; the lengthy and crafted account of Timothy E. Quill's counseling with and providing lethal drugs for "Diane" in the pages of the *New England Journal of Medicine* (*NEJM*) in 1991;[142] the voiced approvals of Quill's actions by notable physicians, including Arnold Relman, the editor of *NEJM* at the time;[143] and the publication of prosuicide publications, not the least of which was Derek Humphry's how-to-end-your-life bestseller, *Final Exit* (1991).

While historians should exercise extreme caution in explicating the forces that empower movements that breathe at their backs, I offer this thesis: that the explosion of interest in and the weighty issues surrounding PAS are, with two provisos, empowered by the concerns previously identified with respect to the victories over patients' rights to refuse treatment and the controversies over euthanasia. Autonomy still held and holds center-stage, because doctor-aided suicide endows patients with greater levels of control over when and how they would end their lives in the face of widespread fears over life prolongation.[144] Accompanying autonomy, however, are physician-centered issues, in particular the far less threatening penalties of the law for suicide-accomplicement than for doctor-administered death,[145] and the fact that the degree of participation by physicians is different for assisted death than for euthanasia.[146]

The first proviso to the view that these were the only dominating factors behind the ferment over PAS is that in spite of significant opposition to the morality of such assistance on the part of doctors and many ethicists,[147] doctors who give this aid can model how suicide assistance *ought* to be done. For many doctors, suicide assistance by empathetic and skilled physicians who seek to maintain trusting and long-term relationships with their patients stands in stark contrast to two unseemly options—the "treatment" provided by a disliked and distrusted physician renegade, Kevorkian, and the do-it-yourself campaign of Humphry and the Hemlock Society. Little love exists between these parties.[148]

The second proviso involves political reality and the medical profession's responsiveness, however belated it might be, to the social demands of the American public. For more than a century the majority of U.S. physicians, with the support of the public, viewed euthanasia as morally untenable. Under the rubric "Aid in Dying" (not Aid in Death) the referenda in the states of Washington and California sought to decriminalize both euthanasia and PAS. These efforts failed. Following the defeat of these efforts, however, a citizen-led initiative in Oregon advanced this euthanasia-free proposition: that adults should have the right "to request and obtain prescriptions from doctors to end their life." Oregon passed this "Death with Dignity Act" in 1994. Although this act cannot become instated as law unless and until controversies over its legality are adjudicated, the voters of Oregon have spoken. How the medical profession will respond, and possibly adjust, to this referendum (and surely others) remains an open question. How it should respond and how it might be able to adjust its traditions to the new public pressures is the subject of this book and a topic within the souls of American doctors.

NOTES

I thank my research assistant, Dr. Sara Clausen, for her library searches and editorial suggestions, both of which contributed immeasurably to my writing this essay.

1. Edwin R. DuBose, "A Brief Historical Perspective," in Ron P. Hamel, ed., *Choosing Death: Active Euthanasia, Religion, and the Public Debate* (Philadelphia: Trinity Press, 1991), pp. 16–26; W. Bruce Fye, "Active Euthanasia: An Historical Survey of Its Conceptual Origins and Introduction into Medical Thought," *Bulletin of the History of Medicine* 52 (1979): 492–502; President's Commission for the Study of Ethical Problems in Medicine and Biomedical and Behavioral Research, *Deciding to Forego Life-Sustaining Treatment* (New York: Concern for Dying, 1983), pp. 15–26 and 231–39; Rita L. Marker et al., "Euthanasia: A Historical Overview," *Maryland Journal of Contemporary Legal Issues* 2 (Summer 1991): 257–98; Stanley Joel Reiser, "The Dilemma of Euthanasia in Modern Medical History: The English and American Experience," in John A. Behnke and Sissela Bok, eds., *The Dilemmas of Euthanasia* (New York: Anchor Books, 1975), pp. 27–49; Harold Y. Vanderpool, "Death and Dying: Euthanasia and Sustaining Life: Historical Aspects," in Warren Thomas Reich, ed., *Encyclopedia of Bioethics*, revised ed. (New York: Simon & Schuster Macmillan, 1995), 554–63; and Jerry B. Wilson, *Death by Decision* (Philadelphia: Westminster Press, 1975), pp. 17–45.

2. Albert R. Jonsen, "To Help the Dying Die—A New Duty for Anesthesiologists?" *Anesthesiology* 78 (February 1993): 225–28.

3. Harold Y. Vanderpool, "Cultural Roots of Medicalized Dying," 1977, unpublished ms.

4. Ezekiel J. Emanuel, "The History of Euthanasia Debates in the United States and Britain," *Annals of Internal Medicine* 121 (15 November 1994): 793–802.

5. William Livingston, "Of the Extravagance of Our Funerals," reprinted in Charles O. Jackson, ed., *Passing: The Vision of Death in America* (Westport, Conn.: Greenwood Press, 1977), p. 46.

6. Emily A. Smith, *The Life and Letters of Nathan Smith, M.B., M.D.* (New Haven: Yale University Press, 1914), pp. 99–100, 140–41.

7. William G. Rothstein, *American Physicians in the Nineteenth Century* (Baltimore: Johns Hopkins University Press), pp. 41–62.

8. The quotation is from Dr. Thaddeus Betts in 1778 by David T. Courtwright, *Dark Paradise* (Cambridge: Harvard University Press, 1982), p. 44.

9. Courtwright, pp. 43–46.

10. Ibid., pp. 56–59, and James Harvey Young, *The Toadstool Millionaires* (Princeton: Princeton University Press, 1961).

11. Courtwright, pp. 45, 56–59.

12. An example of this ideal in 1816 is found in Barbara M. Cross, ed., *The Autobiography of Lyman Beecher* (Cambridge: Harvard University Press, 1961), pp. 215–21.

13. Quoted in Lewis O. Saum, "Death in the Popular Mind of Pre–Civil War America," in Jackson, p. 81.

14. The quotation is from an account of Doctor Joshua Brackett's death in 1802, found in Timothy Alden, *A Collection of American Epitaphs and Inscriptions with Occasional Notes*, vol. 1 (New York: Arno Press, 1977 [1814]), p. 221. For more details on noble and holy dying, see Harold Y. Vanderpool, "The Wesleyan-Methodist Tradition," in Ronald L. Numbers and Darrel W. Amundsen, eds., *Caring and Curing: Health and Medicine in the Western Religious Traditions* (New York: Macmillan, 1986), pp. 336–37.

15. A. Gregory Schneider, "Sentimental Community: The Ritual Drama of Happy Dying among Nineteenth-Century American Evangelicals," 1981, unpublished ms., and Alden, pp. 5–8.

16. See, e.g., the quotations in Saum, p. 82, and Cross, p. 217.

17. Code of Ethics, American Medical Association, 1847, in Reich, p. 2640.

18. The term *euthanasia* was first coined by Francis Bacon (1561–1626); and its historic use denoting physical and mental care short of ever ending life is found, e.g., in the essays of Carl Friedrich Heinrich Marx (1826) and William Munk. See C. F. H. Marx, "Medical Euthanasia," introduced and translated by Walter Cane, *Journal of the History of Medicine and Allied Sciences* 7 (1952): 401–16, and William Munk, *Euthanasia or Medical Treatment in Aid of an Easy Death* (New York: Arno Press, 1977 [1887]), pp. 65–105. Also see Vanderpool, "Death and Dying," pp. 554 and 558.

19. Vanderpool, "Death and Dying," pp. 554–57.

20. Rothstein, pp. 41–121. See also the impressive analysis of Martin S. Pernick, who cautions against singular and simplistic notions of "professionalism." Pernick, *A Calculus of Suffering* (New York: Columbia University Press, 1985), esp. pp. 241–48.

21. Hooker addressed these matters in detail. See Worthington Hooker, *Physician and Patient: A Practical View of the Mutual Duties, Relations and Interests of the Medical Profession and the Community* (New York: Baker and Scribner, 1849), pp. 344–417, quotes from 346–47.

22. Hooker, pp. 351–56. An earlier thoroughgoing critique of popular and evangelical rituals surrounding death was published in a Unitarian journal by an anonymous author: "Erroneous Views of Death," *Christian Examiner* 11 (November 1830): 161–85.

23. Hooker, p. 396, emphasis mine.

24. Ibid., p. 400.

25. Pernick indicates how, in keeping with the tradition revived by Francis Bacon and in contrast to the view of U.S. physicians that the prolongation of life was an absolute value, Hooker and others regarded relief of suffering or

mitigation of pain as an additional duty of physicians. This, of course, is reflected in the AMA's 1847 code. Pernick, pp. 104–20.

26. Marx, p. 407. Munk's belief that dying persons should be "left alone, and allowed to die in peace" (p. 87) led him to oppose both the employment of useless medical interventions (pp. 86–87) and the harassing effects of "exclamations of grief, and the crowding of the family round the bed" (p. 93).

27. In 1860 Samuel Dickson came close to such a discussion by defending the use of chloroform to ease pain even if it might on occasion end in "a prompt and painless termination of life for a succession of cruel and protracted tortures." See Pernick, pp. 110–11. In 1868, John Collins Warren described how he used ether "to ease pain in death," and in one ambiguous text, Warren tells of how a woman patient "received the consolations of religion," and "finally under etheral influence her spirit imperceptibly took its flight." John C. Warren, *Etherization; with Surgical Remarks* (Boston: William D. Ticknor, 1868), pp. 69–74, quotes from 72.

28. Hooker, p. 344.

29. Horace Mann, "Law of Physical Life," *Christian Examiner* 35 (September 1843): 29–30. See also the moral prohibitions of attempting to shorten life either by withdrawing soothing care or by the use of narcotics in Marx, p. 413, and Munk, pp. 94–95, and the strictures against "the heathen stoics" in W. C. Dendy, "On the Physiology of Death and the Treatment of the Dying," *Journal of Psychological Medicine and Mental Pathology* 1 (1848): 120–21.

30. Courtwright, pp. 46–47.

31. Pernick, pp. 125–239.

32. Fye, pp. 495–97.

33. Vanderpool, "Death and Dying," pp. 557–59.

34. Pernick, pp. 233–34.

35. *Euthanasia* denoted the older tradition of doctors' assuaging dying in, e.g., the essays of Frank E. Hitchcock (1889) and Arthur MacDonald (1921) and in editorials in the *Journal of the American Medical Association (JAMA)* as late as 1913. Although articles in *JAMA* toyed with the notion that *euthanasia* should denote doctor-induced death, while the term *euphoria* (as "causing comfort") should denote the older tradition (Louis J. Rosenberg and N. E. Aronstam, "Euthanasia—A Medicolegal Study," *JAMA* [12 January 1901]: 108–10), the term *euphoria* was soon dropped, while the modern usage of euthanasia became standard. Hitchcock, "Euthanasia," *Transactions of the Maine Medical Association* 10 (1889–1891): 30–41; MacDonald, "Death in Man," *Medical Times* 49 (July 1921): 149–58; editorials, *JAMA* 60 (14 June 1913): 1897.

36. "Euthanasia," *Popular Science Monthly* 3 (1873): 90–91. For background, see Fye, pp. 498–99.

37. *Popular Science,* pp. 91–92. For Hume, see Vanderpool, "Death and Dying," p. 558.

38. *Popular Science,* pp. 93–96, quotation from 94.

39. E.g., Arthur MacDonald, "Human Death," *Medical Times* 59 (September 1938): 28–39; Willard L. Sperry, *The Ethical Basis of Medical Practice* (New York: Harper and Brothers, 1950), pp. 154–55; and Marcia Angell, "Euthanasia," *New England Journal of Medicine* 319 (17 November 1988): 1349.

40. The literature here was rather extensive, and included Hitchcock's observations in 1890 that most dying persons exhibit few "signs of severe suffering," Olser's widely read report of investigating the deaths of 500 persons, most of whom died unconscious and unconcerned, and MacDonald's reports that popular beliefs regarding "Death agony" were false. Hitchcock, pp. 32–33; William Osler, *Science and Immortality* (Boston: Houghton Mifflin, 1904), pp. 18–19; and MacDonald, "Death in Man," pp. 154–55.

41. E.g., Rosenberg and Aronstam, 109–10; Sperry, pp. 144–46; Joseph Fletcher, *Morals and Medicine* (Boston: Beacon Press, 1960 [1954]), pp. 144–45.

42. Clark Bell, "Has the Physician Ever the Right to Terminate Life?" *Medico-Legal Journal* 14 (1896): 464–65; "Euthanasia for the Defective and Incurable," *JAMA* 43 (24 September 1904): 896–97; Willard L. Sperry, "Moral Problems in the Practice of Medicine," *New England Journal of Medicine* 26 (23 December 1948): 988; Joseph V. Sullivan, "The Immorality of Euthanasia," in *Beneficent Euthanasia*, ed. Marvin Kohl (Buffalo: Prometheus Books, 1975), pp. 12–33.

43. Abraham L. Wolbarst, "The Doctor Looks at Euthanasia," *Medical Record* 149 (1939): 354; Fletcher, pp. 191–95.

44. A. A. Brill, "Reflections on Euthanasia," *Journal of Nervous and Mental Disease* 84 (July 1936): 1–12, quote from p. 3.

45. Arthur J. Dyck, "Physician-Assisted Suicide: Is It Ethical?" *Trends in Health Care, Law and Ethics* 7 (Winter 1992): 20.

46. Robert N. Wennberg, *Terminal Choices* (Grand Rapids, Mich.: Eerdmans, 1989), pp. 189–90.

47. "Euthanasia Again," *JAMA* 87 (30 October 1926): 1491.

48. "The Moral Side of Euthanasia," *JAMA* 5 (1885): 382–83.

49. This lawyer (Rosenberg) and doctor (Aronstam) rightly identified their position as "utilitarian" in the tradition of "Jeremiah Benton" (actually Jeremy Bentham). Rosenberg and Aronstam, pp. 109–10.

50. "Euthanasia Again," p. 1491. The phrase "right to die" apparently originated in England about this time.

51. Sperry, "Moral Problems," p. 988. For background to the turmoil of the times, see Wilson, pp. 35–38.

52. E.g., William P. Williamson, "Life or Death—Whose Decision?" *JAMA* 195 (5 September 1966): 793–95; Marcia Angell, "Euthanasia," *New England Journal of Medicine* (17 November 1988): 1350–51; and Dennis L. Breo, "MD-Aided Suicide Voted Down," *JAMA* 266 (27 November 1991): 2895–2900. In 1988 the AMA declared that "the intentional termination of the life of one human being by another—mercy killing—is contrary to public policy, medical tradition, and the most fundamental measures of human value and worth." AMA, "Euthanasia," Report 12, June 1988, in *Reports of the Council on Ethical and Judicial Affairs* (Chicago: AMA, 1989), p. 2.

53. Hitchcock, pp. 30–43; MacDonald, "Death in Man," pp. 149–58, and "Human Death," pp. 232–41; Alfred Worcester, *The Care of the Aged, the Dying and the Dead* (Springfield, Ill.: Charles C. Thomas, 1935), pp. 33–61; and Walter C. Alvarez, "Care of the Dying," *JAMA* 150 (13 September 1952): 86–91.

54. The quotations are from MacDonald, "Death in Man," p. 240; and Hitchcock, p. 40.

55. Alvarez, p. 87.

56. Pernick, pp. 104–20

57. Bell (1896), p. 465. See also the description of Simeon E. Baldwin, *The Natural Right to a Natural Death* (Cincinnati: Frank H. Vehr, 1904), pp. 4–5.

58. "Cancer and Conscience," *Time* 78 (3 November 1961): 60.

59. *Transactions of the South Carolina Medical Association*, Charleston, 1879, pp. xiv-xvii. At the same meeting one of Robertson's colleagues told how he had done the same.

60. Sperry, *The Ethical Basis*, pp. 133–34.

61. Sometimes the phrase "hastening death" was used synonymously with or perhaps in partial disguise of euthanasia. See MacDonald, "Human Death," pp. 237 and 240.

62. Gregory Costigan, "Dr. Costigan on Euthanasia," *New York Times*, 6 February 1906, p. 8, col. 7. An example of another physician's views is found in George W. Jacoby, *Physician Pastor and Patient* (New York: Harper and Brothers, 1936), pp. 305–306.

63. "Urges Legal Killing of Hopeless Invalids," *New York Times*, 25 September 1917, p. 8, col. 2.

64. Robert M. Veatch, "Choosing Not to Prolong Dying," *Medical Dimensions* (December 1972): 8.

65. Dr. Walter Kempster quoted in "Fatal Dose to Incurable," *New York Times*, 26 January 1906, p. 1, col. 4.

66. "The Right to Kill," *Time* 26 (18 November 1935): 53–54.

67. Bell (1896), pp. 472–73.

68. "Euthanasia for the Defective," p. 896. See also the defense of suicide for patients whose "suffering is irretrievably hopeless and irremedial" in Bell (1896), p. 465.

69. Sperry, "Moral Problems in the Practice of Medicine," p. 988.

70. Alvarez, p. 91.

71. Rosemary Stevens, *In Sickness and in Wealth: American Hospitals in the Twentieth Century* (New York: Basic Books, 1989), esp. pp. 229–40.

72. President's Commission, pp. 17–18.

73. Arlo S. Hermreck, "The History of Cardiopulmonary Resuscitation," *American Journal of Surgery* 156 (December 1988): 435.

74. Thomas L. Petty, "The Modern Evolution of Mechanical Ventilation," *Clinics in Chest Medicine* 9 (March 1988): 1–10.

75. Barney G. Glaser and Anselm L. Strauss, *Awareness of Dying* (Chicago: Aldine, 1965), p. 202.

76. Ibid., pp. 194–203, quotations from 194, 200, and 203.

77. A quotation from a nursing student in ibid., p. 216.

78. Ibid., pp. 3–115, 204–56; also Donald Oken, "What to Tell Cancer Patients," *JAMA* 175 (1 April 1961): 86–94.

79. Though centered on sociological "awareness" theory, Glaser and Strauss's entire book was about the control of patients and families within the hospital setting. See especially, e.g., pp. 236, 248, 269–70.

80. Ibid., pp. 197, 209–22, and 236, quotes from pp. 197 and 222.

81. Ibid., pp. 223–25.

82. Ibid., quotations from pp. 196, 202, 224, 248.

83. Lawrence A. Kohn, "Thoughts on the Care of the Hopelessly Ill," *Medical Times* 89 (1961): 1180.

84. Anonymous, "A Way of Dying," *Atlantic Monthly*, January 1957, pp. 53–55.

85. Ibid., pp. 53–54.

86. Frank J. Ayd, "The Hopeless Case," *JAMA* 181 (29 September 1962): 1100.

87. Ibid., p. 1101.

88. Pope Pius XII, "The Prolongation of Life" [1958], in Stanley Joel Reiser, Arthur J. Dyck, and William J. Curran, eds., *Ethics in Medicine* (Cambridge: MIT Press, 1977), pp. 501–504.

89. Edward H. Rynearson, "You Are Standing at the Bedside of a Patient Dying of Untreatable Cancer," *CA* 9 (1959): 85–87.

90. For example, William P. Williamson, "Life or Death—Whose Decision?" *JAMA* 197 (5 September 1966): 793–95.

91. Paul Ramsey, *The Patient as Person* (New Haven: Yale University Press 1970), pp. xix-xxii.

92. Ibid., pp. 114–16.

93. Ibid., pp. 119–24, quotations from 119 and 124.

94. Ibid., pp. xi-xvii, 126–32, quotations from xii, xiii, and 126.

95. Ibid., pp. 129, 132.

96. Elisabeth Kubler-Ross, *On Death and Dying* (New York: Macmillan, 1969), p. 9.

97. Peter Steinfels and Robert M. Veatch, eds., *Death Inside Out* (New York: Harper and Row, 1974), p. 1. For the death and dying movement, see Harold Y. Vanderpool, "The Responsibilities of Physicians toward Dying Patients," in J. Klastersky and M. J. Staquet, eds., *Medical Complications in Cancer Patients* (New York: Raven Press, 1981), pp. 124–27.

98. Daniel Callahan, Preface, in Steinfels and Veatch, p. viii.

99. Veatch, "Choosing Not to Prolong Dying," pp. 8–10, 40, quotation from p. 40.

100. Robert M. Veatch, *Death, Dying, and the Biological Revolution* (New Haven: Yale University Press, 1976), esp. pp. 77–203; for Veatch's thinking about the content of living wills and his guidelines for "allowing to die" legislative policy, see pp. 176–203.

101. Ibid., p. 98.

102. Kenney F. Hegland, "Unauthorized Rendition of Lifesaving Medical Treatment," *California Law Review* 53 (August 1965): 860–77.

103. Norman Cantor, "A Patient's Decision to Decline Lifesaving Medical Treatment: Bodily Integrity versus the Preservation of Life," *Rutgers Law Review* 26 (Winter 1973): 228–64, quotations from p. 264.

104. Ezekiel J. Emanuel and Linda L. Emanuel, "Proxy Decision Making for Incompetent Patients," *JAMA* 267 (15 April 1992): 2067–71.

105. President's Commission, pp. 43–90. "Guidelines for the Supportive Care for Dying Patients" were given in Appendix B, pp. 275–97.

106. Ibid., pp. 121–70.

107. Ibid., pp. 8–9, 231–55.

108. Office of the General Council of the American Medical Association, "The Illusion of Patient Choice in End-of-Life Decisions," *JAMA* 267 (15 April 1992): 2101–4.

109. Tom L. Beauchamp and LeRoy Walters, *Contemporary Issues in Bioethics,* 3rd ed. (Belmont, Calif.: Wadsworth, 1989), p. 242. Beauchamp and Walters reprinted parts of the texts of the 1978 Florida *Satz v. Perlmutter* decision (one similar to the Quinlan decision), as well as the 1986 California Court of Appeals *Bouvia v. Superior Court* decision that affirmed the right of a competent but severely physically disabled woman, Elizabeth Bouvia, to refuse tube feeding and hydration, pp. 256–62. For the full text of the Conroy decision, see "In the Matter of Claire C. Conroy," Supreme Court of New Jersey, 98 N.J. 321, 486A. 2nd 1209, January 17, 1985.

110. See especially the chapters by Daniel Callahan, Michael Nevins, and Alan J. Weisbard and Mark Siegler in Joanne Lynn, ed., *By No Extraordinary Means: The Choice to Forego Life-Sustaining Food and Water* (Bloomington: Indiana University Press, 1986), pp. 61–66, 99–107, and 108–16.

111. See the chapters by Joanne Lynn and James F. Childress, Edward J. Bayer, Dan W. Brock, and Brock and Lynn in Lynn, pp. 47–60, 89–98, 117–31, and 202–15.

112. Ramsey, pp. 146–52; Veatch, *Death, Dying,* pp. 7–8, 83–84, 98–101; and President's Commission, p. 24.

113. E.g., Behnke and Bok, *Dilemmas of Euthanasia.* Given the usage of the term at the time, this was natural. In keeping with that usage, one of the authors in Behnke and Bok's book dealt with the morality of "the taking of another's life because of merciful motives to alleviate his pain and suffering," pp. 52–67, while the others focused on termination of treatment. For textbooks, see, e.g., Thomas A. Mappes and Jane S. Zembaty, *Biomedical Ethics* (New York: McGraw-Hill, 1981), pp. 342–98, and Ronald Munson, *Intervention and Reflection: Basic Issues in Medical Ethics* (Belmont, Calif.: Wadsworth, 1988), pp. 157–93.

114. That the holocaust *should* have put the issue to rest is another matter. See, e.g., Veatch, *Death, Dying,* pp. 86–90, and Edmund D. Pellegrino, "Doctors Must Not Kill," in Robert I. Misbin, ed., *Euthanasia: The Good of the Patient, the Good of Society* (Frederick, Md.: University Publishing Group, 1992), pp. 27–41, esp. 35–37. An early recognition of the bearing of the holocaust on euthanasia is found in Kohn, "Thoughts on the Care of the Hopelessly Ill," p. 1180.

115. Fletcher, *Morals and Medicine,* pp. 172–73. For Fletcher's use of the proeuthanasia platforms of the New York campaign, see pp. 185, 187, and 191.

116. Ibid., pp. 177–202.

117. Ibid., pp. 190–207, quotation from 207. Fletcher also discussed the three provisions of the New York State initiative, which he regarded as "model legislation," pp. 187–88.

118. K. R. Eissler, *The Psychiatrist and the Dying Patient* (New York: International Universities Press, 1955), pp. 116–27.

119. Fletcher, "Elective Death," in E. Fuller Torrey, ed., *Ethical Issues in*

Medicine (Boston: Little, Brown, 1968), reprinted in Sandra Galdieri Wilcox and Marily Sutton, eds., *Understanding Death and Dying* (Dominguez Hills, Calif.: California State College, 1977), pp. 352–67.

120. Fletcher, "Ethics and Euthanasia," in Robert H. Williams, ed., *To Live or to Die* (Springer-Verlag, 1973), as reprinted in Robert F. Weir, ed., *Ethical Issues in Death and Dying* (New York: Columbia University Press, 1977), p. 348.

121. Ibid., pp. 349–50, 355–56.

122. Marvin Kohl and Paul Kurtz, "A Plea for Beneficent Euthanasia," in Kohl, *Beneficent Euthanasia,* pp. 233–38.

123. Thomas W. Furlow, Jr., "Euthanasia and the Tyranny of Technology," in Kohl, *Beneficent Euthanasia,* pp. 169–79, quotations from 172, 176–78.

124. "It's Over, Debbie," *JAMA* 259 (8 January 1988): 272.

125. E.g., Willard Gaylin et al., "Doctors Must Not Kill," *JAMA* 259 (8 April 1988): 2139–40.

126. The quotes are from Susan Wilson, "To the Editor," *JAMA* 259 (8 April 1988): 2097.

127. Fletcher, *Morals and Medicine,* pp. 172–210; Marvin Kohl, "Voluntary Euthanasia," in Kohl, *Beneficent Euthanasia,* pp. 130–41; Wilson, p. 2097.

128. Ramsey, pp. 124–64; Arthur Dyck, "Beneficent Euthanasia and Benemortasia: Alternative Views of Mercy," in *Beneficent Euthanasia,* pp. 117–29; and Gaylin, p. 2139.

129. E.g., Don C. Shaw, "To the Editor," and Derek Humphry, "To the Editor," *JAMA* 259 (8 April 1988): 2096.

130. Jonsen, pp. 227–28.

131. See the analysis of Robert W. Wood and Ralph Mero, "Washington State's 'Death with Dignity' Initiative," in Robert H. Blank and Andrea L. Bonnicksen, eds., *Emerging Issues in Biomedical Policy* (New York: Columbia University Press, 1993), pp. 102–16. A very helpful annotated introduction to the extensive literature on euthanasia and physician-assisted suicide is provided by Pat Milmoe McCarrick, "Active Euthanasia and Assisted Suicide," *Kennedy Institute of Ethics Journal* 2 (1992): 79–100.

132. Alexander Morgan Capron, "Even in Defeat, Proposition 161 Sounds a Warning," *Hastings Center Report* 23 (January–February 1993): 32.

133. Jack D. McCue, "The Naturalness of Dying," *JAMA* 273 (5 April 1995): 1039–43.

134. See, e.g., Maria T. CeloCruz, "Aid in Dying: Should We Decriminalize Physician-Assisted Suicide and Physician-Committed Euthanasia?" *American Journal of Law and Medicine* 18 (1992): 378, and C. Gerald Fraser, "Man Allows Friend to Commit Suicide," *New York Times,* 11 December 1977.

135. For example, Glanville Williams, a professor of law in England whose articles were reprinted for U.S. audiences, said that "the obvious solution" to problems over life termination "would be to allow a doctor to assist a person . . . to commit suicide." And Joseph Fletcher argued why he believed that "suicide is the signature of freedom" for persons with severe physical and mental deficiencies. Williams, "Euthanasia and the Physician," in Kohl, *Beneficent Euthanasia,* pp. 145–68, quotation 164, and Fletcher, "In Defense of Suicide"

(1976), reprinted in John Donnelly, ed., *Suicide: Right or Wrong?* (Buffalo: Prometheus Books, 1990), pp. 61–73, quotation from 73.

136. Sissela Bok, "Euthanasia and the Care of the Dying," in *Dilemmas of Euthanasia,* p. 9.

137. Derek Humphry, *Let Me Die before I Wake* (Los Angeles: Hemlock Society, 1984), pp. 1, 131.

138. Humphry, p. 3.

139. See n. 109.

140. See Humphry, p. 5, and the discussion of Marker, pp. 278–80.

141. Ron P. Hamel and Edwin R. DuBose, "Views of the Major Faith Traditions," in Hamel, pp. 85–87. In June 1990 the Rocky Mountain Conference, a regional body of the United Church of Christ, affirmed "the right of persons under hopeless and irreversible conditions to terminate their lives . . . [by] suicide and euthanasia." The predicates for this position parallel those of Joseph Fletcher—"ever-increasing anxieties about a prolonged dying process," "quality of human life" concerns, and opposition to the "biological idolatry" within religious and medical tradition, pp. 89–90.

142. Timothy E. Quill, "A Case of Individualized Decision Making," *New England Journal of Medicine* 324 (7 March 1991): 691–94.

143. "Account of Assisted Suicide in Journal Advances Debate," *Medical Ethics Advisor* 7 (April 1991): 44–47.

144. Note, e.g., how Quill emphasized that his assistance enabled Diane "to maintain dignity and control on her own terms until her death." Quill, p. 693. See also Catherine L. Bjorck, "Physician-Assisted Suicide: Whose Life Is It Anyway?" *SMU Law Review* 47 (1994): 373.

145. Bjork, pp. 371–97, and T. Howard Stone and William J. Winslade, "Physician-Assisted Suicide and Euthanasia in the United States," *Journal of Legal Medicine* 16 (1995): 481–507.

146. Council on Ethical and Judicial Affairs, AMA, "Decisions Near the End of Life," *JAMA* 267 (22 April 1992), pp. 2229 and 2233.

147. E.g., Council on Ethical and Judicial Affairs, p. 2233.

148. E.g., George J. Annas, "Killing Machines," *Hastings Center Report,* March–April 1991, pp. 33–35; Nancy S. Jecker, "Giving Death a Hand: When the Dying and the Doctor Stand in a Special Relationship," *Journal of the American Geriatric Society* 39 (August 1991): 831–35; and Susan M. Wolf, "Final Exit: The End of Argument," *Hastings Center Report* 22 (January–February 1992): 30–33.

Part II

Ethical Assessments and Positions

3

SELF-EXTINCTION
THE MORALITY OF THE HELPING HAND

Daniel Callahan, Ph.D.

What can be said about human suffering? This much at least: No one wants to suffer. No one wants a death marked by suffering. Only tyrants and those who are pathologically cruel want others to suffer. Medicine is dedicated to the relief of suffering, and we proclaim ourselves to be a society that will not knowingly countenance the relievable misery of any group. Suffering not only brings pain, physical and mental (just as pain can bring suffering), it can in its extreme forms seem to rob people altogether of their humanity.

Given so many shared convictions—our mutual agreement that human suffering should be avoided if possible and relieved when it occurs—how can anyone morally oppose physician-assisted suicide (PAS) to save someone from it? Even if one personally opposes it, how in a free and pluralistic society can one legitimately deny it to others, those with a different ethical view? What could be a more private matter than our own life and fate? Who am *I* morally to judge what is bearable or unbearable suffering in others, or to evaluate what others might do to relieve their suffering? Does not common sense, moreover, seem to indicate that if someone is going to die anyway, and do so with needlessly unbearable suffering, PAS offers a merciful way of averting that misery?

For many people, the answers to these now-familiar questions seem almost self-evident. The moral case in favor of PAS appears to draw so obviously upon a store of shared values, a pervasive consensus about freedom and the relief of suffering, that it is sometimes hard to understand why the matter should so trouble others. Is that a matter of prejudice and irrationality? Or moral insensitivity? Or religious dogmatism?

No. It is none of those things, though they may surely be present in some people opposed to PAS. On the contrary, the longstanding historical prohibition of PAS—cultural, medical, and religious—rests upon a solid and enduring insight: that it is dangerous and wrong to sanction and endorse suicide as a way of relieving suffering and equally hazardous to make physicians the helping agents of such an action. I contend that there is no such thing as a right to PAS and that even if some *believe* they have such a right, they should voluntarily waive its exercise because of its dangers to others (much as we should not exercise our legal right of free speech to make nasty and demeaning racist statements).

There are, conventionally, two general philosophical approaches to the morality of euthanasia and PAS. One of them tries to show that those actions are intrinsically wrong—wrong, that is, even if some or all of their consequences may be beneficial. The other approach attempts to demonstrate that the consequences of PAS, its actual results, would be harmful, either directly and immediately or because they would lead us down that famous slippery slope. This tidy kind of dichotomy in moral theory is not helpful. It is hard to imagine how we can ignore consequences in determining what is intrinsically wrong and no less difficult to determine what counts as good and bad consequences without some notion of what is intrinsically right and wrong. Each theory seems, in practice, to need the other even to make good sense.

This is not the place to take up any further that longstanding debate in moral philosophy. For the purposes of this essay, I will adopt what I characterize as an ecological approach to the moral questions. Think of PAS as a seemingly attractive flower that we contemplate planting in the meadow that is our society. Should we do this or not? To answer this question we need, first, to ask whether the plant will take root and flourish in its own right. Will it grow as expected? We must ask, second, what it will do to the other plants in the meadow. How will it affect their flourishing? We must, that is, ask a twofold question: is PAS good in its own terms, and what will be its meaning and implications for the society in which it is introduced?

On the whole, it is that latter question that will most interest me here, but I want at the outset to say something about the intrinsic rightness or wrongness of PAS. What kind of a plant is it that we want to introduce into our societal meadow: good or bad, beneficial or noxious? I believe that PAS is in and of itself noxious. While I am quite prepared to acknowledge that some people may, out of despair over their fate or their suffering, want to commit suicide and am no less prepared to suspend moral judgment about their particular act, it is a wholly different matter to socially endorse and legitimate suicide as an acceptable and routine, even if relatively rare, way of dealing with the problem of an unhappy life. Our common moral intuition that suicide is ordinarily an act of desperation, that it usually bespeaks some degree of treatable depression, and that it ought not to be encouraged, strikes me as entirely valid. It is a way to defend ourselves, and help others defend us, from the despair that life can bring our way; and it is generally recognized that we need to help each other cope with it, not succumb to it. To give a physician, moreover, the power to kill another, even with the permission of that person, or to assist someone to kill himself is to place too much power in the physician's hands, that of a right to take life as a means of eliminating despair.

Euthanasia and Physician-Assisted Suicide: Are They Morally Different?

Quite apart from that argument, however, do I not here confuse and conflate euthanasia and PAS? After all, in PAS the physician does not kill at all. It is the patient who is the direct cause and agent of death. The distinction between euthanasia and PAS is not morally significant. A physician who provides a patient with a deadly drug and instructions about its use to bring about death bears as much responsibility for the death as the patient himself. The doctor is knowingly a part, and a necessary part, of the causal chain leading to the death of the patient. In most jurisdictions, the law holds equally responsible those who are "accessory" to capital crimes: if I give one person the gun with which I know he intends to kill another person, then stand by while he does so, the law will hold me as responsible for the death as the person who pulled the trigger. The same reasoning applies here: doctors who kill directly by injection or give others the pills to kill themselves are fully blameworthy (or praiseworthy if one accepts such actions as ethically acceptable) for what occurs.

I contend, then, that it is wrong to give one person an absolute power over the life of another, whether this power is gained by force or by voluntary means, and whether it is achieved directly or by accessory means. Consenting adult killing, where the parties are in voluntary agreement, is a moral wrong, not mitigated by its voluntary nature nor excusable because of its possibly beneficial consequences. I concede one exception to a general rule against giving people the legal power to kill each other or help each other to die: when that is the only way of saving or protecting the lives of others. But even that exception must be looked at with care and a wary eye. Western societies have allowed one person to kill another under three general circumstances: in self-defense, when that is the only way to protect one's own life; in just warfare, when that is the only way to defend one's country or community; and in capital punishment, when that is believed to be the only way to protect the lives of others. In each case, it should be noted, there is now considerable controversy. The harms, deliberate and accidental, done in the name of capital punishment (unjust executions), just warfare (massacres of civilians and other atrocities), and self-defense (negligent homicides) are notorious. For just that reason, many nations have abolished capital punishment, have denied their citizens the right to own hand guns (even for self-defense), and have become skeptical about the idea of a "just" war (though not enough to make much difference).

Euthanasia and PAS would have the dubious benefit of adding one more socially tolerated reason for one person to kill another or to assist another to kill herself. Given the well-established and longstanding failures and the corruptions of the other accepted reasons why one person may be allowed to kill another, considerable doubt is in order about whether this newest entry into our repertoire of acceptable killing will improve our common lot. In sum, I believe PAS to be wrong in and of itself because of the excessive power it puts in the hands of physicians; and this perception of wrongness is strengthened by the collateral experience of many societies that abuse seems a natural and inevitable component of the exercise of similar powers over the lives of others in a variety of contexts.

Even if one grants that the potential for abuse is considerable, two responses are possible. One of them is that some degree of abuse is a corollary of any legislation for any purpose. Abuse-free legislation is not possible and thus cannot be advanced as a reason to avoid passing laws whose purpose is otherwise taken to be morally acceptable. As a general proposition, that is undoubtedly correct, but we have to ask just what *exactly* it would mean in *this* context to tolerate some degree of abuse. It would mean this: that we would tolerate the deliberate killing of someone (euthanasia) or the deliberate manipulation of someone to kill herself (PAS) to support the freedom of others to be killed or be assisted in killing themselves. We would, in short, be allowing some lives to be unjustly taken in order that others could take their own lives. That would be a most strange and wrongful way of advancing or supporting self-determination: my autonomy would be promoted at the price of the wrongful taking of the life of another.

The other response is that the meaning of our individual right to life is, in actuality, not a positive right to live but, instead, a right not to be killed by others against our will. It is, so to speak, a negative right, which we should be free to waive if we believe that to be in our interest and beneficial to our welfare. From this perspective, it is then argued that we ought to be free to allow a physician to kill us, by waiving our right not to be killed, or to ask a physician to assist us in committing suicide, where we choose to forego our life by our own hand.

It is hard to know what to make of this seemingly arbitrary stipulation of the meaning of a right to life. The basis of the entire modern movement for general welfare rights, whether the right to a job or food or health care, has been based on the assumption that we owe each other more than a mere abstention from killing or harming them. It has been an effort to lay out a framework of positive rights, drawing upon widely shared convictions that we have positive obligations to each other no less than negative, noninterference obligations. Is the right of women not to be raped merely a negative right, which they may waive if they choose? Is the right not to be enslaved no less a right that can be waived if we are made an attractive enough offer to buy our bodies? The cost, in short, of taking our right to life to be merely a right to noninterference, a right not to be killed, is to impoverish the notion of rights and to threaten the expanded range of mutual human obligations that have been advanced in modern times.

A Turning Point?

Let me turn to the social meaning and impact of PAS. I take the desire of some, even many, for the legalization and social legitimation of PAS to be profoundly emblematic of three important turning points in Western thought. The first I have already sketched and will not say more about: the acceptance of PAS would morally sanction what can only be called consenting adult killing, whether the killing of another (euthanasia) or the assisted killing of oneself (PAS).

The second turning point lies in the meaning and limits of self-determination. The acceptance of euthanasia would sanction a view of autonomy holding that individuals may, in the name of their own private view of the good life and the relief of suffering, call upon others—doctors—to help them pursue that life, even at the risk of harm to the common good. This works against the idea that the meaning and scope of our right to lead our own lives must be conditioned by and be compatible with the good of the community, which is more than an aggregate of self-directing individuals.

The third turning point is to be found in the claim being made upon the institution of medicine, that it should be prepared to make its skills available to individuals to help them achieve their private vision of the good life. This puts medicine in the business of promoting the individualistic pursuit of general human happiness and well-being. It would overturn the traditional belief that medicine should limit its domain to promoting and preserving human health and life, redirecting it instead to the relief of that suffering which stems from life itself, not merely from a sick body or mind.

At each of these three turning points, proponents of PAS push us in the wrong direction. Arguments in favor of PAS fall into four general categories, which I will take up in turn: (1) the moral claim of individual self-determination and well-being; (2) the supposed moral irrelevance of the difference between killing and allowing to die; (3) the alleged lack of evidence to show the likely harmful consequences of legalized euthanasia; and (4) the compatibility of euthanasia and medical practice.

Self-Determination

Central to most arguments for PAS is the principle of self-determination. People are presumed to have a right to decide for themselves, according to their own beliefs about what makes life good, how they will conduct their lives. That is an important value, highly and correctly honored. But the question in the PAS context is: what does it mean and how far should it extend? If it were a question of suicide, where a person takes her own life without assistance from another, that principle might be pertinent, at least for debate. But assisted suicide is not that limited a matter. The self-determination in that case can only be effected by the moral and physical assistance of another. Assisted suicide is thereby no longer a matter only of self-determination but of a mutual, social decision between two people, the one to commit suicide and the other to technically facilitate it. Since, moreover, it is presently illegal in most jurisdictions, any change in the law will require the social sanction of a legislature or the courts; that would be a powerful act of legitimation—changing a longstanding set of convictions and laws—and not merely a neutral act of permissibility.

By what warrant, however, are we to make the moral move from my right of self-determination to some doctor's right to assist me—from *my* right to *his* right? From whence comes the doctor's moral license to help someone kill himself? Ought doctors to be able to help people kill themselves as long as a request to do so comes from those who are mentally competent? Is our right to life just like a piece of property, to be given away or alienated if the price is right (happiness, relief of suffering)? And then to be destroyed with our permission once alienated?

In answer to all those questions, I will say this: I have yet to hear a plausible argument why it should be permissible for us to put this kind of power in the hands of another, whether a doctor or anyone else. The idea that we can waive our right to life, then give to another the power to take that life or help us take it, requires a justification yet to be provided by anyone. To simply say that we have a right to delegate the sovereignty over our life to another begs the question. That question is whether someone ought to have the right to take the life of another or assist in its taking simply because someone is willing to hand over or to exercise his sovereignty in that way. Put another way, can one receive from another that kind of delegated right?

There are two possible rationales for such a transfer. One of them is that (a) the very notion of sovereignty over self, of full self-determination, allows us to do with our self what we will, including the transfer of that right to someone else to exercise it in our behalf. The other rationale is that (b) under some circumstances, it may be physically impossible to exercise our right of self-determination, thus requiring the assistance of another to make the right efficacious.

(a) *The sovereignty of the self.* I will consider the first rationale, that of our right to transfer to another our right of self-determination, by offering two analogies, situations where civilized societies have denied an absolute sovereignty of self. Slavery was long ago outlawed on the ground that one person should not have the right to own another, *even with the other's permission.* Why? Because it is a fundamental moral wrong for one person to give over his life and fate to another, whatever the good consequences, and no less a wrong for another person to have that kind of total, final power. Like slavery, dueling was long ago banned on similar grounds: even free, competent individuals should not have the power to kill each other, whatever their motives, whatever the circumstances. Consenting adult killing, like consenting adult slavery or degradation, is a strange route to human dignity.

There is another problem as well. If doctors, once sanctioned to carry out euthanasia or PAS, are to be themselves responsible moral agents—not simply hired hands with lethal injections or deadly pills at the ready—then they must have their own *independent* moral grounds to kill or assist those who request such services. What do I mean? As those who favor euthanasia are quick to point out, some people want it because their life has become so burdensome it no longer seems worth living. The doctor will have a difficulty at this point. The degree and intensity to which people suffer from their diseases and their dying,

whether they find life more of a burden than a benefit, has little directly to do with the nature or extent of their actual physical condition.
Physical and mental suffering are, by themselves, utterly poor predic-
tors of a desire for suicide. Three people, moreover, can have the same
grave medical condition, but only one will find the suffering unbearable. People suffer, but suffering is as much a function of the values of
individuals as it is of the physical or psychological causes of that suffering. Inevitably in that circumstance, the doctor will in effect be treating
the patient's values. To be responsible, the doctor would have to share
those values. The doctor would have to decide, on her own, whether
the patient's life was "no longer worth living."

But how could a doctor possibly know that or make such a judgment? Just because the patient said so? I raise this question because in
Holland at a euthanasia conference, the Dutch doctors present agreed
that there is no objective way of measuring or judging the claims of
patients that their suffering is unbearable. And if it is difficult to measure suffering, how much more difficult to determine the value of a
patient's statement that her life is not worth living?

However one might want to answer such questions, the need to ask
them, to inquire into the physician's responsibility and grounds for
medical and moral judgment, points out the social nature of the decision. Euthanasia and PAS are not private matters of self-determination. They are acts that require two people to make either act possible
and a complicit society to make either act acceptable.

(b) *Inability to exercise self-determination.* I turn to the second
rationale for a right of physicians to help another commit suicide, that
of the physical inability of some patients to exercise their right of self-
determination, as, for instance, with ALS or quadriplegia. Here the
issue is somewhat different. Can it be said, first, that we have a right
to commit suicide to such an extent that a physical inability to do so
constitutes an impediment to the exercise of that right? Second, if we
grant such a right, does that entail a corresponding right on the part of
physicians to assist us in committing suicide?

Suicide is legal in the United States, in the sense that there is no law
forbidding it. Does that fact entail that there is a right to suicide? Not
necessarily. Many acts are permitted that are not understood to be
rights; that is, we have no special claim to perform those acts, only the
permission of society to perform them. We are free to use our power
of vision and hearing, but there is no constitutional or other right to
them. We are free to eat in restaurants rather than at home, but no one
claims that there is a right to do so. Suicide seems to fall into this
category. The permissiveness of society in not forbidding me to commit
suicide does not translate into a positive right to do so; we cannot, that

is, call upon the power of the state to help us commit suicide or to require others to honor our decision to do so. This conclusion follows whether the person committing suicide is physically capable of doing so or not; that is irrelevant. Suicide, then, falls into that gray zone of acts that are permitted by the state but not given the privileged place of an accepted right.

Given this situation, I conclude that no one can claim that another has an obligation to help her commit suicide. No one, that is, can claim that there is a right to commit suicide and thus an obligation on the part of someone to assist us in doing so. What if, however, a doctor is willing to assist, even if not obliged to do so? Ought such assistance be permitted if a person who desires to commit suicide is physically unable to carry it out? This question, however, cannot be answered apart from our overall moral evaluation of assisted suicide. I have argued that self-determination as a moral principle is not sufficient to make a *prima facie* case for physician-assisted suicide. As the case of voluntary slavery makes clear (or legal prohibitions against the sale of organs) we do not grant unlimited rights to people to do what they will to or with their bodies simply because they are their bodies. A right of self-determination does not, that is, entail that every way of exercising that right must be equally protected, much less assisted. To say, then, that those who are physically unable to commit suicide have a claim upon doctors to help them, or that doctors have an obligation to help them, or that they *may* help them—each of those claims begs the question; and that question is whether we ought (a) to extend the right of self-determination to encompass physician-assisted suicide or (b) at least permit it in the case of those who are physically unable to commit suicide.

We can answer neither of those questions solely in terms of a right to self-determination. The reason for that is evident: if there is no *prima facie* right of self-determination to commit suicide, there can be no right either to the help of another to do so; and this would be true even if we are unable to commit suicide on our own. The question before us is not whether there is a right to PAS but whether we want to permit it as social policy. Self-determination as a principle does not automatically entail that conclusion.

Killing and Allowing to Die

I have argued that there is *no essential moral difference* between the direct killing of a patient, euthanasia, and directly assisting a patient to kill himself (i.e., providing him the means to do so). Now it has been held by some that there is no moral distinction between killing a person

and allowing that person to die by virtue of the termination of life-pre-
serving treatment. Can it, therefore, be argued that there is also no
moral difference between (a) directly killing a patient (euthanasia), (b)
terminating life-saving treatment on a dying patient (allowing to die),
and (c) assisting a dying person to kill herself (PAS)? Consider the case
of a victim of ALS, dependent upon a respirator but able to control
some hand movements, who considers the following choices: (a) being
killed by a physician's injection; (b) having the respirator turned off; (c)
and being given a pill in order to commit suicide. Are these equivalent
moral actions, such that it is morally irrelevant whether the choice is
(a), (b), or (c)?

The argument I want to make is that (a) and (c) are morally equivalent, but that (b) is not. I want, that is, to say that while euthanasia and
PAS are moral equivalents—for it will be the action of another (a
doctor) or of oneself aided by another (PAS) that is the physical *cause*
of death—turning off the respirator is different. In the latter case it will
be the underlying ALS that is the cause of death. We may want to make
the moral judgment that it is wrong to turn off the respirator of someone suffering from ALS even if that patient is dying, but it would be a
mistake to equate the morality of the physician's act in so doing with
nature's act in ending life.

Since it has become all too common to conflate euthanasia, assisted
suicide, and allowing to die, it is important to see why the distinction
between killing and helping to kill another, on the one hand, and allowing to die, on the other, are morally different. Consider one broad implication of what the erasure of the distinction between these two
categories implies: that death from disease has been banished, leaving
only the actions of physicians in terminating treatment as the cause of
death. Biology, which used to bring about death, has apparently been
displaced by human agency; doctors end life, not nature.

What is the mistake here? It lies in confusing causality and culpability and in failing to note the way in which human societies have overlaid natural causes with moral rules and interpretations. Causality (by
which I mean the direct physical causes of death) and culpability (by
which I mean our attribution of moral responsibility to human actions)
are confused under three circumstances.

They are confused, first, when the action of a physician in stopping
treatment of a patient with an underlying lethal disease is construed as
causing death. On the contrary, the physician's omission can only
bring about death on the condition that the patient's disease will kill
him in the absence of treatment. We may hold the physician morally
responsible for the death if we have morally judged such actions
wrongful omissions. But it confuses reality and moral judgment to see

an omitted action as having the same causal status as one that directly kills. A lethal injection will kill both a healthy person and a sick person. A physician's omitted treatment, by contrast, will have no effect on a healthy person. Turn off the machine on me, a well person, and nothing will happen. The same action will only bring the life of a sick person to an end because of an underlying fatal disease.

Causality and culpability are confused, second, when we fail to note that judgments of moral responsibility and culpability are human constructs. By that I mean that we human beings, after moral reflection, have decided to call some actions right or wrong and to devise moral rules to deal with them. When physicians could do nothing to stop death, they were not held responsible for it. When, with medical progress, they began to have some power over death—but only its timing and circumstances, not its ultimate inevitability—moral rules were devised to set forth their obligations. Natural causes of death were not thereby banished. They were, instead, overlaid with a medical ethic designed to determine moral culpability in deploying medical power.

To confuse the judgments of this ethic with the physical causes of death—which is the connotation of the word *kill*—is to confuse nature and human action. People will, one way or another, die of some disease; death will have dominion over all of us. To say that a doctor "kills" a patient by allowing this to happen should only be understood as a moral judgment about the licitness of his omission, nothing more. We can, as a fashion of speech only, talk about a doctor killing a patient by omitting treatment he should have provided. It is a fashion of speech precisely because it is the underlying disease that brings death when treatment is omitted; that is its cause, not the physician's omission. It is a misuse of the word *killing* to use it when a doctor stops a treatment he believes will no longer benefit the patient—when, that is, he steps aside to allow an eventually inevitable death to occur now rather than later. The only deaths that human beings invented are those that come from direct killing—when, with a lethal injection, we both cause death and are morally responsible for it. In the case of omissions, we do not cause death even if we may be judged morally responsible for it.

This difference between causality and culpability also helps us see why a doctor who has omitted a treatment he should have provided has "killed" that patient while another doctor—performing precisely the same act of omission on another patient in different circumstances—does not kill her but only allows her to die. The difference is that we have come, by moral convention and conviction, to classify unauthorized or illegitimate omissions as acts of "killing." We call them "killing" in the expanded sense of the term: a culpable action that permits the real cause of death, the underlying disease, to proceed to its lethal conclusion. By contrast, the doctor who, at the patient's request, omits or terminates unwanted treatment does not kill at all. Her underlying disease, not his action, is the physical cause of death; and we have agreed to consider actions of that kind to be morally licit. He thus can truly be said to have "allowed" her to die.

If we fail to maintain the distinction between killing and allowing to die, moreover, there are some disturbing possibilities. The first would be to confirm many physicians in their already too-powerful belief that when patients die or when physicians stop treatment because of the futility of continuing it, they are somehow both morally and physically responsible for the deaths that follow. That notion needs to be abolished, not strengthened. It needlessly and wrongly burdens the physician, to whom should not be attributed the powers of the gods. The second possibility would be that in every case where a doctor judges medical treatment no longer effective in prolonging life, a quick and direct killing of the patient or assisting the patient to commit suicide would be seen as the next most reasonable step on grounds of both humaneness and economics. I do not see how that logic could easily be rejected.

Calculating the Consequences

I have tried to show that physician-assisted suicide and euthanasia are intrinsically wrong because of the excessive power they would put in the hands of physicians, a wrongness that is independent of the voluntary desire of a patient to give them such power. There are also a number of important consequentialist reasons for judging PAS to be morally wrong. Like all such reasons, they depend upon the unwanted events actually taking place; in that sense, consequentialist arguments rest on probabilities. If they are not likely to happen, then they lose their moral force as arguments. I need, then, to show (a) that a legalization of PAS and a social legitimization of the practice *could* have bad consequences and that (b) those consequences are highly certain to take place. In this case, it will be easier to show the possibility of bad consequences than their certainty of occurring. There has been little experience anywhere with PAS and thus there is nothing immediately at hand to draw upon to calculate directly the probabilities of different outcomes. Nonetheless, I believe we can imagine easily enough what some of the harmful consequences might be, and we can also reasonably extrapolate from the Dutch experience with euthanasia to indirectly calculate some probabilities of what is likely to happen with accepted PAS.

Three consequences seem fully plausible: the inevitability of some significant abuse of any law; the difficulty of precisely writing, then enforcing, any law; and the inherent slipperiness of the moral reasons for legalizing PAS in the first place, pushing us in dangerous directions.

Why is abuse inevitable? One reason is that almost all laws on delicate, controversial matters are to some extent abused. This happens because not everyone will agree with the law as written and will bend it or ignore it if they can get away with it. Yet even if it is likely that all or most laws will be abused to some extent, there are good reasons to think that laws attempting to regulate PAS will particularly invite abuse.

Here we have one major social experiment to draw upon, that of the effect of efforts in the Netherlands to regulate euthanasia and PAS. What can we learn about the success of regulatory efforts in the Netherlands, where euthanasia and PAS have been permitted by the courts when certain criteria have been met: a free choice, a considered and persistent request, unacceptable suffering, consultation with another physician, and accurate reporting on the cause of death?

What has been the Dutch experience? The best information on this subject comes from a survey commissioned by the Dutch government's Commission on Euthanasia appointed in January 1990. The survey, directed by Professor P. J. van der Maas, encompassed a sample of 406 physicians, and two other studies, which, when taken together, led to the following estimate. The official results showed that based on that sample, out of a total of 129,000 deaths, there were some 2,300 cases of voluntary ("free choice") euthanasia and 400 cases of assisted suicide. In addition and most strikingly, there were some 1,000 cases of intentional termination of life without explicit request, what the Dutch call "nonvoluntary euthanasia." In short, out of 3,300 euthanasia deaths, nearly one-third were nonvoluntary. Unfortunately, there is no analysis or discussion of the 400 PAS deaths, but if it is the case that such a large proportion of all euthanasia deaths are nonvoluntary, we can reasonably infer that at least some of the PAS cases probably involved some abuse of physician power as well, most likely the well-placed suggestion and insinuation or a casual attitude toward the patient's competence and psychological state.

Is the same result likely in the United States? Here one can only speculate, of course, but there is no special reason to believe a different, less damaging pattern would emerge here. The rationale advanced for the Dutch nonvoluntary cases, that of "necessity," or *force majuere*—that is, that euthanasia was the only ethically possible choice in some heartrending cases, whatever the law might say—could just as easily be advanced in this country. It would be no less difficult for physicians to claim, as they do in Holland, that the patients had at sometime in the past said things to indicate they wanted euthanasia and that such statements should be sufficient. There is some plausibility to this contention, just as it is plausible in my judgment to terminate treatment on a dying patient who had at some time in the past informally told others or a doctor that he would not want treatment continued under certain conditions. Unfortunately, among the 1000 estimated nonvoluntary cases in the Netherlands, there were some where the patient was competent and could have been asked but was not. Here it is apparently the case that the doctors take it upon themselves to judge when continued life is not tolerable, invoking past statements on occasion but, if they are lacking, simply making unilateral judgments even when consent (or nonconsent) would be possible. Could this happen in the United States? Why not?

Apart from those abuse problems, there is a more profound worry. There is no way, even in principle, to write or enforce a meaningful law that can guarantee effective procedural safeguards. The reason is obvious yet almost always overlooked: the euthanasia or PAS transaction will ordinarily take place within the boundaries of the private and confidential doctor-patient relationship. No one can possibly know what occurs in that context unless the doctor or the patient chooses to reveal it. In Holland, fewer than 50 percent of the physicians report their acts of euthanasia, and those who do not enjoy almost complete legal impunity. There is no reason why the situation should be any better elsewhere. Doctors will have their own reasons for keeping euthanasia secret, and some patients will have no less a motive for wanting it concealed.

I would mention, finally, that the moral logic of the motives for euthanasia and PAS contain within them the ingredients of abuse. The two standard motives for euthanasia and assisted suicide are said to be our right of self-determination and our claim upon the mercy of others, especially doctors, to relieve our suffering. These two motives are typically spliced together and presented as a single justification. Yet if they are considered independently—and there is no inherent reason why they must be linked—they reveal serious problems. It is said that a competent, adult person should have a right to euthanasia for the relief of suffering. But why must the person be suffering? Does not that stipulation already compromise the principle of self-determination? How can self-determination have any limits? Whatever the person's motives may be, why are they not sufficient? Those laws that would limit PAS to terminal illness or to insupportable chronic illness already arbitrarily limit self-determination. It would be easy to challenge that arbitrary limitation if we are to be consistent in supporting self-determination. And it would surely be reasonable for those who are handicapped or otherwise physically incapable of committing suicide to demand euthanasia on the grounds that the law did not afford them equal rights and equal protection. A legal acceptance of PAS, that is, would surely pave the way for a legal acceptance of euthanasia.

Consider next the person who is suffering but not competent, who is perhaps demented or mentally retarded. The standard argument would deny euthanasia to that person, as lacking the capacity for self-determination. But why? If a person is suffering but not competent, then it would seem grossly unfair to deny relief solely on the grounds of incompetence. Are the incompetent less entitled to relief from suffering than the competent? Will it only be affluent, middle-class people, mentally fit and savvy about the medical system, who can qualify? Do the incompetent suffer less because of their incompetence? It is precisely this kind of reasoning that has led Dutch doctors, in the name of "necessity," to carry out euthanasia on the incompetent in the absence of any permission.

Considered from these angles, there are no good moral reasons to limit euthanasia or PAS once the principle of taking life or helping another to take her life has been legitimated. If we really believe in self-determination, then any competent person should have a right to be killed by a doctor for any reason that suits him and no less to be assisted in suicide. If we believe in the relief of suffering, then it seems cruel and capricious to deny it to the incompetent. There is, in short, no reasonable or logical stopping point once the turn has been made down the road to euthanasia or PAS, which could soon turn into a convenient and commodious expressway.

Euthanasia and the Purposes of Medicine

A fourth kind of argument one often hears both in the Netherlands and in this country is that euthanasia and assisted suicide are perfectly compatible with the aims of medicine. I would note at the very outset that a physician who participates in another person's suicide already abuses medicine. Apart from depression (the main statistical cause of suicide), people commit suicide because they find life empty, oppressive, or meaningless. Their judgment is a judgment about the value of continued life, not only about health (even if they are sick). Are doctors now to be given the right to make judgments about the kinds of life worth living and to give their blessing to suicide for those they judge wanting? What conceivable competence, technical or moral, could doctors claim to play such a role? Are we to medicalize suicide, turning judgments about its worth and value into one more clinical issue?

Yes, those are rhetorical questions, yet they bring us to the core of the problem of euthanasia, PAS, and medicine. The great temptation of modern medicine, not always resisted, is to move beyond the promotion and preservation of health into the boundless realm of general human happiness and well-being. The root problem of illness and mortality is both medical and philosophical or religious. Why must I die? can be asked as a technical, biological question or as a question about the meaning of life. When medicine tries to respond to the latter, which it is always under pressure to do, it moves beyond its proper role. Medicine has no special insight into the meaning of life or the meaning of a life marked by suffering and death.

It is not medicine's place to lift from us the burden of that suffering which turns on the meaning we assign to the decay of the body and its eventual death. It is not medicine's place to determine when lives are not worth living or when the burden of life is too great to be borne. Doctors have no conceivable way of evaluating such claims on the part of patients, and they should have no right to act in response to them. Medicine should try to relieve human suffering, but only that suffering which is brought on by illness and dying as biological phenomena, not that suffering which comes from anguish or despair at the human condition.

Doctors ought to relieve those forms of suffering that medically accompany serious illness and the threat of death. They should relieve pain, do what they can to allay anxiety and uncertainty, and be a comforting presence. As sensitive human beings, doctors should be prepared to respond to patients who ask why they must die or die in pain. But here the doctor and the patient are at the same level. The doctor may have no better answer to those old questions than anyone else and certainly no special insight from his training as a physician. It would be terrible for physicians to forget this and to think that in a swift, lethal injection or in the provision of suicide pills, medicine has found its own technical answer to the riddle of life.

Physicians ought not to abandon their critically ill, suffering patients. They should accompany them to the end. But it is not abandonment for a physician to refuse to step over that line which separates the medical struggle against pain, suffering, and death from the active pursuit of death, to positively seek death as the answer to the problem of life. That is to fundamentally compromise the nature of medicine, to mistake its skill with the lethal tools of death as a warrant for the bringing of death to relieve a patient of the burden of life. But would this be true even in those cases where it was the earlier actions of the physician that perhaps brought on the pain and suffering of a critical or terminal illness? Do not physicians have a duty to relieve that suffering which was caused by their treatment?

This seems a false conclusion. If patients understand that doctors do not have a moral license to commit euthanasia or engage in PAS and also give their informed consent to treatment, they can hardly blame the physician if, despite good intentions, the treatment does not turn out well. Nor does it follow that because a doctor was a causal source of pain and suffering, doctors should be able to directly kill patients or help them kill themselves by way of reparation. Medicine is an uncertain art and a less than perfect science. There is no call for reparation when it fails, nor is unavoidable pain and suffering to be understood as a failure of medicine. Human bodies must fail and eventually die. It can hardly be made an obligation on the part of medicine to be held responsible for that biological state of affairs. Nor can it be a right of patients to claim that doctors must set the world right when it goes wrong.

A final word. It is not within the power of medicine—and probably never will be—to master life and death and to control nature. It *ought* never to be within the moral power of medicine to use its skills to bring about death, whether directly or indirectly. A medicine that took on that role would soon corrupt itself, inevitably falling into abuse and assuming a kind of power it ought not to have; and it would inevitably corrupt the rest of us as well, turning to medicine to relieve us of the weight and meaning of life. Medicine does not and cannot have that kind of wisdom, and it surely would not gain it by acting as our agent in death.

4

PHYSICIAN-ASSISTED SUICIDE IS SOMETIMES MORALLY JUSTIFIED

Dan W. Brock, Ph.D.

There are two central and distinct moral issues about physician-assisted suicide.[1] First, is physician-assisted suicide morally justified in any individual cases? Second, would it be ethically justified for public and legal policy to permit physician-assisted suicide? This chapter is concerned only with the first of these questions, and I shall argue the affirmative answer. The second question is addressed in other chapters in this volume; the affirmative case for a public policy permitting physician-assisted suicide is in my view more complex and less decisive, though nevertheless also sound. But my concern will be broader than the first question in one important respect. The argument that I shall make applies in nearly all essentials to voluntary active euthanasia as well as physician-assisted suicide, and I shall begin by indicating why I believe the two are not importantly different morally. (For brevity and unless explicitly indicated otherwise, I shall hereafter use "assisted suicide" to refer to physician-assisted suicide and "euthanasia" to refer to voluntary active euthanasia.)

In the recent bioethics literature some have endorsed assisted suicide but not euthanasia, even in individual cases and not only for public policy.[2] Moreover, the policy proposals that in the last few years have been brought to legislatures or to the public in state referenda in nearly all cases have applied only to assisted suicide and not to euthanasia. Are they sufficiently different that the moral arguments that apply to one often do not apply to the other? First, what is the difference between assisted suicide and euthanasia? A paradigm case of assisted suicide is a patient's ending his or her life with a lethal dose of a medication requested of and provided by a physician for that purpose. A paradigm case of euthanasia is a physician's administering the lethal dose, often because the patient is unable to do so. The only difference that need exist between the two is the person who actually administers the lethal dose—the physician or the patient. In each, the physician plays an active and necessary causal role in providing the lethal dose. In each, the intent of the patient and physician is to pursue a course of action that will end in the patient's death.

In assisted suicide the patient acts last (for example, Janet Adkins pushed the button after Dr. Jack Kevorkian hooked her up to his suicide machine), whereas in euthanasia the physician acts last by performing the physical equivalent of pushing the button. In both cases, however, the choice rests fully with the patient in the sense that neither will take place without the patient's desire for them; of course, in each the physician must also be willing to play his or her role. In both the patient acts last in the sense of retaining the right to change his or her mind until the point at which the lethal process becomes irreversible. How could there be a substantial moral difference between the two based only on this small difference in the part played by the physician in the causal process resulting in death? Of course, it might be held that the moral difference is obvious and important—in euthanasia the physician kills the patient, whereas in assisted suicide the patient kills him- or herself. But this is misleading at best. In assisted suicide the physician and patient act together to kill the patient. To see this, suppose a physician supplied a lethal dose to a patient with the knowledge and intent that the patient will wrongfully administer it to another. We would have no difficulty in morality or the law recognizing this as a case of joint action to bring about another's death, or to kill, for which both are responsible. The physician is involved in killing in both assisted suicide and euthanasia, and so we will have to address the morality of killing later in this chapter.

If there is no significant, intrinsic moral difference between assisted suicide and euthanasia, it is also difficult to see why public or legal policy should permit one but not the other; worries about abuse or about giving anyone dominion over the lives of others seem also to apply equally to either. Some argue that because in assisted suicide the patient must take the final physical act that results in his or her death, there is greater certainty of the patient's voluntary resolve to die than when the physician performs that act. In some cases this may be true, but there are also cases of euthanasia in which the voluntary resolve of the patient to die is not in significant doubt. However, I shall not pursue the policy issue here, but I shall take the arguments developed below about individual cases of physician-assisted suicide to apply both to assisted suicide and to euthanasia.

My concern here will be only with *voluntary* cases of assisted suicide or euthanasia, that is, with cases in which a clearly competent patient makes a fully voluntary and persistent request for assisted suicide or euthanasia. Perhaps the assumption of voluntariness is implicit in the very concept of physician-assisted suicide, either in the condition that the patient performs the final physical act of using the means to end his or her life or in the notion of the physician assisting the patient, but I have said that my argument applies to active euthanasia as well, and voluntariness is not implicit there. Involuntary euthanasia, in which a competent patient explicitly refuses or opposes receiving euthanasia, and nonvoluntary euthanasia, in which a patient is incompetent and unable to express his or her wishes about euthanasia, are both possible but will not be my concern here. Finally, I will be concerned with assisted suicide and euthanasia where the motive of those who perform them is to respect the wishes of the patient and to provide the patient with a "good death"; only in such cases is the physician's participation morally justified.

A last introductory point is that I will be examining only secular arguments about assisted suicide and euthanasia, though of course many people's attitudes to them are inextricable from their religious views. Even if an individual's religious and moral views on this question are deeply connected, the moral justification for his or her position cannot consist simply in an appeal to religious authority. If the individual claims to offer a moral position on the issue, I believe that position must be stated and defended with arguments that do not presuppose or appeal to the authority of a particular religion and its beliefs and principles. The content of the moral reason or argument offered in secular terms can be the same as the content of the reasons that particular religions offer for their tenets and positions, but it must be offered as persuasive in its own terms, not only from within the standpoint or authority of the particular religion. (I also take this secular focus to be appropriate for public policy in a pluralistic society like our own; public policy should not be based on religious views reasonably rejected by a substantial portion of the society, though, since public policy is not my concern here, I shall not pursue or defend this claim.) Even if the position I will defend here is correct that assisted suicide and euthanasia are sometimes morally justified, I will take that to mean only that they would be morally permissible and justified in those circumstances. This is compatible with a position that I would also support, that anyone who has serious religious objections to them need not ask for them for him- or herself nor take any part in them when asked to do so by others.

The Central Ethical Argument for Assisted Suicide and Euthanasia

The central ethical argument for assisted suicide and euthanasia is familiar. It is that the very same two fundamental ethical values supporting the consensus on patients' rights to decide about life-sustaining treatment also support the ethical permissibility of assisted suicide and euthanasia in some circumstances. And this implies that acceptance of assisted suicide and euthanasia is not as radical a moral departure from the current consensus and practice giving patients the right to decide to forgo life support, as is commonly supposed. These values are individual self-determination or autonomy and individual well-being. By self-determination, as it bears on assisted suicide and euthanasia, I mean people's interest in making important decisions about their lives for themselves according to their own values or conceptions of a good life and in being left free to act on those decisions. Self-determination is valuable because it permits people to form and to live in accordance with their own conception of a good life, at least within the bounds of justice and consistent with not preventing others from doing so as well. In exercising self-determination people exercise significant control over their lives and thereby take responsibility for their lives and for the kinds of persons they become. A central aspect of human dignity and the moral worth of persons lies in individuals' capacity to direct their lives in this way. The value of exercising self-determination presupposes some minimum of decision-making capacities or competence, which thus limits the scope of assisted suicide or euthanasia supported by self-determination; it does not apply, for example, in cases of serious dementia or treatable clinical depression that impair the individual's decision-making capacity.

Individual self-determination has special importance in choices about the time and manner of one's death, including assisted suicide and euthanasia. Most people are very concerned about the nature of the last stage of their lives. This reflects not just a fear of experiencing substantial pain or suffering or of being abandoned by loved ones when dying, but also a desire to retain dignity and control to the extent possible during this last period of life. Death is today increasingly preceded by a long period of significant physical and mental decline, due in part to the technological interventions of modern medicine designed to stave off death. Many people adjust to their disability and dependency and find meaning and value in new activities and ways. Others find the impairments and burdens in the last stage of their lives at some point sufficiently great to make life no longer worth living. For some patients near death, maintaining the quality of one's life, avoiding great pain or suffering, maintaining one's dignity, and ensuring that others remember us as we wish them to become of paramount importance and outweigh merely extending one's life. But there is no single, objectively correct answer for everyone regarding when, if at all, one's life when critically or terminally ill becomes, all things considered, a burden and unwanted. If self-determination is a fundamental value, then the great

variability among people on this question makes it especially important that individuals control to the extent possible the manner, circumstances, and timing of their dying and death.

The other main value that supports assisted suicide and euthanasia
is individual well-being. It might seem that protecting and promoting
individual well-being must always conflict with a person's self-determination when the person requests assisted suicide or euthanasia, but
it is important to understand why this is not so. Life itself is commonly
understood to be a central good for persons, often valued for its own
sake, as well as necessary for the pursuit of all other goods within a life.
But when a competent patient decides to forgo all further life-sustaining treatment, then the patient, either explicitly or implicitly, commonly decides that the best life possible for him or her with treatment
is of sufficiently poor quality that it is worse than no further life at all.
Life is then no longer considered a benefit by the patient but has now
become without value or meaning and a burden. The same judgment
underlies a request for assisted suicide or euthanasia—continued life
is then seen by the patient as no longer a benefit, but now a burden.
Especially in the often severely compromised and debilitated states of
many critically ill or dying patients, there is no objective standard but
only the competent patient's judgment of whether continued life is no
longer a benefit.

Of course, sometimes conditions such as clinical depression call into
question whether the patient has made a competent choice, either to
forego life-sustaining treatment or to seek assisted suicide or euthanasia, and then the patient's choice need not be evidence that continued
life is no longer a benefit for him or her.[3] Just as with decisions about
treatment, a determination of incompetence can warrant not honoring
the patient's request for assisted suicide or euthanasia; in the case of
treatment, we then transfer decisional authority to a surrogate, though
in the case of assisted suicide or voluntary euthanasia a determination
that the patient is incompetent to make that choice means that neither
should take place.

The value or right of self-determination of patients does not entitle
them to compel physicians to act contrary to physicians' own moral or
professional values. Physicians are moral and professional agents
whose own self-determination or integrity should be respected as well.
If performing assisted suicide or euthanasia becomes legally permissible but conflicts with a particular physician's reasonable understanding of his or her moral or professional responsibilities, the care of a
patient who requests assisted suicide or euthanasia should be transferred to another. But the ethical issue with which I am concerned here
is the moral permissibility or justification of performing either assisted

suicide or euthanasia by those who do not have moral or professional objections to it.

Most opponents of assisted suicide and euthanasia do not deny that there are some cases in which the values of patient self-determination and well-being support them. Instead, opponents commonly offer two kinds of arguments against assisted suicide and euthanasia which they take to outweigh or override this support. The first kind of argument is my concern here—that in any individual case where considerations of the patient's self-determination and well-being do support assisted suicide or euthanasia, they are nevertheless always ethically wrong or impermissible. The second kind of argument is that even if in some individual cases assisted suicide or euthanasia may not be ethically wrong, it nonetheless would not be ethically sound or wise public and legal policy to permit them. While I do not pursue this second kind of argument here, it is important to distinguish it so that it is clear that the position I defend here, that assisted suicide and euthanasia are morally justified in some individual cases, is not determinative of whether public and legal policy should ever permit them.

Assisted Suicide and Euthanasia Are Deliberate Killing of an Innocent Person

In order to state the argument of the opponent of assisted suicide and euthanasia in its strongest form and to avoid unnecessary complexity in exposition, I shall focus in this section on euthanasia. The claim that any individual instance of euthanasia is a case of deliberate killing of an innocent person is, with only minor qualifications, correct. Unlike forgoing life-sustaining treatment, commonly understood as allowing to die, euthanasia is clearly killing, understood as depriving of life or causing the death of a living being. While providing morphine for pain relief at doses where the risk of respiratory depression and an earlier death may be a foreseen but unintended side effect of treating the patient's pain, in a case of euthanasia the patient's death is deliberate or intended even if in both the physician's ultimate end may be respecting the patient's wishes. If the deliberate killing of an innocent person is wrong, euthanasia would be nearly always impermissible.

In the context of medicine, the ethical prohibition against deliberately killing the innocent derives some of its plausibility from the belief that nothing in the currently accepted practice of medicine is deliberate killing. Thus, in commenting on the "It's Over Debbie"[4] case in which a resident deliberately gave a patient a lethal dose of morphine, four prominent physicians and bioethicists, led by Willard Gaylin, could entitle their paper "Doctors Must Not Kill."[5] The belief that doctors do not kill requires the corollary belief that forgoing life-sustaining treatment, whether by not starting or by stopping treatment, is allowing to die, not killing. Common though this view is, I shall argue that it is confused and mistaken. Typical cases of stopping life-sustaining treatment are killing, not allowing to die, although they are cases of ethically justified killing. But if so, that shows that an unqualified ethical prohibition of the deliberate killing of innocent persons is indefensible and must be revised.

Why is the common view mistaken that stopping life-sustaining treatment is allowing to die and not killing? Consider the case of a patient terminally ill with amytrophic lateral sclerosis disease (ALS, or Lou Gehrig's disease). She is completely respirator dependent with no hope of ever being weaned from the respirator. She is unquestionably competent but finds her condition intolerable and persistently requests to be removed from the respirator and allowed to die. Most people and physicians would likely agree that the patient's physician should respect the patient's wishes and remove her from the respirator, though this will certainly cause the patient's death. The common understanding is that the physician thereby allows the patient to die. But is that correct?

Suppose the patient has a greedy and hostile son who mistakenly believes both that his mother will never decide to stop her life-sustaining treatment and that even if she did her physician would not respect her wishes and remove her from the respirator. Afraid that his inheritance will be dissipated by a long and expensive hospitalization, he enters his mother's room while she is sedated, extubates her, and she dies. Shortly thereafter the medical staff discovers what he has done and confronts the son. He replies, "I didn't kill her, I merely allowed her to die. It was her ALS disease that caused her death." I think this would rightly be dismissed as transparent sophistry—the son went into his mother's room and deliberately killed her. But, of course, the son performed just the same physical actions, did just the same thing, with all the same consequences for the patient, that the physician would have done. If that is so, then doesn't the physician also kill the patient when he extubates her and stops the respirator?

I underline immediately that there are important ethical differences between what the physician and the greedy son do. First, the physician acts with the patient's consent, whereas the son does not. Second, the physician acts with a good motive—to respect the patient's wishes and self-determination—whereas the son acts with a bad motive—to protect his own inheritance. Third, the physician acts in a social role through which he is legally authorized to carry out the patient's decision to stop treatment, whereas the son has no such authorization. These and perhaps other ethically important differences show that what the physician did was morally justified, whereas what the son did was morally wrong. What they do *not* show, however, is that the son killed while the physician allowed to die. One can either kill or allow to die with or without consent, with a good or bad motive, within or outside a social role that legally authorizes one to do so.

The difference between killing and allowing to die that I have been implicitly appealing to here is roughly the difference between acts and omissions resulting in death.[6] Both the physician and the greedy son act in a manner intended to cause death, do cause death, and so both kill; neither allows to die. One reason this conclusion is resisted is that on a different understanding of the distinction between killing and allowing to die, what the physician does is allow to die. In this account, the mother's ALS is a lethal disease whose normal progression is being held back or blocked by the life-sustaining respirator treatment. Removing this artificial intervention is then viewed as standing aside and allowing the patient to die of her underlying disease. I have argued elsewhere that this alternative account is deeply problematic, in part because it seems to have the unacceptable implication that what the greedy son also does is to allow to die, not kill.[7] Here I want to note two other reasons why the conclusion that stopping life support is killing is resisted.

The first reason is that killing is often understood, especially within medicine, as unjustified or wrongful causing of death; in medicine it is thought to be done only accidentally or negligently. It is also increasingly widely accepted that a physician is ethically justified in stopping life support in a case like that of the ALS patient. But if both of these beliefs are correct, then what the physician does cannot be killing and so instead must be allowing to die. Killing patients is not, to put it flippantly, understood to be part of a physician's job description. What is mistaken in this line of reasoning is the assumption that all killings are *unjustified or wrongful* causings of death. Instead, some killings are ethically justified, including most instances of stopping life support.

Another reason for resisting the conclusion that stopping life support is often killing is that it is psychologically uncomfortable. Suppose the physician had stopped the ALS patient's respirator and had made the son's claim, "I didn't kill her, I merely allowed her to die. It was her ALS disease that caused her death." The clue to the psychological role here is how naturally the "merely" modifies "allowed her to die." The characterization as allowing to die is meant to shift felt responsibility away from the agent—the physician—and to the lethal disease process that the physician merely allowed to proceed to the patient's death.

Other language common in death and dying contexts plays a similar role; "letting nature take its course" or "stopping prolonging the dying process" both seem to shift responsibility from the physician who stops life support to the fatal disease process. However psychologically helpful these conceptualizations may be in making the difficult responsibility of a physician's role in the patient's death bearable, they nevertheless are confusions. Both physicians and family members can instead be helped to understand that it is the patient's decision and consent to stopping treatment that limits their responsibility for the patient's death and which shifts that responsibility to the patient.

Many who accept this understanding of the difference between killing and allowing to die as the difference between acts and omissions resulting in death have gone on to argue that killing is not in itself morally different from allowing to die.[8] In this account, very roughly, one kills when one performs an action that causes the death of a person (e.g., we are in a boat, you cannot swim, I push you overboard, and you drown), and one allows to die when one has the ability and opportunity to prevent the death of another, knows this, and omits doing so, with the result that the person dies (e.g., we are in a boat, you cannot swim, you fall overboard, I don't throw you an available life ring, and you drown). Those who see no moral difference between killing and allowing to die typically employ the strategy of comparing cases that differ in these and no other potentially morally important respects. This will allow people to consider whether the mere difference that one is a case of killing and the other of allowing to die matters morally, or whether instead it is other features that make most killings worse than most instances of allowing to die. Here is such a pair of cases.

> *Case 1.* A very gravely ill patient is brought to a hospital emergency room and sent up to the ICU. The patient begins to develop respiratory failure that is likely to require intubation very soon. At that point the patient's family members and long-time physician arrive at the ICU and inform the ICU staff that there had been extensive discussion about future care with the patient when he was unquestionably competent. Given his grave and terminal illness as well as his state of debilitation, the patient had firmly rejected being placed on a respirator under any circumstances, and the family and physician produce the patient's advance directive to that effect. The ICU staff do not intubate the patient, who dies of respiratory failure.

> *Case 2.* The same as Case 1 except that the family and physician are slightly delayed in traffic and arrive shortly after the patient has been intubated and placed on the respirator. The ICU staff extubate the patient, who dies of respiratory failure.

In Case 1 the patient is allowed to die, in Case 2 he is killed, but it is hard to see why what is done in Case 2 is significantly different morally than what is done in Case 1. It must be other factors that make most killings worse than most allowings to die, and if so, assisted suicide and euthanasia cannot be wrong simply because they are killing instead of allowing to die.

A Rights Approach to the Morality of Killing

Suppose that both my arguments are mistaken. Suppose that killing is worse than allowing to die and that withdrawing life support is not killing, although assisted suicide and euthanasia are. Assisted suicide and euthanasia still need not for that reason be morally wrong. To see this, we need to determine the basic principle for the moral evaluation of killing persons. What is it that makes paradigm cases of wrongful killing wrongful? One very plausible answer is that killing denies the victim a very great good over whose possession he or she should have control—continued life or a future. Our continued life or future is typically the object of one of our strongest desires. It can be thought of as a dispositional or standing desire, which typically becomes an occurrent desire, occupying an important place in one's conscious desires and plans, when one's life is threatened. Moreover, continued life is a necessary condition for being able to pursue and achieve any of one's other plans and purposes; loss of life brings the frustration of all of these plans and purposes as well. In a nutshell, wrongful killing typically deprives a person of a great and valued good—his or her future and all that the person wanted and planned to do in that future. It is important to see that there is another distinct moral idea at work in this account of the wrongness of killing besides that killing typically deprives the victim of a very great good, on which nearly all other goods for that person depend. The other idea is that one's life is a good over which, at least within limits, a person him- or herself should retain control.

Sometimes these two moral ideas or values can be in conflict, as, for example, when an apparently competent patient makes an informed and voluntary choice to refuse life-sustaining treatment that would restore the patient to full function and a life that most people would consider a life well worth having. Here the patient is exercising his or her right of control over his or her life and what is done to his or her body to give up the apparently very great good of continued life. If we cannot come to understand why the patient reasonably does not value that continued life or cannot find serious impairments in the patient's decision making or cannot persuade the patient to accept the treatment, then we may be forced to decide which value is more important, preserving the good of the patient's life or respecting the patient's right of control over his or her own life, that is, his or her self-determination or autonomy.

Public policy, as expressed in the law, gives competent patients the right to refuse any treatment, including life-sustaining treatment, and thereby gives greater weight to respecting the patient's right of control or self-determination regarding his or her own life. The law's resolution of this conflict in favor of self-determination recognizes not only the deep place of that value in our moral, cultural, and legal traditions but also the circumstance that when a competent individual rejects life-sustaining treatment he or she either no longer finds continued life a good or finds the means of gaining it unacceptable (for example, when Jehovah's Witness patients reject life-sustaining blood products). Our moral and cultural traditions, however, do not speak with one voice about how these values should be weighed when they are in conflict. Reasonable people can and do disagree about how this conflict should be resolved when an apparently worthwhile life is being given up by a competent patient.

In a comparable case in which a person with an apparently worthwhile life sought assisted suicide or euthanasia, most physicians and most persons probably would refuse to take part. But that is not at all the typical case in which assisted suicide or euthanasia is sought; nor is it the kind of case in which I am arguing that they are morally permissible and justified. Instead, in the typical and relevant case others view the competent individual's decision as quite reasonable, that continued life is no longer a good because that life is so filled with suffering and bereft of possibilities for the activities and experiences that make life valuable and meaningful. In such cases, the morally great good of continued life and the respect owed the patient's self-determination are not in conflict because continued life is no longer a great good but is now reasonably judged by the patient to be a burden and without value. Some physicians who give great weight to patient self-determination might be willing to participate in assisted suicide even when they cannot accept the patient's judgment that his or her life is no longer worth living. But many others would be willing to participate in assisted suicide or euthanasia only if they either share or at least view as reasonable the patient's judgment that his or her life is no longer worth living. In such cases, no significant good for the patient need be sacrificed in order to respect the patient's self-determination.

A natural expression of my account of the wrongness of killing is that people have a moral right not to be killed.[9] But the right not to be killed, like other rights, should be understood as waivable when the person makes a competent decision that continued life is no longer wanted or a good but is instead worse than no further life at all, and so wishes to die. In this rights view of the wrongness of killing, assisted suicide and euthanasia are properly understood as cases in which the person killed has waived his or her right not to be killed, thereby making the physician's action not a violation of that right.

This rights view of the wrongness of killing is not, of course, universally shared. Many people's moral views about killing have their origins in religious beliefs that human life comes from God and cannot be justifiably destroyed or taken away, either by the person whose life it is or by another. I noted earlier that I would be addressing only secular moral arguments regarding assisted suicide and euthanasia, and so will only reiterate two points made there. First, in a pluralistic society like our own with a strong commitment to freedom of religion, public policy should not be grounded in religious beliefs which many in that society reject. Second, if the position about the wrongness of killing rests on theological premises that many persons can and do reasonably reject, then those persons will have been given no reason why they should regard such killing as wrong.

The rejection of the rights view of the wrongness of killing, however, does not always have a religious basis. Some people believe it is always morally wrong deliberately to take an innocent human life—what is sometimes called a duty-based view on taking human life. The "innocence condition" may permit killing in self-defense or even in capital punishment under some interpretations, but not when a person seeks assisted suicide or euthanasia. If this moral prohibition does not derive from God, however, it is difficult to see what its moral basis can be. That basis can be neither that life is a very great good that should never be destroyed nor that one individual should never claim dominion over the life of another. As we have seen, sometimes the killing of an innocent person, in particular assisted suicide and euthanasia, does not conflict with but is instead supported by these two values. These are the moral values that support the rights account, not the duty account, of the morality of killing.

The Good Consequences of Some Assisted Suicide and Euthanasia

I have largely addressed the question of whether assisted suicide and euthanasia are in some cases morally permissible. I have argued that it is most importantly the patient's moral right to self-determination, ether with the waiving of his or her right not to be killed, that grounds that moral permissibility. However, the moral case in support of assisted suicide and euthanasia is in some instances considerably stronger than "mere permissibility"; they are then not just permissible but justified. On most accounts of "moral permissibility," an action may be morally permissible even if it would be better if an agent did not do it or if doing it would be wrong.[10] But assisted suicide and euthanasia are not merely permissible in this sense; they are in some cases morally justified with strong moral reasons in support of them. We can see this best if we ask what other good consequences assisted suicide or euthanasia could produce besides the obvious one of granting to patients who seek them what they want.

Perhaps the most important good consequence of physician-assisted suicide or voluntary active euthanasia concerns patients whose lives while they are dying are filled with severe and unrelievable pain or suffering. When there is a life-sustaining treatment which, if forgone, will lead relatively quickly to death, then doing so can bring an end to these patients' suffering without recourse to assisted suicide or euthanasia. For patients with no life-sustaining treatment that can be withheld or withdrawn, however, assisted suicide or euthanasia may be the only release from their otherwise prolonged suffering and agony. This argument from mercy has always been the strongest argument for assisted suicide or euthanasia in those cases to which it applies.[11]

The moral importance of relieving great pain and suffering is less controversial than is the frequency with which patients are forced to undergo untreatable agony that only assisted suicide or euthanasia could relieve. If we focus first on suffering caused by physical pain, it is crucial to distinguish pain that *could* be adequately relieved with modern methods of pain control, though it in fact is not, from pain that is relievable only by death.[12] For a variety of reasons, including some physicians' discomfort with prescribing large amounts of narcotics for fear of hastening the patient's death, as well as the lack of a publicly accessible means for assessing the amount of the patient's pain, many patients suffer pain that could be but is not relieved.

Specialists in controlling certain types of pain, for example the pain of terminally ill cancer patients, argue that there are very few patients whose pain could not be adequately controlled, though sometimes at the cost of so sedating them that they are effectively unable to interact with other people or their environment. Thus the argument from mercy in cases of physical pain can probably be met in the great majority of cases by providing adequate measures of pain relief. This should be a high priority, whatever one's view about assisted suicide or euthanasia—the relief of pain and suffering has long been, quite properly, one of the central goals of medicine.

Dying patients often undergo substantial psychological suffering, however, that is not fully or even principally the result of physical pain.[13] The knowledge about how to relieve this suffering is much more limited than in the case of relieving pain, and efforts to do so are probably more often unsuccessful. If the argument from mercy is extended, as it properly can be, to patients experiencing great and unrelievable psychological suffering, the numbers of patients to which it applies is much greater. In these cases, assisted suicide or euthanasia may be the only release from the patient's suffering.

A second good consequence of some instances of assisted suicide or euthanasia is that once death has been accepted, it is often more humane to end life quickly and peacefully, as can be done by assisted suicide or euthanasia, when that is what the patient wants. Such a death will often be seen as better than a more prolonged one in which the patient may be robbed of his or her dignity. People who suffer a sudden and unexpected death by dying quickly or in their sleep from a heart attack or stroke, for example, are often considered lucky to have died in this way instead of by a more drawn-out process. We care about how we die in part because we care about how others remember us, and we hope they will remember us as we were in "good times" with them and not as we might be when disease has robbed us of our dignity as human beings. As with much in the treatment and care of the dying, people's concerns differ in this respect, but for at least some people, assisted suicide or euthanasia will be a more humane death than what they have often experienced with other loved ones and might otherwise expect for themselves.

This aim of providing a patient with a better death is relevant to the objection to assisted suicide or euthanasia, that they are never necessary because it is always possible to withdraw or withhold nutrition and hydration from a patient, which will result in the patient's death without recourse to the active and more controversial interventions of assisted suicide or euthanasia. In some cases patients are not being fed or hydrated by artificial means, and so this alternative would require withholding ordinary food and water from an initially conscious patient.[14] There are, for good reasons, strong social and moral inhibitions to doing this, but even when it is possible it may not be seen merely as forgoing life-sustaining treatment but instead as killing the patient. Doing so in some cases would also result in suffering to the patient until consciousness is lost after about a week. This additional suffering would sometimes attend the withdrawal of artificially provided nutrition and hydration as well. In some cases, the cost of restricting the steps that can be taken in order to hasten death to forgoing of life-support would be a substantially worse death for the patient. The issue should not be whether we can find a treatment to forgo so as to avoid the need for assisted suicide or euthanasia but which means of hastening death will result in the death that is most humane and most in accord with what the patient wants.

Should Physicians Take Part in Assisted Suicide or Euthanasia?

Finally, I want to consider an objection to assisted suicide or euthanasia that is specifically to *physicians* ever performing them. Permitting physicians to perform assisted suicide or euthanasia, it is said, would be incompatible with their fundamental moral and professional commitment as healers to care for patients and to protect life. Moreover, if assisted suicide or euthanasia by physicians became common, patients would come to fear that a medication was intended not to treat or care but instead to kill and would thus lose trust in their physicians. This position was forcefully stated in the paper cited earlier by four prominent physicians and bioethicists:

> The very soul of medicine is on trial. . . . This issue touches medicine at its moral center; if this moral center collapses, if physicians become killers or are even licensed to kill, the profession—and, therewith, each physician—will never again be worthy of trust and respect as healer and comforter and protector of life in all its frailty.[15]

These authors go on to make clear that while they oppose permitting anyone to perform assisted suicide or euthanasia, their special concern is with physicians' doing so:

> We call on fellow physicians to say that they will not deliberately kill. We must also say to each of our fellow physicians that we will not tolerate killing of patients and that we shall take disciplinary action against doctors who kill. And we must say to the broader community that if it insists on tolerating or legalizing active euthanasia, it will have to find nonphysicians to do its killing.[16]

If permitting physicians to kill would undermine the very "moral center" of medicine, then almost certainly physicians should not be permitted to perform assisted suicide or euthanasia. But how persuasive is this claim? Patients should not fear, as a consequence of permitting *voluntary* assisted suicide or euthanasia, that their physicians will substitute a lethal injection for what patients want and believe is part of their care. If assisted suicide and euthanasia are restricted to cases in which they are truly voluntary, then no patient should fear getting either unless he or she has voluntarily requested them. Moreover, the central concern of patients to control their care when dying that has driven the debates over life-sustaining treatment decisions, the development of advance directives, and now assisted suicide and euthanasia, casts further doubt on this purported erosion of patients' trust of their physicians. The fear of loss of control should be lessened, not strengthened, if assisted suicide and euthanasia are permitted. Doing so would extend to dying patients control over their own dying in circumstances where there is no life-sustaining treatment to be withheld or withdrawn, or where waiting for death from forgoing treatment will provide the patient with a substantially worse death.

Might Gaylin and his colleagues, nevertheless, be correct in their claim that the moral center of medicine would collapse if physicians were to become killers? This question raises what at the deepest level should be the guiding aims of medicine, a question that obviously cannot be fully explored here. But I do want to say enough to indicate the direction that I believe an appropriate response to this challenge should take. In spelling out what I called the positive argument for assisted suicide and euthanasia, I suggested that two principal values—respecting patients' self-determination and promoting their well-being—underlie the consensus that competent patients or the surrogates of incompetent patients are entitled to refuse any life-sustaining treatment and to choose from among available alternative treatments. It is the commitment to these two values in guiding physicians' actions as healers, comforters, and protectors of their patients' lives that should be at the "moral center" of medicine, and these two values *support* physicians' performance of assisted suicide or euthanasia when their patients make competent requests for them.

What should not be at that moral center is a commitment to preserving patients' lives as such without regard to whether those patients want their lives preserved or judge their preservation a benefit to them. In recent years, vitalism has been increasingly rejected by physicians and, despite some statements that suggest it, is almost certainly not what Gaylin and colleagues intended. One of them, Leon Kass, has elaborated elsewhere the view that medicine is a moral profession whose proper aim is "the naturally given end of health," understood as the wholeness and well-working of the human being; "for the physician, at least, human life in living bodies commands respect and reverence—*by its very nature.*"[17] Kass continues, "the deepest ethical principle restraining the physician's power is not the autonomy or freedom of the patient; neither is it his own compassion or good intention. Rather, it is the dignity and mysterious power of human life itself."[18] I believe Kass is in the end mistaken about the proper account of the aims of medicine and the limits on physicians' power, but this difficult issue will certainly be one of the central themes in the continuing debate about physicians' roles in assisted suicide and euthanasia.

It is worth adding in conclusion that there are at least three reasons for restricting the performance of assisted suicide or euthanasia to physicians only. First, physicians would inevitably be involved in some of the important procedural safeguards necessary to a defensible practice of assisted suicide or euthanasia, such as ensuring that the patient is well informed about his or her condition, prognosis, and possible treatments and ensuring that all reasonable means have been taken to improve the quality of the patient's life. Second, physicians have access to and knowledge about (or can gain that knowledge with training) the necessary means and methods for carrying out assisted suicide or euthanasia effectively, and so can be instrumental in avoiding failed attempts by the patient to take his or her own life that only worsen the patient's condition. Third, one necessary protection against abuse of any legalization of assisted suicide or euthanasia is to limit who is given authority to perform them so that those persons can be held accountable for their exercise of that authority. Physicians, whose training and professional norms give some assurance that they would perform assisted suicide or euthanasia responsibly, are an appropriate group of persons to whom that authority might be reasonably restricted. But this is to take us beyond the case for which I have argued here, that assisted suicide and euthanasia are morally justified in some individual cases, and to the subject of the last section of the book, whether it would be wise public policy to permit them.

NOTES

1. This chapter is a substantially revised version of my earlier paper "Voluntary Active Euthanasia," *Hastings Center Report* 22 (March–April 1992): 10–22, which was reprinted in my *Life and Death: Philosophical Essays in Biomedical Ethics* (Cambridge: Cambridge University Press, 1993).

2. Sidney H. Wanzer et al., "The Physician's Responsibility toward Hopelessly Ill Patients," *New England Journal of Medicine* 310 (1984): 955–59.

3. There is evidence that physicians commonly fail to diagnose depression; see Robert I. Misbin, "Physicians Aid in Dying," *New England Journal of Medicine* 325 (1991): 1304–7.

4. Anonymous, "Its Over Debbie," *JAMA* 259 (1988): 272.

5. Willard Gaylin et al., "Doctors Must Not Kill," *JAMA* 259 (1988): 2139–40.

6. Bonnie Steinbock and Alastair Norcross, eds., *Killing and Letting Die*, 2d ed. (New York: Fordham University Press, 1994).

7. Dan W. Brock, "Forgoing Food and Water: Is It Killing?" in Joanne Lynn, ed., *By No Extraordinary Means: The Choice to Forgo Life-Sustaining Food and Water* (Bloomington: Indiana University Press, 1986).

8. James Rachels, "Active and Passive Euthanasia," *New England Journal of Medicine* 292 (1975): 78–80; Michael Tooley, *Abortion and Infanticide* (Oxford: Oxford University Press, 1983). In my paper "Taking Human Life," *Ethics* 95 (1985): 851–65, I argue in more detail that killing in itself is not morally different from allowing to die and defend the strategy of argument employed in this paragraph in the text.

9. Dan W. Brock, "Moral Rights and Permissible Killing," in John Ladd, ed., *Ethical Issues Relating to Life and Death* (Oxford: Oxford University Press, 1979).

10. Jeremy Waldron, "A Right to Do Wrong," *Ethics* 92 (1981): 21–39.

11. James Rachels, *The End of Life* (Oxford: Oxford University Press, 1986).

12. Marcia Angell, "The Quality of Mercy," *New England Journal of Medicine* 306 (1982): 98–99; M. Donovan, P. Dillon, and L. Mcguire, "Incidence and Characteristics of Pain in a Sample of Medical-Surgical Inpatients," *Pain* 30 (1987): 69–78.

13. Eric Cassell, *The Nature of Suffering and the Goals of Medicine* (New York: Oxford University Press, 1991).

14. James L. Bernat, Bernard Gert, and R. Peter Mogielnicki, "Patient Refusal of Hydration and Nutrition: An Alternative to Physician-Assisted Suicide or Voluntary Active Euthanasia," *Archives of Internal Medicine* 153 (1993): 2723–28.

15. Gaylin et al.

16. Ibid.

17. Leon R. Kass, "Neither for Love nor Money: Why Doctors Must Not Kill," *Public Interest* 94 (1989): 25–46; see also his *Toward a More Natural Science: Biology and Human Affairs* (New York: Free Press, 1985) chaps. 6–9.

18. Kass, "Neither for Love nor Money," p. 38.

Part III

Medical Practices and Perspectives

5

PHYSICIAN-ASSISTED SUICIDE IS *NOT* AN ACCEPTABLE PRACTICE FOR PHYSICIANS

Ira R. Byock, M.D.

As the end of the twentieth century approaches, Western medicine is experiencing momentous, some would say cataclysmic, shifts in financing, systems of care, ethics related to allocation of resources, rights, and futility of care. Society is also grappling with the very notions of health and disease that give shape to clinical practice. Care at the end of life is a crucial focus due to the disproportionate resources it consumes, the multiple ethical dilemmas it presents, and the documented prevalence of serious clinical deficiencies in terminal care.[1] In recent years public services, including health care services for the elderly and chronically ill, have been scaled back. Within the political process, health care is understood as a commodity and it makes economic sense to invest at the beginning rather than at the end of life.[2] The hospice movement has constituted one response to this state of affairs. However, more than two decades after hospice's entry into the health care world, serious problems persist and the surrounding health care crisis has intensified. The assisted suicide movement has emerged as a radical response and, increasingly, physicians are among its most articulate spokespersons.

Can medicine as a profession ever have a legitimate role to play in facilitating the suicide of patients? In arguing that it must not, I will not diminish the extent of the crisis that exists or minimize the extent of change that is required within society and within the medical profession.

It is not possible to consider professional standards for medical practice separately from the actual practice of individual physicians. Nor is it possible to consider the impact on the community of the avail-

ability of sanctioned physician assistance with suicide without acknowledging the experience of individual patients and families. Public policy,
professional standards, and bedside therapeutics are inextricably entwined and each merits attention. However, the focus of the present
argument will be that as a matter of public and professional policy,
physician-assisted suicide (PAS) should be rejected as a sanctioned
practice. As such this chapter will not attempt to develop general
arguments against suicide, nor will it address the social or legal consequences of mercy killings that lie outside of a sanctioned professional
sphere, including mercy killings by a clinician who consciously steps
beyond his or her professional role in taking the life-ending action.

Several attitudes seem to characterize the cultural mindset during the
current debate about PAS. These attitudes are represented by the following statements:

1. Each person is fundamentally an individual, distinct from others
and the community.

2. At times severe physical distress among the dying cannot be alleviated.

3. Physician-assisted suicide is a wholly personal and private act and,
thus, strictly a matter between a patient and his or her physician.

4. For persons who are dying, avoidance of suffering is the only hope.

5. Being ill, frail, and dependent on others is undignified.

6. In discussing the legalization of physician-assisted suicide society
is addressing the problem of suffering among the dying.

These attitudes will be sequentially examined in light of "first
principles": the essential nature of dying, the fundamental values of
society, and the canons of ethical behavior within the community and
within professional practice. In so doing, the current cultural and professional premise toward terminal care will be challenged. The meaning of physician-assisted suicide will be contrasted with the meaning of
care. The notion of beneficence will be expanded in light of empiric
knowledge of the range of the human experience of dying and of the
therapeutic potential of care for the dying. An integrated model of
social and professional ethics will be presented which balances the
language of individual rights and the principle of autonomy with the
language of mutual responsibility and the principle of beneficence. A
realistic, achievable model for end-of-life care emerges that is ethically
consistent with historical social and professional values and can yield
reliable and gratifying clinical results.

Medicine as a Profession

Much of what has been written about PAS in recent years has concerned the contemporary social context of end-of-life care and the potential scope of medical care for the dying in the future. In seeking to understand the various implications of physicians either being enabled to assist patients with suicide on the one hand or prohibited from doing so on the other, it is useful to begin by reflecting on the fundamental nature of professions within society.

As civilization developed through the centuries, the professions gradually became recognized as loci of expertise and specialized services within society.[3] Practitioners of medicine, as well as counselors of law and religion, were not initially drawn to their vocations by expectations of respect, special compensation, or other social privilege but rather out of a sense of calling. One meaning of the word *profession* is "the body of persons engaged in a calling."[4] In recognition for the dedication and discipline required and in appreciation for the value of the specialized service afforded to society, members of the professions were gradually accorded favored status within the social structure.

Given this sense of having been called that motivated the work of a profession, it is understandable that members of the profession were held—actually held themselves—to a higher than ordinary standard of conduct and practice. For medicine this is reflected in the prohibitions within the Hippocratic Oath regarding the performance of abortion, euthanasia, and assistance in suicide as well as the admonition to refrain from sexual relations with patients or members of their family.

Over the history of civilizations the congealing of practitioners as formal professions has extracted from the larger society a significant measure of independence in the setting of standards of conduct and of practice and in the determination of quality of service provided.[3,5] Historically, societies have supported this autonomous notion of professional integrity through the creation of formal mechanisms for the credentialing and licensing of professionals and in restricting from practice those not admitted to the profession. Furthermore, societies have traditionally looked to the professions for leadership in guiding action and public policy within their purview.

The medical profession developed around the need to care for those who were injured, ill, suffering, or dying. Among the highest values of medicine are the preservation of life and the alleviation of suffering. The modern medical model is built upon the problems of illness and injury, and its beneficent goals include saving lives or prolonging them, restoration of function, and alleviation of physical distress. In addition to the beneficence principle of acting to the good of patients, the prevailing biomedical model includes the principles of nonmaleficence, autonomy, truth-telling, justice in the distribution of health care resources, and maintenance of professional standards of practice.[6–9]

The medical profession has conducted the current debate regarding the issue of PAS within the confines of the prevailing model of biomedical ethics and the therapeutic model of medicine. Autonomy has become the dominant principle in the debate. Built upon the historic opinion of Justice Benjamin Cardozo in the 1914 case of *Shloendorff v. New York Hospital,* the accumulation of judicial decisions, legislation, and professional position papers during the last half of the twentieth century reflects the existing consensus that autonomy conveys to patients or their legal surrogates the right to refuse any medical care offered and the right to choose between indicated options for care that are available.[6,8,10–14] Proponents of PAS assert that autonomy should now be extended to include the right of specific categories of persons to receive assistance in suicide from willing licensed professionals.

The need to maintain established professional standards of medical practice has acted to balance autonomy within the construct of biomedical ethics. Patients may request any variety of services from physicians, from antibiotics for viral pharyngitis to laetrile for widely metastatic cancer. In order to preserve integrity of medical practice, physicians have not only the right but also the responsibility of declining to comply with some requests by autonomous patients.

Yet professional integrity is also not an absolute principle; medical practice always takes place within a contemporary social context and professional standards may change over time. While professional standards can help moderate rapid shifts in practice due to extreme social conditions such as occur during times of famine, economic depression, or war, the profession of medicine must remain responsive to the society it serves and should, optimally, provide leadership in areas of critical public policy. It has recently been argued that since it is proper for the notion of professional integrity for medicine to adapt in response to changes in society, it is now acceptable to incorporate the act of assisting with suicide within the practice of medicine.[15]

It is my contention that a self-enforcing interplay between the prevailing therapeutic clinical model and the prevailing biomedical ethical model exists and that this interplay has acted to severely constrict the debate on PAS. Unexamined, the prevailing interpretations of medical ethics and medical care of the dying jointly threaten to limit the potential of medicine to contribute in valuable ways to the care of dying persons.

When the models of medicine and biomedical ethics are applied to care for the dying, the only beneficent goal that seems to apply is relief of physical distress. The choice offered to autonomous patients who are living with far-advanced illness is that between continued life-prolonging medical interventions and death, the unspoken consequence of refusal. "Comfort care" is a common, almost apologetic term applied to the lowered intensity of medical care accorded terminally ill patients who do refuse cure-directed—and, ultimately, futile—medical interventions. The language of contemporary medicine portrays the bias toward curative intervention. It remains common for the category of terminally ill patients to be referred to as "hopeless" or "helpless," particularly within articles by physician proponents of legalizing physician-assisted suicide.[16-19] Indeed, from a perspective that views life prolongation and relief of physical distress as all that can be hoped for, a terminally ill person whose suffering derives from the impending loss of family, friends, and life itself does appear hopeless and beyond any capacity to help.

But is this truly the case? Perhaps it is the dominant therapeutic and ethical models which must change. The six attitudes identified earlier reflect common assumptions underlying the current debate regarding PAS. Each of these assumptions will be presented in the form of a declarative statement and will be challenged in the process of developing an expanded clinical and ethical premise for appropriate end-of-life care.

Assumption One: Each Person Is Fundamentally an Individual, Distinct from Others and the Community

Modern biologic and physical sciences have revealed that we live in a quantum world of profound, fundamental interconnection. However, the contemporary mindset continues to reflect Cartesian and Newtonian assumptions that isolate mind from body and one being from another.

Respect for the individual is a cornerstone of American history and culture and pervades other Jeffersonian democracies. In matters concerning social justice and the equitable allocation of public resources it is often proper to consider each person as an individual; however, several lines of research from archeology, anthropology, and social biology support a view of humans as fundamentally social beings.[20-22] Available evidence strongly suggests that the early primates lived in clans and that early humanoid species were clan or tribal animals. Without rudimentary family and community structure these species would not have survived and the species we recognize as *Homo sapiens* would never have come into being. Individually, each human infant and toddler has a remarkably long period of dependency which requires at least a minimum of family structure for normal development. Erik Erikson's model of development, now supported by substantial observational studies and an accepted part of child psychiatry and the behavioral medicine components of pediatrics and family practice, holds that supportive interactions with family and others are a requisite to normal development.[20,23]

Each adult human being maintains physiologic responsiveness to others. Research designs in which participants were unwittingly made to witness a feigned injury or seizure have consistently documented immediate and profound neurohumoral and cardiovascular changes in response to apparent danger or injury to another human being.[22] More familiar is the effect that an inconsolable, crying infant has on airline passengers or diners in an otherwise quiet restaurant. Irritability rises and there is an instinctive sense that someone should respond. The impact on others is not explained by the volume of the sound, for a crying infant in a restaurant will reliably diminish appetites while the same decibels of discordant street noise would pass virtually unnoticed. An even more dramatic example from daily experience is the releaser effect of a baby's plaintive cry on a lactating woman aisles away in a department store; the let-down response provides a clear physiologic example of persistent human connection.

From a social perspective as well, "humanness" has little meaning in isolation, out of the context of relationship with others. In modern times even the most reclusive of hermits maintains a variety of relations with society for at least part of his or her clothing or food as well as for basic information (i.e., news and weather forecasts). At a minimum, reclusive persons depend on the local social structure for protection from others who might prey upon them and for general safety needs, including emergency medical services and fire and police protection.

Extremes of age and periods of ill health are predictable times of heightened physical and emotional dependency. During the course of most people's lives there will be times and situations in which they are primarily the providers of care for others and other times and situations in which they are primarily the recipients of care. Throughout life some people tend to be more or less dependent upon others; there is wide variation with regard to this personality trait. Some couples and families tend to be emotionally dependent on one another to an unhealthy extent and may merit diagnostic labels of "enmeshed" or "co-dependent." However, some degree of mutuality and of interdependence is a fundamental aspect of the human condition. These inherent, fundamental human qualities of mutuality and interdependence deserve recognition within the ethical and therapeutic models of medicine. There is precedent in both realms.

Ethical Implications of Mutuality and Interdependence

In a 1978 article entitled "The Ethics of Terminal Care," Harold Vanderpool asserted,

> Being part of a community is essential for the development of consciousness and individuality and is characterized by communication, mutuality, and the ethical ideals of fidelity, gratitude, reciprocity, justice, and love.... These four fundamental features of human worth—respect for the individual, inclusion in community, concern for the body, and considerations of a broader purpose—are offered as ethical guidelines for terminal care.[24]

More recently, Dan Brock and Norman Daniels outlined a set of principles that can serve to guide policy decisions and choices about the central features of health care reform proposals and can provide a tool for an ethical assessment of whatever new health care system results. The most basic underlying values they identified are equality, liberty, justice, and community:

> We are members not only of a national community but also of many other communities that flourish within our society: religious, racial and ethnic, as well as the neighborhoods, towns and cities in which people share a sense of common life. *Fundamental to all these different communities is a shared concern and responsibility for one's fellow members, especially those suffering misfortune and in need of help.* [emphasis added][25]

Fundamental to the values of every culture and religion is a rudimentary contract that concerns mutual responsibility. Society firmly recognizes an obligation on the part of the whole and its members to respond in a helpful fashion to those who are suffering or experiencing profound human need. When the concept of responsibility is applied to considerations of suffering, incurable illness, and the end of life, there is indeed an aspect of obligation that pertains. This is part of the very fabric of society, as fundamental to the social structure as is the rule of law, prohibition against violence, and respect for the safety needs of others. As members of society, what constitutes our fundamental obligation—our responsibility—to a dying person, not only to a loved one or neighbor but even to a dying stranger?

In attempting to develop an ethical model for terminal care that incorporates these fundamental values, pertinent questions arise. What are the essential needs of persons as they die and, even more fundamentally, what is the nature of the human condition in the process of dying?

It is a fundamental, almost axiomatic, feature of the human condition during the process of dying that most people are frail and in need of care. Indeed, the concept of responsibility to our fellow human beings as death approaches seems embodied in the notion of care.

Caring is at the center of one human being's ability to respond to another. The dictionary defines the verb *care* in its infinitive form, *to care for*: "to take thought for, provide for, look after, take care of."[26] As such the verb *care* incorporates a quality of continuance.

Reflecting on the basic needs of people as they die, a list of the essential constituents of human care can be elaborated. This list of the fundamental components of care for the dying is not intended to forge new social principles for behavior but rather to help us discern basic features of the social construct. Care for the dying includes at a minimum the following:

- the provision of shelter from the elements,
- the provision of hygiene,
- assistance with elimination,
- the offering of food and fluid,
- the keeping of company (nonabandonment),
- bearing witness (recognizing the essential value of each individual), and
- the relief of suffering.

In the provision of these services members of society collectively say to the other, "We will keep you warm and dry. We will keep you clean. We will help you with your bowels and your bladder. We will always offer you food and water. We will be with you. And we will bear witness to your pain, your struggles and your sorrows, your disappointments and your triumphs; we will listen to the stories of your life, and we will remember the story of your passing."

Finally, of course, we say to the other, "We will do whatever we can, with as much skill and expertise as is available, to lessen your discomfort." This last component of care is uniquely within the medical profession's purview and forms medicine's primary responsibility to society's members as they die. While delegating to the caring professions the responsibility to alleviate suffering, society retains the general and fundamental responsibility for care.

It seems ironic that the proscription against euthanasia has held as strongly as it has throughout human history, since it is only recently that the most effective symptom-relieving modalities have come into being. This irony is exemplified by another assumption that powerfully shapes the current debate on legalization of physician-assisted suicide.

Assumption Two: At Times Severe Physical Distress among the Dying Cannot Be Alleviated

This assertion is made or inferred so often that it has come to be accepted as fact. Even the Clinical Practice Guideline "Management of Cancer Pain" issued by the Agency for Health Care Policy and Research, developed to correct misunderstandings and deficiencies in clinical practice, opens with the following statement: "Pain control in people with cancer remains a significant problem in health care even though cancer pain can be managed effectively in up to 90 percent of patients."[27] In truth, there are no biologic or pharmacologic limits on the ability to control physical suffering associated with dying.

The reticence to use absolutes such as "all," "none," "always," and "never" in matters of medicine is understandable and it is essential in clinical writing that the context of unequivocal statements be carefully specified. In the experience of the author and many palliative medicine colleagues, physical distress among the dying can *always* be alleviated. This statement assumes that basic human needs are met and access to competent medical care exists and, therefore, excludes situations of war or extreme social deprivation. Furthermore, the assertion is carefully restricted to physical suffering and to the terminally ill. Physician proponents of assisted suicide disagree. The authors of an article entitled "Care of the Hopelessly Ill: Proposed Clinical Criteria for Physician-Assisted Suicide," state:

> Those who have witnessed difficult deaths in hospice programs are not reassured by the glib assertion that we can always make death tolerable, and patients fear that physicians will abandon them if their course becomes difficult or overwhelming in the face of comfort care. In fact, there is no empirical evidence that all physical suffering associated with incurable illness can be effectively relieved.[28]

Similarly, in the process of arguing that the principle of professional integrity can be extended to include physician assistance with suicide, Franklin Miller and Howard Brody assert:

> Some hospice physicians and ethicists opposed to such assistance have argued that it [physical suffering] always amounts to incompetent medical practice, because competent palliative care provided by well-trained hospice clinicians obviates the need to relieve suffering by lethal means. We believe that clinical experience fails to support this claim. Not all patients can receive adequate relief of pain or suffering even under conditions of optimal palliative care.[15]

It is undeniably true that physical suffering is not always adequately controlled even in current hospice settings; however, the contention that physical suffering exists "even under conditions of optimal palliative care" extends beyond empiric observation to imply theoretical limitations. It is illogical to use the existence of a problem to argue against the possibility of a solution. Care is not "optimal" if significant physical distress is allowed to exist unabated. Alleviation of pain, dyspnea, and agitation associated with terminal illness is not always readily achieved and may require formidable interventions involving the services of multiple consultant physicians, nurse specialists, and clinical pharmacologists. At times it is expensive. Commonly, in order to meet the needs of patients as they die, palliative care, whether practiced in a hospice program or nonhospice setting, becomes a form of intensive care. This portrayal describes optimal palliation of physical distress and is effectively modeled by a small but growing number of hospice and palliative care programs.

Hospice care is not practiced in a world of Platonic ideals but rather in the real world of the late twentieth century. As with trauma care, acute cardiac care, and mental health services, funding, resources, knowledge, and clinical competence of hospice and palliative care programs vary widely, and the corresponding quality of care varies widely and, regrettably, often is less than optimal. Nevertheless, the National Hospice Organization recently approved a monograph written by the Ethics Committee entitled *Proactive Responses to the Euthanasia/Assisted Suicide Debate* that contains the statement, "Symptoms can be controlled and physical suffering can *always* be alleviated." This defines a practice standard toward which member programs must strive.[29]

Certainly until someone documents a patient for whom general anesthesia is ineffective, there exists empiric evidence that "all *physical suffering* associated with incurable illness can be effectively relieved." Published reports of the use of subanesthetic doses of barbiturates to treat the most difficult instances of pain or terminal agitation document remarkably positive results.[30–31] Guidelines for the use of such agents must be refined and made widely available. At least within affluent Western nations, when physical suffering among the dying occurs, the deficiency is not one of resources or technology but rather of will and commitment. During curative or life-prolonging phases of medical therapy, extreme means of life-saving often are appropriate; similarly, extraordinary means of symptom control at times are required during the palliative phase of care.

The use of medication with the primary intention of inducing deep sedation for the management of otherwise unrelieved pain, dyspnea, or terminal agitation is extraordinary care. Fortunately, with meticulous attention to principles of palliative medicine such measures are infrequently needed.[30-34] When they are needed they must be used. In this way practitioners of medicine can fulfill a commitment to patients that care will continue for them and that they will not be allowed to suffer physical agony in their dying.

In debates on legalizing PAS and euthanasia the issue of sedation as medical management of otherwise uncontrolled physical suffering often is met with a response from legalization proponents that may be paraphrased, "If physicians are willing to sedate someone into unconsciousness, why not assist them in suicide or directly euthanize them?" The fact of such questions represents a tacit acceptance that the notion of uncontrollable terminal distress is itself unfounded.

However, the distinction between sedation and euthanasia does merit consideration. Miller and Brody articulate this reservation:

> Deep sedation to counteract refractory suffering is a possible option; however, this will not be satisfactory for patients who want to remain alert without suffering intolerably. Some patients may prefer to end their lives at home than to be hospitalized and persist in a sedated state pending death. Furthermore, it is not clear that relieving terminal suffering by inducing unconsciousness, which may hasten death, is morally superior to voluntary physician-assisted death.[15]

The prevailing biomedical models of therapeutics and ethics provide few tools for exploring important differences between the two actions. Significant differences become apparent by considering the meaning of the physician's actions and by examining the meaning and potential value of sedation as an extraordinary symptom-alleviating measure within the context of a community ethic of end-of-life care.

The Influence of Physician Attitude and Expertise on the Inclination of the Patient Regarding Suicide

The relationship of a physician to a patient with far-advanced disease does not conform to the Cartesian metaphor of a watchmaker's relationship to a broken watch. Physicians practice within a context of mutuality that has emotional as well as clinical components. Attention must be accorded the real possibility that a physician's inability to perceive an alternative means of responding to a dying patient's distress comprises an important factor contributing to suicidal ideation on the part of the patient.[35-36] Another potential factor influencing a patient's

disposition regarding suicide is the treating physician's level of palliative medical expertise; where one physician may see a patient's pain
syndrome as intractable and thus consider the patient helpless, another
may recognize the syndrome as an indication for a neurolytic block,
spinal anesthesia, urgent radiotherapy, high dose opioid infusion, or
other intensive palliative interventions.

The psychology of requests for assistance in suicide has just begun
to be studied. There are substantive concerns regarding the impact that
a patient's suffering and feelings of depression and hopelessness can
have on the physician, as well as the impact that the physician's emotional history—including previous experience with the death of a loved
one, recent experience of multiple losses, personal values or emotional
depression—and current feelings of sadness, grief, frustration, helplessness, fatigue and previous personal experience may have on the
patient.[35-36] Authenticity and intimacy are to be encouraged within the
physician-patient relationship; professional guidelines for conduct
exist specifically to establish clear boundaries within which a safe environment is created that encourages these attributes of the clinical relationship.

Concerns of this nature are not confined to opponents of legalizing
PAS. Dutch psychologist René Diekstra, a principal architect of the
permissive policy on assisted suicide in the Netherlands and a strong
proponent for legalization, recalls his experience on a committee
"established in 1982 under the auspices of the Dutch Association for
Voluntary Euthanasia and the Dutch Humanist Association, to assist
health care workers who are confronted with a request for assistance
with suicide."

> The members of the committee often were left with the impression that
> had the professional not had the opportunity to consult with others
> about potential assistance with suicide, he or she might have provided
> such assistance, not because no alternatives to suicide were available but
> because of a certain type of emotional involvement in or commitment
> with the patient. Sometimes it appeared that the professional had, so to
> speak, prematurely translated their own feelings of powerlessness or
> helplessness with regard to the patient's condition into the rationality,
> or even the unavoidability, of the patient's suicide.[37]

Of note, no such committee exists in the protocols of the Netherlands today, nor is one envisioned within provisions of any proposed
state legislation in the United States.

Assumption Three: Physician-Assisted Suicide Is a Wholly Personal and Private Act and Thus Strictly a Matter between a Patient and His or Her Physician

The contention that PAS is fundamentally a personal act forms a central tenet of proponent arguments. In an opinion overturning a Washington State law that prohibited assisting a person in suicide, U.S. District Judge Rothstein asserted, "There is no more profoundly personal decision, nor one which is closer to the heart of personal liberty, than the choice which a terminally ill person makes to end his or her suffering and hasten an inevitable death."[38]

The fact that this rationale has acquired the status of an assumption in many people's minds reflects a general social ethic that emphasizes individuality to the virtual exclusion of mutuality and interdependence. Within this world view, norms for social interaction are based on respect for individual rights, such as the rights of privacy and of protection from intrusion. The primacy of individuality within contemporary culture finds expression in the emphasis on the principle of autonomy in biomedical ethics. Paternalistic abuses in the name of beneficence during the first half of the twentieth century engendered in the 1960s and subsequent decades a reaction in which the principle of autonomy ascended to become the highest value in clinical ethics. The interpretation of autonomy in biomedical ethics that emerged closely parallels the social rights of privacy and protection from intrusion; autonomy is understood as the right to refuse any medical care offered and the right to choose between available treatment alternatives.[8-9,39]

On these points, proponents and opponents of PAS agree. Patients who possess decision-making capacity and those who have clearly expressed their preferences in formal advance directives and through surrogates have the right to refuse any medical care offered. This interpretation of autonomy does not directly inform ethical thought regarding the question of a general right to suicide. If a right to suicide exists, it is not absolute, for there is consensus that at least in situations such as severe depression in the physically healthy person, society can assert a legitimate interest in preserving life that places limits on the person's actions. Of note, in these instances physicians, in concert with emergency medical personnel under their authority, are the social agents who assert society's directive to save the life of a person who wished to die.

If consideration of the right to end one's own life is restricted to persons with a far-advanced, life-limiting illness, whether by inhaling carbon monoxide, taking an overdose, or refusing to eat, the matter is of philosophical more than practical significance. The courts have ruled that even a feeding tube can be refused by a competent adult.[11] Other than addressing protection of life insurance benefits in this context, no legal changes are required. In the context of terminal illness, causing one's own death at least theoretically can be a purely personal and private act.

However, refusing life-prolonging treatment, suicide, and physician assistance with suicide are distinct categories of action. In common with members of other professions, physicians always act as agents for the larger society within the purview of their professional expertise. Contemporary physicians receive training from society's highly subsidized medical education programs; they are licensed by boards of medicine and certified by specialty boards duly recognized by society's accrediting bodies. Furthermore, physicians are reimbursed by society for the specialized work that they do. In return, physicians are expected to act with higher than normal standards toward patients who are in an inherently vulnerable role.

Judge Rothstein's decision, with the rationale it reflects, dismisses the distinction between the taking of one's own life and the conscripting of the lethal assistance of a physician. Proponents of legalization point to cases such as that of Timothy Quill's "Diane" as examples of the need for protection for a caring physician.[40] As reflected in the narrative report of the case, Dr. Quill's personal struggle and willingness to put himself at risk constitute factors that contribute a sense of legitimacy to his action. In taking the action he did, Quill consciously stepped outside the accepted role of the physician and acted more as a friend to Diane than as a professional.

It is illogical to conclude, however, that the legitimacy of the specific act requires general acceptance of the legitimacy of PAS. As an analogy, the existence of a stable and happy marriage that began as a therapeutic relationship between patient and psychiatrist does not argue persuasively for relaxing the general proscription against physicians having sex with their patients, even when those relations are apparently consensual. Physicians are held to a higher professional standard of practice that contravenes such actions. Transgressions deserve serious attention; exceptions to the general proscription can be recognized on a case-by-case basis, rather than prospectively. In this regard it has been suggested that the medical failure to adequately control symptoms could form the basis for legal and professional defense against the offense of assisting a patient in suicide.[41–42] It is noteworthy that Dr. Quill was not indicted and that there have not been any successful prosecutions of physicians for assisting in a patient's suicide in recent decades.

Physician-assisted suicide is not a purely personal and private act. When it does become legally available, PAS will represent a new social service available to those who meet the requisite criteria. Physicians will perform such assistance under guidelines, they will be scrutinized in such action and, very likely, will be paid for the service. Whether by court decision, legislation, or plebescite, this component of medical service will be imposed on the profession by the larger society.

In opposing PAS as a proposed service of society, it is necessary to articulate another vision within which the medical profession can respond in a robust, effective manner to suffering among the dying. An alternative social ethic based on mutuality, which emphasizes mutual responsibility and interdependence and which includes a fundamental responsibility to provide care to those most in need, can provide the basis for an expanded clinical role. However, beyond meeting patients' most basic human needs, the rudiments of care, the human community possesses an ability to respond to those who are dying that is limited only by its collective imagination. The fourth assumption exemplifies the manner in which therapeutic imagination can be critically restricted.

Assumption Four: For Persons Who Are Dying, Avoidance of Suffering Is the Only Hope

Within the prevailing cultural mindset, dying is thought of as a time of inherent discomfort and almost inevitable emotional depression. The best that can be hoped for in one's dying is avoidance or alleviation of suffering. This narrow view does not conform to what we know of the range of human experience with the dying process.

Reflecting this cultural mindset, physicians typically approach the dying patient by defining a set of medical problems to be addressed. Yet dying is fundamentally a personal experience, the experience of life coming to an end, and it is literally a part of living. Hospice and palliative care clinicians regularly encounter patients and families who speak of the value and importance *for them* of this time of life. While needless suffering among the dying at times appears to be pervasive and deserves to be the focus of corrective action, accounts of dying persons (or their families) who express feelings of enhanced well-being have long been documented in biographic literature and are being substantiated with increased frequency in the palliative care literature.[43-49] These phenomena demand scrutiny by the professions of psychology and clinical medicine.

As with every other phase of human life, the subjective experience with dying ranges from agony to bliss; for the majority of people it falls somewhere in between. When the basic needs for shelter, nourishment, hygiene and companionship are met and at least a modicum of medical attention is directed toward control of symptoms, the dying experience encompasses much more than avoidance of pain and suffering. People who are fortunate enough to be cared for in a fairly comprehensive manner as they die are able to accomplish important goals and achieve a sense of completion—at times satisfaction—and readiness which underlies Elizabeth Kubler-Ross's stage of acceptance and is observed by others as the person being "at peace."[50] Such favorable experiences are not exclusive of antecedent suffering; indeed, symptoms which have been brought under control were once uncontrolled and emotional distress which has been resolved was once unresolved. Typically, the sense of compelling importance and value that people express in the time of their dying occurs *in addition to* some degree of physical discomfort, personal sense of loss, and profound sadness.

For example, the mother of a man who died in his thirties from AIDS sent me the following letter, the last her son ever wrote her:

> Dear Mom,
>   This last part of my life could have been very unpleasant, but it wasn't. In fact, in many ways, it has been the best part of my life. I've had the opportunity to get to know my family again, a chance very few people have or take advantage of. I've enjoyed a life full of adventure and travel. . . . But I probably never would have slowed up enough to really appreciate all of you if it hadn't been for my illness. That's the silver lining in this very dark cloud. . . . When you get down to it, I'd have to live several hundred years to fulfill all the dreams I've had. I have done pretty well with the time allotted me, so I have no regrets. . . . If anyone ever asks you if I went to heaven, tell them this: I just came from there.[51]

Another example. During a successful psychiatric hospitalization necessitated by bizarre behavior caused by a combination of cerebral metastases, extreme anger, and rigid emotional denial of his impending death, a fifty-three-year-old father of three told me, "Doc, somebody should have done this to me twenty years ago. This has been the most wonderful experience of my life."[46]

Beneficence in care for the dying requires meeting the fundamental physical and human needs of persons, but it need not stop there. The principle of beneficence must be reexamined in light of what we know of the range of the human condition as death approaches. Beyond symptom management, the ability to act for the good of our patients (and their families) extends to help with the alleviation of personal suffering and to the preservation of personal opportunity.

While neither of these roles is well modeled by contemporary medical practice of terminal care, both have precedent within the medical profession.

Personal suffering associated with dying is at once intensely individual and predictably universal. Persons who are dying frequently express a loss of hope and self-worth; they may experience themselves to be undignified and a burden on their families and society. While each person's experience is intensely unique, the commonality of issues allows for effective clinical intervention in a high proportion of cases. There is a myth that psychotherapy among the dying is complex because of the myriad of issues involved. In practice the therapeutic approach is usually straightforward and requires mostly the commitment to try. It begins by listening, meeting the person where he or she is. Active listening that is attentive and reflects what Carl Rogers referred to as "unconditional positive regard" invites trust and security from which feelings of deeper concern, fears, and sorrow can be expressed. Suffering often derives from the loss of meaning and feelings of impending disintegration.[52–53] With skillful clinical support these issues can be addressed; clinicians will not have definitive answers, but it is not the clinician's answers that matter. What matters is the willingness—the commitment—to stand with the patients, helping them in seeking their own answers. This level of comprehensiveness, which palliative medicine borrows from and builds on developmental psychotherapy, can facilitate subjective growth of the person even as parts of the self are completed and released.[46–47,54]

Clinical experience in counseling persons who are suffering as they die reveals that personal suffering is not analogous to physical pain, which exists on a continuum from complete comfort through minor irritation to the extreme of physical agony. Despite its severity, suffering that is existential or spiritual in nature may be separated by the thinnest membrane from relief and well-being. The suffering that derives from an experienced loss of dignity, feelings of being a burden and of being without hope, invites clinical intervention.

Presentation of a Case

Mr. S., a forty-nine-year-old man with advanced ALS who was described as suffering and had been voicing suicidal ideation, was seen for a single consultation at a residential hospice. Craig, a close friend of the patient, was in attendance. Mr. S. denied any pain and had only occasional dyspnea associated with isolated episodes of choking while eating. He was depressed over the progression of his disability and the loss of activities and relationships, as well as the impending loss of life itself. He feared suffocating but expressed that his real suffering derived from having become a burden to his family and even to the nurses who had to feed and toilet him. "I'm not good to anyone anymore. I just wish I could get this over. It is so undignified!"

The basic facts of family, place of birth, and personal history were elicited, allowing Mr. S. to tell his story. He spoke of his children, his career that had been cut short, and the adventures he had enjoyed with male friends. The depth of the tragedy that this illness and dying represented was acknowledged and a degree of therapeutic rapport was discerned. The physician then further acknowledged to Mr. S. that his dying was placing burdens on his family and friends but emphasized that in changing their schedules to be by his side, in providing physical care and even in grieving, family and friends were doing what they needed to do for themselves.

> Dr.: "If it were Craig in this bed, you would do the same thing, wouldn't you?"
>
> Mr. S.: "Yes, I'd be with him." Mr. S. voice was hoarse from his illness and from having begun to tear.
>
> Dr.: "It is a fact that as people are dying they often need to be cared for as they did in infancy and young childhood. Caring for babies and toddlers is a burden, but it is also a blessing for families. Families create and sustain themselves around the care of the youngest and the care of their dying loved ones. Your role at present may be the hardest of all, to passively accept the care that your family and friends need to give you. Never for a moment believe that this time has no value."
>
> Mr. S. was quiet, Craig was holding his arm and confirming, "What the doctor is saying is right. We love you and we have to take care of you." Both he and Mr. S. were softly crying.
>
> Dr.: "I cannot tell you how to feel, but it's important to me for you to know that I do not consider you to be undignified. You are simply dying and you are only human. A baby is not undignified in his or her physical dependence, neither are you undignified because you are no longer able to care for yourself. The nurses and aides here do not feel awkward in caring for your body and you need not feel embarrassed in receiving care. It is our pleasure to do so."

This session lasted less than an hour, yet it represented a turning point in the patient's hospice course. Mr. S.'s anger and frustration gave way to sadness and acceptance of himself and of the loving care he was given. His dependence remained a source of mild annoyance and grist for his dry, self-deprecating humor; however, during the last two weeks of his life Mr. S. expressed a sense of well-being, self-acceptance, and serenity. Two weeks later he died quietly with family and friends present.

While the brief nature of this clinical encounter and the degree of subsequent change will invite skepticism of its implications to clinical policy and practice, it must be remembered that Mr. S. resided—before and after the consultation—within an environment of family, friends, and hospice providers that constituted a microculture of a caring, loving community. Without this context, the clinical intervention would have been unlikely to have had significant impact.

Too often in case conferences, nonphysical suffering in a dying patient is labeled anxiety or situational depression and primarily treated with anxiolytics or antidepressant medications. Counseling for these conditions is considered inherently complex and esoteric. Psychiatric consultation may be advised or the matter dismissed with vague references to psychosocial support. In palliative care practice, actual complexity of counseling varies from patient to patient, but personal suffering of this nature routinely proves to be comprehensible and approachable. The issues with which people struggle characteristically concern meaning, worth, dependence, burden, forgiveness, reconciliation. The clinical work that can assist a person to find his or her own way through their particular membrane is delicate but reliable. It is not mystical—and it can be taught.

The encounter with Mr. S. also illustrates a fifth assumption that merits challenge.

Assumption Five: Being Ill, Frail and Dependent on Others Is Undignified

The loss of dignity is frequently expressed by people who are dying and is tightly bound to feelings of being a burden, low self-esteem, and loss of any sense of worth. Avoidance of indignity is consistently cited in proponent arguments regarding PAS. If patients' experience of indignity is to become a medical indication for assistance with suicide, it is imperative that it be understood. Dignity is a notion that derives from those aspects of life that members of society collectively decide to invest with value. The word *dignity* is derived from the Latin *dignitas*, meaning "honorableness, grandeur, esteem and high rank." In a literal sense, society, via its members, determines what is dignified. Dignity is reflected in those styles of living, modes of behavior and aspects of life which society invests with value. What is considered dignified changes over time and varies between cultures and subcultures. Dominant Western notions of dignity are tied to prevailing views of physical beauty; to the values of youthfulness, independence, and self-control; and to the quantity and quality of one's possessions. In this context, being ill, old, and debilitated or being dependent on others seems "inherently" undignified.

This prevailing cultural assumption contributes tangibly to the frequency and extent of personal suffering at life's end. While efforts to preserve function and faculties of patients with far-advanced disease continue, it would also seem valuable to challenge this notion of dignity. In this matter the medical profession has an opportunity to make a contribution by fulfilling a traditional role of professions within society: that of providing leadership and value clarification in matters within the profession's realm of expertise.

The profession of medicine has an opportunity to help mature cultural values in a way that recognizes the worth of the many frail and chronically ill persons within our communities. As members of a profession, physicians can declare that the patients for whom we care are not undignified by their illness, physical appearance, dependency, or dying. The caring professions can demonstrate respect for the dignity of persons who consciously allow themselves to be cared for as a gift to their loved ones who need to provide care as a healthy expression of their grieving.[32] Existing hospice and palliative care programs can serve as a model for this stance.

Assumption Six: In Discussing the Legalization of Physician-Assisted Suicide, Society Is Addressing the Problem of Suffering among the Dying

The fallacy of this final assumption must be recognized before the medical profession can directly address and effectively respond to the crisis of end-of-life care. The supposition that in adding this one last step to our clinical algorithms we will have fixed the problem has diverted attention from the core problems within medical practice and medical education of conceptualization of and approach to end-of-life care. Current proposals to legalize PAS include provisions that specifically exclude large categories of persons from consideration. These exclusions are presented as necessary safeguards to abuse and unwise extension of assisted suicide; however, the categories of people excluded are at least as vulnerable to suffering as they die as those eligible.

Dying persons whose suffering would be left unaddressed by all of these proposals include children, people with significant developmental disability, people with serious psychiatric illness, people who are alert but "locked in," and people who are paralyzed and thus unable to participate in the suicidal act. Unless society with the medical profession can effectively respond to suffering within these groups in alternative ways, it will become mandatory to extend the service of PAS or euthanasia to them. Indeed, once PAS is made available to one group, the social ethics based on rights will necessitate such extensions and they can be predicted from the Netherlands experience.[55-58]

In their proposed guidelines for PAS, authors Christine Cassel, Timothy Quill, and Diane Meier present as an example of the need for legalization "a fiercely independent retired factory worker, quadriplegic from amytrophic lateral sclerosis, who no longer wants to linger in a helpless, dependent state waiting and hoping for death." The authors then propose guidelines for legal medically assisted suicides that require self-administration of the lethal drug and which, thus, disqualify this patient from consideration.[16,41] Instead, for suffering persons unable to self-administer the necessary medication they offer the following statement:

> Such persons, who meet agreed-on criteria in other respects, must not be abandoned in their suffering; a combination of decisions to forgo life-sustaining treatments (including food and fluids) with aggressive comfort measures (such as analgesics and sedatives) could be offered, along with a commitment to search for creative alternatives.[16]

As noted, care of this nature is available in relatively few programs. A major commitment would be required in order for care at the level of comprehension and quality described to be reliably available to patients who did not qualify for physician assistance with suicide. Is it to be a standard only for people who are disqualified from physician assistance with suicide? As a society and profession, when can we adopt this description as a standard for care for all?

If legalized, guidelines for PAS would undoubtedly be expanded to include patients who are physically unable to perform the life-ending act and to those who are minors, mildly retarded, or mentally ill. It is consistent with autonomy-based biomedical ethics to further extend such rights to people who are currently demented or unresponsive but who have previously requested such assistance in formal advanced directives.

Furthermore, experience in the Netherlands suggests that the rationale on which current proposals are based would lead, inevitably, to extensions of the "right" to assistance in suicide being broadened to include people who suffer emotional depression but who are not terminally ill.[59] This extension was long foreseen by architects of the Dutch policy:

> Approximately 10–15% of all cases of severe depressive disorders are not amenable to available methods of treatment and patients suffering

from such disorders may after many years and modalities of treatment come to a realistic assessment of their bad prognosis. If then the only possibility of preventing death by suicide of a person who is not psychotic nor mentally retarded is by "psychiatric imprisonment," assisted suicide might be considered the "least of all possible tragedies."[37]

Toward a Role for the Profession of Medicine within a Rebalanced Social Ethic

The crisis of end-of-life care presents an opportunity for the profession of medicine to take strong corrective action and, in so doing, assert a traditional leadership role concerning the values of care for fellow members of society in their times of illness and suffering, in their time of dying and their time of grief.

While medicine cannot unilaterally transform the general culture's mindset with regard to death, dying, and end-of-life care, it can model for society a caring ethic in which rights of privacy and freedom from intrusion are balanced with genuine respect for mutual responsibility. While acknowledging the real world in which clinicians live and practice, an aligning vision for palliative care can be a world in which, to paraphrase medical ethicist Laurie Zoloth-Dorfman, people are born into the expectant arms of community and die from the reluctant arms of community.[60] Here the meaning of care and PAS can be seen in stark contrast. Care, as modeled by hospice, incorporates continuance as a fundamental principle by extending services through the dying process to include bereavement support to family as a core service. The meaning of care entails a commitment on the part of the clinician(s) to keep trying and an openness to the possibility of value emerging within whatever life remains. The meaning of acceding to a patient's request for a lethal prescription includes the tacit agreement that the person is hopeless and otherwise helpless.

In this time of crisis in end-of-life care, medical ethics is challenged to incorporate the biological fact of human interdependence and mutuality. In so doing the profession of medicine has an opportunity to articulate an ethic of a caring community. For persons with far-advanced disease, autonomous rights of refusal of treatment and choice must be balanced by offering robust choices for care that include the type of care exemplified by state-of-the-art hospice programs. Such care recognizes the fundamentally personal nature of dying, for the person and family, and extends beyond symptom management to preserve and gently nurture personal opportunity at the end of life.

Provision of basic human needs and comprehensive care for all persons (with their families) as they die would require unwavering commitment on the part of the clinical professions and far-reaching changes in health care. These changes are, perhaps, only slightly less dramatic than the changes that legalized PAS would present. Unlike PAS, however, the expansion of beneficence within clinical and ethical models reflects historical professional values.

Individually, as applied to medical ethics and care by providers for specific patients, as well as on the scale of society, as applied to social ethics and care by the community for its dying members, the principle of beneficence merits reexamination. In pediatric medicine as well as the pediatric component of family medicine, beneficence refers to more than life prolongation and relief of suffering. There is an understanding that medical beneficence toward the neonate and young child must include *preservation of opportunity* for the person to grow and develop normally.[21,61] Thus the medical student and intern studying neonatal assessment and learning the components of the pediatric health maintenance clinical visit is taught to attend to more than issues of nutrition, bowel function, and skin care. It is necessary to pay attention to the quality of interactions between the baby and the mother and father. Is the baby being talked to, played with? If so, in what ways?

In the early decades of the twentieth century in the U.S. mortality of orphaned infants in foundling homes reached 75 to 90 percent in the first two years of life. By the mid-1940s mortality had been reduced, but the effect of *hospitalism* on infants and toddlers resulted in universal and profound developmental delay. Utilizing exacting observational methodology, René Spitz conducted comparative studies of care between prison nurseries in which mothers were able to care for their children until age one and foundling homes in which care was provided by nursing staff.[61] Hygiene, nutrition, preventive medical care, and infectious precautions were at least comparable in the foundling home. While health and near-normal development of children prevailed within the prison nursery, over 25 percent of the children in the foundling home died by age two and one-half years, and without exception the foundling home residents were shown to have severe developmental delay.[61]

Disturbing parallels can be drawn to the current institutional care of the infirm, advanced elderly. Nursing homes for care of the most physically dependent members of our communities, including many of those who are dying, remain inadequately staffed; aide positions within the nursing home industry are filled by entry-level workers who are underpaid and who enjoy no stature within the medical profession or the human resource professions. Care of nursing home residents is commonly depersonalizing.[62–64] Residents are frequently left unattended and untouched unless it is time for them to be fed or they are needing to be changed. Hospice care is available to only a small fraction of people who die each year, barely more than one in ten Americans.[65] Programs to extend hospice services to nursing home residents are tentative and imperiled by the priority of controlling costs. In the United States the current medical system routinely results in patients and families becoming impoverished during treatment of chronic progressive illness.[1]

When beneficence is lacking, as it is presently, autonomy is unbalanced and the ethical perspective is distorted. The support for autonomy represented by assisted suicide disguises a withdrawal of resources and an admission of failure on the part of society. In the full meaning of the principle, autonomy asserts the value of each person being creatively involved in developing his or her plan of care. For autonomy to be genuinely honored by a caring community and the caring professions, persons must be offered authentic alternatives from which to choose. The example of a dyspneic seventy-five-year-old patient with extensive pulmonary metastases who has lived alone and has no local family illustrates the dilemma faced by far too many dying patients: the current choice is between hospitalization with the attendant charade of life-prolonging therapy and nursing home placement with a virtual abandonment by the medical system and the community. Contemporary society must develop an effective, uncompromising response to intolerable suffering. This issue is larger and distinct from the question of whether to provide medical assistance in suicide. While medicine has an integral role to play in society's response to the suffering of its dying members, that role need not extend to providing assistance in suicide and euthanasia.

Medical Practice in the Context of Legalized Assistance with Suicide

These arguments notwithstanding, efforts to legalize PAS will continue and, given the growing numbers of Americans who favor such action, the view that this "right" should be honored will likely prevail by legislation, referendum, or judicial decision. Once PAS is legal, its availability will affect all clinicians who care for the terminally ill. As a right, PAS will, of course, be accessible to all patients who meet specified criteria. Individually as clinicians and collectively as a profession, physicians will have to decide how to respond. The discussions and policy debates in Oregon following passage of Measure 16 illustrate that the responses from health care systems, including hospice programs, can range from discharge of patients who voice suicidal intent, to referral to licensed physicians willing to provide assistance, to incorporation of PAS within medical plans of care.[66-68]

The social and professional ethical framework presented can serve to guide clinical policy and practice in a manner which honors the new "right" to such service while preserving core values and principles of medical ethics and while continuing to serve patients who are suffering in their dying. Once assistance with suicide or euthanasia becomes legal, physicians and hospice programs can and, I believe, must allow patients or their families to contact licensed providers of those services and should not obstruct a qualified patient's receipt of such services. As physicians we can choose not to participate but we *must not* abandon our patients.

Even after the decision to pursue assistance in suicide, persons who are dying have need of care. At very least they have need for continued symptom management in the interval between the decision and demise. Thus the hallmarks of this suggested orientation toward the patient who qualifies for and seeks legally sanctioned assistance in suicide are noninterference, nonparticipation, and nonabandonment. Ethically and clinically, this stance is closely comparable to the accepted orientation of hospice providers toward a dying person who consciously refuses food and fluid.[69]

Within an ethical construct in which autonomy is balanced by social responsibility, another perspective on the meaning of a patient's suicide is revealed. Social responsibility is a reciprocal concept that conveys mutual obligation. Within a community ethic that values care for the infirm, elderly, and dying, each person can be seen as retaining rudimentary responsibilities even as they die: to allow oneself to be cared for, to express one's needs and, perhaps, to tell one's story. The choice of suicide represents a clear statement by the patient that care has nothing left to offer; it is a rejection of care. In asserting his or her autonomous right to refuse care, the patient choosing suicide constricts the contract of social responsibility.

While nonabandonment is asserted as a key feature of a caring orientation toward the dying patient, continued involvement might appear inconsistent with recognition that the persistent demand for assistance in suicide is a rejection of care. The construct of community and clinical ethics presented suggest that clinicians must remain involved and continue to offer whatever components of care the patient will accept. To withdraw care would reinforce people's perception that their life and personhood has no value, that they are hopeless, worthless, and entirely burdensome. By remaining involved, clinicians can demonstrate on both a professional and personal level that they do *care.* A founder of the modern hospice movement, Dr. Cicely Saunders, defined a core principle of palliative care: "You matter because you are you. You matter to the last moment of your life, and we will do all we can not only to help you die peacefully, but also to live until you die."[70] In its ethics and practice, medicine would do well to reflect on those words.

Rejection of assisted suicide by the medical profession must not become an endorsement of the tragic status quo. By acknowledging the fact of life-long human mutuality and the full range of human experience at life's end, medicine can contribute to maturing the culture with regard to dying. Building upon the best of hospice care, the profession is challenged to exert strong leadership in setting and achieving high standards for end-of-life care. If this challenge is met, within a single generation dying can cease being thought of as a time of agony and despair. Gradually, the experience of dying can come to be understood as a part of full and healthy living, as a time of caring, and as a time of remarkable opportunity for persons, families, and communities.

NOTES

1. K. Covinsky, L. Goldman, E. Cook, et al., "The Impact of Serious Illness on Patients' Families," *JAMA* 272 (December 21, 1994): 1839–44.

2. Bruce Jennings and M. J. Hanson, "Commodity or Public Work? Two Perspectives on Health Care," *Bioethics Forum* (Fall 1995): 3–11.

3. Michael D. Bayles, "The Professions," *Professional Ethics* (Belmont, Calif.: Wadsworth, 1981), pp. 7–11.

4. *Oxford English Dictionary,* 2d ed., vol. 12 (1989), pp. 572–73.

5. E. C. Hughes, "Professions," *Daedalus* 92 (Fall 1963): 655–68.

6. Sidney H. Wanzer et al., "The Physician's Responsibility toward Hopelessly Ill Patients," *New England Journal of Medicine* 310 (1984): 955–59.

7. J. E. Ruark and T. A. Raffin, "Initiating and Withdrawing Life Support," *New England Journal of Medicine* 318 (1988): 25–30.

8. President's Commission for the Study of Ethical Problems in Medicine, *Making Health Care Decisions* (Washington, D.C.: U.S. Government Printing Office, 1982), pp. 1–12 and 493–545.

9. The Hastings Center, a Report by. *Guidelines on the Termination of Life-Sustaining Treatment and the Care of the Dying* (Bloomington: Indiana University Press, 1987).

10. *In re: Bartling (1984),* 163 Cal. App. 3d 186:220–27.

11. *Bouvia v. Superior Court (Glenchur),* 179 Cal. App. 3d 1127, 225 Cal. Rptr. 297 (Ct. App. 1986).

12. *Right-To-Die Law Digest,* Right-To-Die Case & Statutory Citations, State-By-State Listing (New York: Choice In Dying, Inc., March 1994).

13. J. W. Ross, *Handbook for Hospital Ethics Committees,* American Hospital Association, 1986.

14. AMA Council on Ethical and Judicial Affairs, "Guidelines for the Appropriate Use of Do-Not-Resuscitate Orders," *JAMA* 265 (April 10, 1991): 1868–71.

15. F. G. Miller and Howard Brody, "Professional Integrity and Physician-Assisted Death," *Hastings Center Report,* May–June 1995, pp. 8–17.

16. Timothy E. Quill, Christine K. Cassel, and D. E. Meier, "Care of the Hopelessly Ill: Proposed Clinical Criteria for Physician-Assisted Suicide," *New England Journal of Medicine* 327 (1992): 1380–84.

17. Christine Cassel and D. Meier, "Morals and Moralism in the Debate over Euthanasia and Assisted Suicide," *New England Journal of Medicine* 323 (1990): 750–52.

18. S. H. Wanzer, D. D. Federrman, R. E. Cranford, et al., "The Physician's Responsibility toward Hopelessly Ill Patients: A Second Look," *New England Journal of Medicine* 320 (1989): 844–49.

19. S. H. Wanzer, "Euthanasia: The Argument in Favor, from the Euthanasia Debate, Point and Counterpoint," *Clinical Report on Aging,* vol. 2 (American Geriatrics Society, 1988).

20. S. Guisinger and S. J. Blatt, "Individuality and Relatedness—Evolution of a Fundamental Dialectic," *American Psychologist* 49 (February 1994): 104–11.

21. J. Bowlby, "Developmental Psychiatry Comes of Age," *American Journal of Psychiatry* 145 (January 1988): 1–10.

22. M. L. Hoffman, "Is Altruism Part of Human Nature?" *Journal of Personality and Social Psychology* 40 (1981): 1121–37.

23. Erik H. Erikson, *The Life Cycle Completed, a Review* (New York: Norton, 1982).

24. Harold Y. Vanderpool, "The Ethics of Terminal Care," *JAMA* 238 (February 27, 1978): 850–52.

25. Dan W. Brock and N. Daniels, "Ethical Foundations of the Clinton Administration's Proposed Health Care System," *JAMA* 271 (April 20, 1994): 1189–96.

26. *Oxford English Dictionary,* 2d ed., vol. 12 (1989), p. 894.

27. A. Jacox, D. B. Carr, and R. Payne, "Management of Cancer Pain," *Clinical Practice Guideline,* no. 9, Agency for Health Care Policy and Research, Rockville, M.D. (AHCPR publication no. 94-0592, 1994).

28. Quill, Cassel, and Meier, "Care of the Hopelessly Ill."

29. *Proactive Responses to the Euthanasia/Assisted Suicide Debate,* the National Hospice Organization, 1995 (in press).

30. R. D. Truog, C. B. Berde, H. E. Mitchell, and C. Grier, "Barbiturates in the Care of the Terminally Ill," *New England Journal of Medicine* 327 (1992): 1678–81.

31. W. R. Greene and W. H. Davis, "Titrated Intravenous Barbiturates in the Control of Symptoms in Patients With Terminal Cancer," *Southern Medical Journal* 84 (March 1991): 332–37.

32. Ira R. Byock, "Consciously Walking the Fine Line: Thoughts on a Hospice Response to Assisted Suicide and Euthanasia," *Journal of Palliative Care* 9 (1993): 25–28.

33. N. I. Cherny and R. K. Portenoy, "Sedation in the Management of Refractory Symptoms: Guidelines for Evaluation and Treatment," *Journal of Palliative Care* 10 (1994): 31–38.

34. B. M. Mount and P. Hamilton, "When Palliative Care Fails to Control Suffering," *Journal of Palliative Care* 10 (1994): 24–26.

35. H. Hendin, "Selling Death and Dignity," *Hastings Center Report*, May–June 1995, pp. 19–23.

36. Steven Miles, "Physician-Assisted Suicide and the Profession's Gyrocompass," *Hastings Center Report*, May–June 1995, pp. 17–19.

37. R. F. W. Diekstra, "Assisted Suicide and Euthanasia: Experiences from the Netherlands," *Annals of Internal Medicine* 25 (1993): 5–9.

38. *Compassion in Dying, Inc., et al. v. State of Washington*, Ninth Circuit U.S. Court of Appeals Case No. 94-35534.

39. Tom L. Beauchamp and J. F. Childress, *Principles of Biomedical Ethics*, 3d ed. (Oxford: Oxford University Press, 1979).

40. Timothy E. Quill, "Death and Dignity: A Case of Individualized Decision Making," *New England Journal of Medicine* 324 (1991): 691–94.

41. Howard Brody, "Assisted Death—A Compassionate Response to a Medical Failure," *New England Journal of Medicine* 327 (1992): 1384–88.

42. Ira R. Byock, "The Euthanasia/Assisted Suicide Debate Matures," *American Journal of Hospice and Palliative Care* 10 (March–April 1993): 11.

43. Terry Tempest Williams, *Refuge* (New York: Pantheon Books, 1991).

44. Ken Wilber, *Grace and Grit: Spirituality and Healing in the Life and Death of Treya Killam Wilber* (Boston: Shambhala, 1991).

45. Ronald Bergen, *Anthony Perkins: A Haunted Life* (London: Little, Brown, 1995).

46. Ira R. Byock, "When Suffering Persists . . . ," *Journal of Palliative Care* 10 (1994): 8–13.

47. M. Kearney, "Palliative Medicine—Just Another Specialty?" *Palliative Medicine* 6 (1992): 39–46.

48. P. Kelley and M. Callanan, *Final Gifts* (New York: Poseidon Press, 1992).

49. C. Saunders, *St. Christopher's in Celebration* (London: Hodder & Stoughton, 1988).

50. E. Kubler-Ross, *On Death and Dying* (New York: Macmillan, 1969).

51. C. Goethe, personal communication.

52. E. J. Cassell, "The Nature of Suffering and the Goals of Medicine," *New England Journal of Medicine* 306 (1982): 639–45.

53. Victor E. Frankl, *Man's Search for Meaning* (New York: Washington Square Press, 1984).

54. Ira R. Byock, "The Nature of Suffering and the Nature of Opportunity at the End of Life," *Clinics in Geriatric Medicine* 12, no. 2 (May 1996): 237–51.

55. C. F. Gomez, *Regulating Death: Euthanasia and the Case of the Netherlands* (New York: Macmillan, 1991).

56. H. Hendin, "Assisted Suicide, Euthanasia, and Suicide Prevention: The Implications of the Dutch Experience," *Suicide and Life-Threatening Behavior* 25 (1995): 193–204.

57. L. Pijnenborg, P. J. Van der Maas, et al., "Life-Terminating Acts without Explicit Request of Patient," *Lancet* 341 (May 8, 1993): 1196–99.

58. J. J. M. Van Delden, L. Pijnenborg, and P. J. Van der Maas, "The Remmelink Study Two Years Later," *Hastings Center Report,* November–December 1993, pp. 24–27.

59. G. Kaufmann, "State v. Chabot: A Euthanasia Case from the Netherlands," *Ohio Northern University Law Review* 20, no. 3 (1994).

60. Laurie Zoloth-Dorfman, "Euthanasia: A Religious Response," presentation at the National Hospice Organization's First National Conference on Spiritual, Bereavement, and Psychosocial Aspects of Hospice Care, San Francisco, August 17, 1995.

61. René Spitz, "Hospitalism: An Inquiry into the Genesis of Psychiatric Conditions in Early Childhood," *Psychoanalytic Study of the Child* 1 (1946): 53–74.

62. Anna Mae Halgrim Seaver, "My World Now," *Newsweek,* June 27, 1994, p. 11.

63. L. Close, C. L. Estes, K. W. Linkins, et al., "A Political Economy Perspective on Frontline Workers in Long-Term Care," *Generations* 18 (1994): 23–27.

64. W. H. Crown, "A National Profile of Homecare, Nursing Home, and Hospital Aides," *Generations* 18 (1994): 29–33.

65. *The National Hospice Organization Reports: 1994–1995 Hospice Statistics (as of July 1995),* National Hospice Organization, 1995.

66. C. Holden, S. Paquette, and Ira R. Byock, "Where and When Physician-Assisted Suicide Might Be Legalized: The Changing Reality for Hospice," panel presentation at the National Hospice Organization's 17th Annual Symposium and Exposition, Phoenix, November 6, 1995.

67. C. S. Campbell, J. Hare, and P. Matthews, "Conflicts of Conscience, Hospice and Assisted Suicide," *Hastings Center Report,* May–June 1995, pp. 36–43.

68. Ira R. Byock, "Opportunities for Growth at the End of Life," presentation at Oregon State Hospice, Salishan, April 21, 1995.

69. Ira R. Byock, "Patient Refusal of Nutrition and Hydration: Walking the Ever-Finer Line," *American Journal of Hospice and Palliative Care* (March–April 1995): 8–13.

70. S. Stoddard, *The Hospice Movement* (New York: Vintage, 1978), p. 120.

6

ASSISTING IN PATIENT SUICIDES *IS* AN ACCEPTABLE PRACTICE FOR PHYSICIANS

Howard Brody, M.D., Ph.D.

Some discussions in medical ethics suffer from a gap between ethical theory and the realities of clinical practice. For example, there have for many years been ethical pronouncements that physicians ought to tell the cancer patient the truth about her diagnosis; but only much more recently has there appeared sensitive, sensible advice to practitioners about exactly *how* to disclose a dire diagnosis in such a way as to minimize harm while showing maximal respect for the patient's values and preferences.[1-2] Similarly, for all the ethical injunctions on the appropriateness of withholding or withdrawing life-sustaining medical therapy at the request of a patient or surrogate, precious little has been written about the best way clinically to manage such a withdrawal—and the process turns out to be more complex and nuanced than many would have thought.[3]

It may be that the apparently interminable and intractable debate over the ethics of physician-assisted suicide (PAS) has similarly suffered from its abstract nature and our inability to picture all the details of how the practice of PAS might be incorporated into clinical practice. In the U.S., two physicians have come forward with detailed descriptions of their activities and with detailed prescriptions for the clinical use of PAS—and one of them has been judged by most medical observers to be a flawed "role model."[4-5] The vast majority of the unknown number of U.S. practitioners who have assisted or offered to assist in patients' suicides have done so outside the glare of publicity and without reporting their activities to peers.

It might be that actual data of practical clinical experience would do nothing to resolve the debate—just as the opposing sides in the euthanasia debate show themselves fully capable of looking at precisely the same data on practices in the Netherlands and reaching diametrically opposed conclusions. But it might also be the case that some practical experience would allow us to judge which of the ethical arguments are substantial and which are purely speculative and inconsequential. In the fall of 1994, it appeared that we would see an experiment of this sort occurring in Oregon; but as of now, that state's law remains mired in the courts with no foreseeable hope of implementation, especially since the recent decision by the Ninth Circuit Court of Appeals (*Compassion in Dying v. State of Washington*) has been appealed to the U.S. Supreme Court.

Lacking this sort of real-world laboratory, what are we to make of the ethical arguments regarding physicians' involvement in their patients' suicides? Bearing in mind Harris's law, which states that any philosophy which can be expressed in a nutshell probably belongs there, we can summarize the major arguments for and against physician involvement. The arguments in favor are, I believe, relatively straightforward:

1. Physicians have a moral obligation to use medical means to relieve their patients' suffering. In most cases, excellent palliative care will relieve suffering without hastening death. In a few cases, prolonged life will be incompatible with relief of suffering; and in those few cases physicians might have to use the medical means at their disposal to shorten life directly.

2. Physicians also have a moral obligation to respect the autonomous choices of their patients. Some few patients, even when provided with excellent palliative care, will autonomously select PAS as their preferred option. Physicians should honor that request in those cases.

3. While abuses of PAS can readily be envisioned and indeed would be likely to occur in at least a few cases if we were to legalize PAS, appropriate safeguards can provide adequate protection against abuse for the vast majority of cases.[6] Physicians are often best placed to apply and implement those safeguards.

4. A physician caring for a terminally ill patient ought to be able to promise the patient that she will be there by the patient's side until the end, no matter what twists the road may take along the way. Since some few patients will experience unbearable suffering and will autonomously request PAS, refusal to even consider the PAS option amounts to a form of patient abandonment.

5. Some physicians, perhaps even a majority, will legitimately refuse to become involved in PAS due to personal moral or religious views.

But the personal morality of these individual physicians must not be confused with the obligations of the profession as a whole. A system which would allow PAS by those physicians who are willing to perform it and would allow those opposed to refuse to participate will promote the values of relief of suffering and respect for patient choice without compromising the moral integrity of any physician.[7]

6. The historical injunction against prescribing deadly drugs must be tempered by an appreciation of the vastly different circumstances of death in many modern patients. Medical technology usually keeps patients alive through the early stages of serious disease, precisely when many patients in earlier times died relatively quickly. Medicine thus allows patients today to enter the chronic and terminal phases of illnesses, during which suffering and loss of useful function may be extensively protracted well before death occurs. Medicine is thus indirectly responsible for the predicament of many suffering, terminally or chronically ill patients; it cannot turn its back upon them when they request relief of their suffering even at the price of shortening life.[8]

While these arguments seem to make a strong case for physician approval of and involvement in PAS, the opposing arguments are also quite weighty:

1. Opposition to PAS is not merely a matter of personal moral choice. Any proper understanding of *professional* integrity would require physicians to see that they can never be true to their role as healers while directly causing or participating in the patient's death.[9]

2. Safeguards are illusory. As soon as PAS becomes a routine practice, abuses are bound to occur, probably in considerable numbers. To think that safeguards would work is to take a highly idealized view of medical practice in the U.S.; the realities of practice (especially among the poor and among stigmatized groups such as persons with disabilities, HIV positive patients, etc.) are far different.[10]

3. While defenders of PAS assume that a reasonable system of hospice and palliative care options is in place and available, this is not so; and endorsement of PAS may further delay the day when our health system makes a true commitment to access to good palliative care.

4. Perhaps as a matter of social policy, a small number of patients should be allowed to choose suicide in the face of advanced medical illness; and others should be allowed to assist them. But we should be extremely wary of *physicians* being placed in the role of the helpers. Just as inappropriate "medicalization" has made other social problems worse instead of better, we should be wary of the medicalization of terminal suffering and the assumption that physicians and drugs provide the proper answer to the human anguish of facing terminal

illness and death. And we should be wary of this even if it were to develop that PAS does not constitute a violation of the physician's professional integrity.[11]

5. Assisting a patient's suicide is, on its face, admission of incompetence. Proper care of dying patients, with close attention to their physical, emotional, and spiritual needs, will almost always reveal ways to relieve suffering and so to dissuade the patient from suicide. To assist the patient's suicide is to take the easy way out and to fail to put enough time and energy into the case to be able to render truly competent terminal care.[12]

I wish to offer a cautious endorsement of PAS as a clinical option for U.S. physicians. But I will arrive there by a somewhat circuitous route. It is hard to give full attention to the "pro" arguments when the opposing arguments appear to demand considerable respect and allegiance. It will therefore be more to the point to proceed by addressing the opposing arguments. Only if they can be shown to be quite a bit weaker than they first appear will it be worthwhile even to consider supporting PAS.

Professional Integrity

This objection to physician involvement in assisted suicide has somewhat greater implications for medical practice than for public policy. If society decides that the benefits of assisted suicide are substantial and the risks are manageable, then rational policy would require legalizing the practice with appropriate safeguards. But, presumably, society would allow individuals to opt in or out of the role of assisting and would require no one to assist a suicide if that act violated conscience. Physicians might then, as a group, argue that their professional integrity would be violated by participation in this policy and inform society that some other group would have to be identified for this role. Nurses, pharmacists, and other health professionals might make analogous claims.

If society viewed the involvement of physicians as highly desirable in order to achieve the benefits and safeguard against abuse, it could of course mandate physician participation as a condition of licensure. But no proposal this draconian has yet been put forth.

An argument from professional integrity may be easily misunderstood, in part because the concept is seldom appealed to today in most debates about medical ethics. First, it may be helpful to distinguish between personal and professional integrity. On this model, physicians arrive at their medical training with some existing values drawn from their religious and philosophical viewpoints and commitments and then subscribe to some additional values as a consequence of *professing* medicine as a calling or career. In a pluralistic society, we would not expect all physicians to bring the same set of personal moral values into medical practice. But, assuming that physicians were to engage in extended and searching dialogue about their role and the nature of their practice, we might imagine them someday reaching reasonable consensus about the core moral commitments that make up their *professional* identity.

For example, when observers of medicine today attack physicians who seem totally dedicated to making money and correspondingly unmindful of the real needs and interests of their patients, it seems implausible to imagine that whether one is a caring professional or purely profit-oriented could legitimately vary according to one's personal religious views, as would be the case in whether a physician will or will not perform sterilizations. Instead the charge seems to be that physicians *ought to have* adopted a moral stance which places profit-making in lower priority than serving one's patients, as a consequence of entering the profession and undergoing professional education.

Thus we should understand the professional integrity argument to mean not that some physicians will as a personal matter have religious or philosophical objections to assisting a patient's suicide. Instead it is asserted that one cannot be a physician of integrity and assist a suicide in one's professional role, even if one's personal philosophy strongly favors the suicide option in terminal illness. (Analogously, some medical codes of ethics would submit today that a physician, *as a private citizen,* might favor capital punishment and vote to extend its practice; but the ethical physician cannot *as a physician* participate in state executions by assisting in the injection of lethal drugs.)[13]

A second misunderstanding arises from the comment above about "extended and searching dialogue." It might be the case that physicians today are quite divided about the ethics of PAS and that strong advocates can be found on both sides of the issue. That may merely mean, however, that the issue is a complex and divisive one and that the profession has not yet had sufficient time to work through its implications carefully. One may assert that in the future, the vast majority of well-intentioned physicians will come to see that the practice violates professional integrity. Thus an argument from professional integrity is not vitiated by current lack of consensus.

Finally, the remark about "extended and searching dialogue" might give rise to a different objection. Some would say that one hardly needs extended investigation to conclude that PAS violates professional integrity; one simply has to read the Hippocratic Oath, and there it is, plain as day. But I do not wish to defend a view of professional integrity which states that one's moral obligations can simply be read off a list which has been passed down through the centuries. I take it that traditional moral commitments must always be reinterpreted and reexamined as the social context and environment changes. Medicine can best be viewed as a *responsive tradition,* in which some of its ethics at any given time is derived from the historical continuity of the practice, while some is derived from a responsiveness to current social needs and concerns.[14] These two factors are always in tension; one can lose one's professional integrity either by being too hidebound or too faddish. So I take the question of whether the traditional prohibition of "deadly drugs" should preclude PAS in today's world as one requiring thoughtful investigation and discussion, not one susceptible to a pat answer.

With this understanding of what professional integrity is and how one may come to understand it, F. G. Miller and I have summarized elsewhere both an account of the elements of professional integrity and arguments as to why some cases of PAS would not violate professional integrity.[7] Briefly, we argue that the proper goals which define medical practice include healing, preventing illness, and helping the dying patient to achieve a peaceful and dignified death. We also suggest that the physician of integrity pursues those goals by medically approved means—she does not practice incompetent medicine, cause harm disproportionate to benefit, fraudulently misrepresent medical knowledge, or abandon the vital interests of her patients.

At first glance, PAS, while perhaps defensible as promoting the goal of achieving a peaceful and dignified death, would seem to violate many if not all of the means requirements. Suicide assistance might be incompetent medicine if palliative care could better relieve suffering while prolonging life; the harm of death might seem disproportionate to any benefit of relieving suffering; and an early death might appear to violate rather than serve any conceivable patient interests. Miller and I claim, however, that if suicide assistance could be restricted to the narrow class of patients who *both* autonomously request this help *and* have demonstrated that their suffering cannot be relieved by any other practicable medical means, then no violation of physician integrity occurs. Specifically, we argue that the patient and not the physician should be the one to determine in such a setting when an earlier death represents a lesser harm, and a better way of serving the patient's own interests, than would prolonged life with protracted suffering.

It is also worth noting that this proposed model of physician integrity does not create a moral *right* to suicide assistance on the part of the patient and thus falls short of the goals of some libertarians and strong advocates for patient autonomy. The model holds that PAS *would,* in a great number of cases, be contrary to the physician's integrity; and so physicians should never be obligated to provide it "on demand" but only after very detailed and searching study of a particular case—which would almost always entail a serious trial of other palliative care efforts first. A patient's "right" to assistance might undermine this requirement of physician integrity. Physicians must retain discretion in doubtful cases and sometimes refuse to assist a patient, even when the physician might agree that if he were in the patient's shoes, suicide might be a rational option.

I take the model of physician integrity outlined briefly here to establish at least a prima facie case for PAS being within the bounds of integrity in some selected cases. No doubt opponents of PAS could find fault with various aspects, either of the model itself, or of our suggested application. But until such an alternative model or application has been elaborated in some detail, it will not do to invoke "physician integrity" as a sort of mantra, as if the words themselves were sufficient to demonstrate that physicians ought not morally to assist their patients' suicides.

Adequacy of Safeguards

The account just given of professional integrity relies very heavily on clinical safeguards, to assure that the patient's choice of suicide is voluntary and consistent over time, and that reasonable palliative care alternatives have been tried and have failed. If these safeguards cannot be satisfied in clinical practice, then it follows generally that physicians should not assist in suicide.

The New York Task Force on Life and the Law[10] concluded a detailed study by rejecting PAS on these grounds. They suggested that so far, all proposals for the adequacy of safeguards presuppose a state of medical practice more idealized than what is widely available in the U.S. Specifically, ensuring voluntary and consistent patient requests for suicide would often require consultation with a psychiatrist who is skilled in distinguishing between a treatable depression and the effects of aging or chronic illness.[15] Ensuring an adequate trial of palliative care would generally require a skilled hospice specialist or team, capable of determining, for instance, whether the failure to get adequate relief from a certain medication arose from the incorrigibility of the symptom or from the use of too low a dose or the wrong route of administration of the medication. But physicians with these skills are all too often not available even to well-off Americans with excellent health insurance. The situation is even less favorable for needier patients and those lacking third-party coverage.

These observations are extremely important; and the final conclusion might be that assisted suicide is morally acceptable in principle but should never be practically implemented in the U.S. until there have been major reforms in access to quality health care for all citizens, a point to which I shall return in the conclusion.

Nonetheless, a possible argument for the cautious legalization of PAS in selected localities today might rely upon a regulatory system which makes skilled clinical consultation a precondition for legalized suicide assistance. One such proposal envisions teams of palliative care consultants which would include both hospice specialists and psychiatrists skilled in diagnosing depression among the terminally and chronically ill.[16] A patient's personal physician could legally assist a patient's suicide but only after consultation with this team and the agreement of the team that (1) the patient was rationally and voluntarily requesting suicide and (2) the patient was unlikely to get any significant relief of suffering from further palliative care measures. The clinical focus of this process helps to ensure that a personal physician seeking legal approval to assist a suicide gets much more than a bureaucratic rubber stamp. She would get expert clinical consultation; and in many if not most cases the result of the consultation would probably be some recommendations for palliation which had not yet been tried.[17]

Critics of this proposal have suggested that this would prove yet another charade. Today, it appears, those physicians who assist patients' suicides do so secretly, outside the law. If it were difficult or time-consuming to consult with this palliative team, or indeed if the team was likely to give a response which was not to the patient's liking, then there is every reason to believe that physicians would simply bypass the team and continue to operate in secret, without effective safeguards. Moreover, as hospice physicians tend as a group to be opposed to assisted suicide, it might well be the case that those with the needed skills would simply refuse to serve on such teams.[18]

Admittedly, if physicians with the requisite skills refused to supervise the safeguards, no system of professional safeguards could be implemented. I have argued above that at least physicians refusing to serve in this capacity could *not* cite professional integrity as the reason for their refusal.

The objection from the currently illicit nature of PAS is more revealing. It shows that opponents of legalizing PAS sometimes wish to have it both ways. On the one hand, they tend to argue against legalization as if the current rate of suicide assistance in the U.S. is zero. That means that if the practice is legalized and some abuses occur, then the fault for the inappropriate deaths can be laid at the doorstep of the advocates for legalization. On the other hand, when it suits their purpose, they can admit that today, cases of assisted suicide (we have no good statistics how many, but the number is likely not negligible) occur outside the scrutiny of society and the law. The opponents of PAS are silent on the question of how many of those cases would count as abuses of the proposed safeguards and whether the extralegal, underground nature of the practice today might not produce at least as many if not more abuses than would legal supervision.

Moreover, opinion polls suggest that fewer physicians would oppose the practice of suicide assistance if it were legalized.[19-21] That seems to suggest that there is some likelihood that physicians would make use of consultant teams if this were the approved legal (and professional) mechanism. If the teams were clinically helpful, that would probably increase compliance further.

Assisted Suicide and Hospice

The previous section has addressed both the need for adequate palliative care as one of the safeguards that would make PAS acceptable; and also the fact that many within the hospice and palliative care communities have been most vocal in opposing PAS. This opposition arises in part from a feeling that support for PAS is a rejection of palliative care and partly from the fear that future support of suicide assistance as a legal option would necessarily undermine financial and political support for the expansion of hospice.[22-23]

It is true that hospice and palliative care have for too long been the poor stepchildren of U.S. medicine, underfunded and underappreciated. This seems to be changing, even if more slowly than we would wish, as the profession wakes up to its failures in the management of pain and other symptoms in terminal illness.[24-25]

The possible future scenario which worries hospice supporters is that with PAS available as a quick and cheap way to deal with terminal suffering, third parties will lack the will to pay for the sometimes expensive and protracted care that would constitute excellent symptom palliation and emotional support. The "option" of assisted suicide would soon, through the back door, become a financial requirement.

Another possible scenario, however, is the establishment of the palliative care team as the society's and the profession's preferred regulatory device to ensure that suicide assistance is restricted to those patients who are the morally appropriate candidates. That scenario would end up strengthening hospice, since almost all patients would have to undergo a trial of hospice care before being viewed as potential candidates for suicide assistance and the vast majority, one hopes, would end up being so satisfied with the palliative approach that they would soon withdraw the request for suicide. If there would be, under that scenario, the political will to legalize PAS, there ought to be the will also to ensure better funding for hospice programs, at least to the extent required to show that no one is seeking assisted suicide because hospice is not available. Moreover, those who now oppose legalizing PAS would presumably have a very strong motive to monitor the practice closely and to raise considerable protest as soon as anyone is assisted in suicide who would appear to have been a good candidate for palliative care instead. In this way political opponents of PAS could end up supporting the expansion of hospice to a much greater degree than is now the case.

Of the two scenarios, it seems that the second is at least as plausible as the first; and so the policy fears of some in the hospice community seem a weak reason to oppose a policy of legal PAS.

Medicalization

In the 1960s, some social critics began to attend seriously to the abuses of power that occur when the medical profession usurps matters which had previously been left to the discretion of individuals or of other social institutions.[26–27] The "medicalization" problem is one which deserves to be taken seriously, no less because its effects are often subtle and gradual.

Steven Miles, in a recent commentary, has applied this line of criticism to PAS.[11] He suggests that one might envision a social practice of suicide assistance in those instances previously alluded to—a voluntary, rational choice in the face of otherwise unrelieved suffering. A patient might rationally choose the suicide option in that limited set of cases. Since flawed execution might cause even further suffering or a physical disability (such as an inability to swallow pills) might interfere with the most painless suicide plan, both the patient and her loved ones might want the suicide to be assisted by others. But the responsibility for assisting would logically lie with the circle of close, intimate family and friends. These are the people that most would want to have present around the bedside during one's last moments; and these are the people, in most cases, who could best determine whether the request was apparently rational and in character or was somehow being coerced by circumstances.

In this ideal model of suicide assistance, the role of the physician would be relegated to confirming the diagnosis and the possible treatment options and to making the materials needed for a painless death available for the family's use with appropriate instructions. The need for legal oversight could be met by having the patient and family go before a judge and obtain a court order permitting the suicide assistance. But *physician*-assisted suicide seems on this view to be an odd way of designing the social practice. Why place the physician in charge? Are we assuming it to be a natural law rather than an artificial restriction that certain drugs and equipment are available only on a physician's prescription? Or are we making the illicit assumption that a morally dubious practice is somehow being cleansed simply because a white coat is on the scene?

Suicide assistance by intimate associates rather than by physicians also would have the advantage of negating most concerns over integrity. If it turned out on careful analysis that professional integrity is incompatible with direct suicide assistance, then this social policy allows physicians to remain true to their assigned role even while patients retain the assisted suicide option. And even if a physician's conscientious refusal to assist a suicide is a matter of purely personal and not professional integrity, then still this policy will minimize the number of physicians facing such conflicts of conscience.

The medicalization criticism, then, forces us to question an assumption which is all too often taken for granted in this debate—that if assisted suicide of any sort is to be legalized, it ought to be, and will be, PAS. Can any arguments in favor of physician participation then be provided, once we have eliminated unwarranted assumptions and examined the alternative models? Why might persons *want* their physicians to be involved in this practice—once we have looked at the relationship between medicine and society in the cold light of day, and have refused to attribute to physicians any expertise which they do not, or ought not, possess?

In some cases, of course, patients will want their physicians to assist because the physician has become over the years an intimate family friend. But that is a special case and falls under the model just delineated; it is the friendship and not the physicianship that gives the doctor a justified role in the end-of-life plan.

I believe that the best answer to the "medicalization" challenge is that rational people, who might be contemplating the option of assisted suicide, would especially want two things. First, they would want to be sure that they were not choosing an early death out of a medical failure to manage their symptoms adequately. Second, if they ended up choosing death, they would want to be sure that the means they selected actually work—specifically, that they are not left alive but lingering on with even worse suffering than before. Moreover, rational people would want their families and friends to be comfortable on both points, and not to feel an undue weight of responsibility for having to assure these things by themselves.

The clinical nuances of palliative care dictate that no specialist can simply interview a patient or review a chart, determine what course of palliative care would be best, estimate its likelihood of success, then walk away. The physician or caregiver has to work closely in tandem with the patient and family over time to see whether doses need to be adjusted, whether anticipated side effects of one drug can be treated effectively with a second drug, and whether the approach needs to be changed in a week or a month as the patient's underlying disease advances and enters a new phase. This clinical fact seems to pose a stark choice—either the physician becomes very closely involved, to the point where she becomes in effect a member of the patient's intimate circle during the terminal phase of illness, or else the patient is effectively denied whatever comfort and caring a hospice approach might offer. Admittedly, given the team organization of the ideal hospice program, the caregiver who assumes this role might well be a nurse rather than a physician; but in principle the question about lay versus professional domination of the life of the dying patient remains the same in either case.

Moreover, the few case studies we have available from publicized assisted suicides in the U.S. all suggest that the patient and family may come to depend very heavily upon the physician's input to ensure that the method of suicide assistance chosen will actually work and will produce a reasonably quick, dignified, and painless death. Rightly or wrongly, lay people assume that physicians know about these matters; and the experience in the Netherlands suggests further that physicians could, if they wished, come very quickly and easily to know as much about these matters as is needed. (Whatever other charges opponents of euthanasia lay against the Dutch medical profession, making botched attempts at euthanasia or assisted suicide is not one of them.) Physicians know full well that the "expertise" required to effectuate death by an overdose of medication is well within the ability of any intelligent layperson to grasp. But those physicians may seriously underestimate the emotional vulnerability of patients and especially family members during the critical time when these tasks must be carried out. A professional who is used to being at the bedside of critically ill and dying patients is much less likely than a family member to be overwhelmed by a sudden, incapacitating panic: *wait a minute, it's no longer just something we have talked about ... I am really going ahead and doing this . . . I have never done such a thing before in my life . . . what if something goes wrong?*

Hospice workers are fully aware of the "911 reflex," when families who have been extensively counseled about what the patient's death at home will be like and have also been counseled carefully that calling for emergency medical assistance would probably result in the patient receiving undesired interventions and being transferred to the hospital at a time when this is least suitable, still panic and call 911 when the patient seems to be near death. Even if the patient's and family's desire, in asking the physician to be a part of the supervision of the suicide assistance, is merely to be sure that one responsible person at the scene is a professional who can be depended upon *not to panic,* then the desire is still fully understandable and worthy of sympathetic support.

An obvious rebuttal, harking back to a previous point of contention, is that this defense of physician involvement assumes an ideal form of medical practice. Physicians, after all, can botch assisting a death, just as they can botch any other procedure. Physicians may be uninformed about palliative care techniques and may be neglectful and unavailable just when the dying patient needs the most careful attention. But those factors do not argue against the legitimacy of a patient's request that the *physician,* and not only the family, assist with the suicide. Where medical practice is flawed, and if the procedure is allowable on other grounds, then the solution is improved practice and not refusing to allow the procedure. A recent, highly publicized case in which a surgeon cut off the wrong leg led to legitimate calls for a review of how medicine works to prevent errors, but not for outlawing surgical amputation.

Incompetence

The final objection, that assisting a suicide is de facto admission of clinical incompetence, has already been addressed in passing in the preceding discussion. That this is true in *some* cases can hardly be doubted, and that the general standard of palliative competency in the U.S. medical profession is abysmally deficient has been too clearly documented to be worthy of any further debate. That it is true in *all* cases would require the unsupported and probably unsupportable assertion that palliative care technologies, unlike any other known medical technology, work 100 percent of the time. This objection boils down in the end to the question of whether the practice of assisted suicide can be effectively regulated so as to assure that it is used only as a last resort, a point which is properly controversial but which has already been discussed.

Conclusion

While I have tended to dismiss the argument from incompetence in the preceding section, the notion of incompetent practice actually helps to frame the debate over assisted suicide in an extremely helpful, if indirect, fashion. I have suggested elsewhere that the best way to look at assisted suicide is as a "compassionate response to a medical failure."[28] The death of a patient is not in itself a sign of medical failure, however much this irrational view may have been impressed upon U.S. physicians during their training (and as an outgrowth of malpractice fears). But a patient who is suffering so much that he freely and "rationally" requests death when so many means to palliate suffering are available to caregivers *is* evidence of medical failure.

Medical failure may arise out of incompetent practice or may arise from forces outside the control of even the best physician. Whether acquiescence in assisted suicide is a sign of incompetence, therefore, hinges upon whether the physician knew about the potential for palliation and has tried all reasonable medical approaches, including appropriate nursing and psychological and spiritual support.

Imagine an analogous case: it is agreed that competent medical management of a certain disease involves prompt surgery. A physician is found to be managing a patient with this disease with a combination of drugs. That situation is prima facie evidence of incompetence. But the physician can rebut the charge of incompetence by showing that he had consulted with a very good surgeon, who explained the peculiar circumstances which made this particular patient not an acceptable surgical candidate.

Similarly, a physician who assists a suicide ought to be ready to respond to a professional accusation of incompetence, and the best way to do so is to have in place the regulatory system mentioned above— consultation with a team of skilled palliative care consultants. (*Knowing* that they will have to face an accusation of incompetence, I would argue, creates in physicians precisely the sense of trepidation which *ought* to accompany contemplating assisting a suicide.)

The debate over legalizing assisted suicide thus turns in large part on whether such a system of professional regulation and consultation could be put in place. Those who deny that it could, citing serious systemic inadequacies in the U.S. in its management of health care, have a number of strong arguments in their favor.

Some have argued that before we could permit assisted suicide, we would first have to ensure that all Americans had access to decent health care regardless of ability to pay; and next we would have to ensure that that package of "decent" health care included up-to-date, compassionate hospice management in all geographic locations. In some cases this argument is simply disingenuous, being based not merely on the notion that these things will never come to pass but indeed on the knowledge that the political forces that most strongly oppose assisted suicide are also working against accomplishing these more general goals.

I think it nonetheless wrong to dismiss such objections out of hand; and it may indeed be true that the realities of clinical practice across the U.S. today will simply not admit of the necessary safeguards that would make suicide assistance professionally prudent. I would like to see a trial of the practice carried out before I would conclude that this is the case. And if it is the case, it is hardly a cause for celebration, even among the foes of assisted suicide; it is rather a sad commentary on the present state of U.S. medical practice.

NOTES

1. R. Buckman, *How to Break Bad News: A Guide for Health Care Professionals* (Baltimore: Johns Hopkins University Press, 1992).

2. Timothy E. Quill and P. Townsend, "Bad News: Delivery, Dialogue, and Dilemmas," *Archives of Internal Medicine* 151 (1991): 463–68.

3. M. J. Edwards and S. Tolle, "Disconnecting a Ventilator at the Request of a Patient Who Knows He Will Then Die: The Doctor's Anguish," *Annals of Internal Medicine* 117 (1992): 254–56.

4. Jack Kevorkian, *Prescription: Medicide: The Goodness of Planned Death* (Buffalo: Prometheus Books, 1991).

5. Timothy E. Quill, "Death and Dignity: A Case of Individualized Decision Making," *New England Journal of Medicine* 324 (1991): 691–94.

6. M. Battin, "Voluntary Euthanasia and the Risks of Abuse: Can We Learn Anything from the Netherlands?" *Law, Medicine and Health Care* 20 (Spring–Summer 1992): 133–43.

7. F. G. Miller and Howard Brody, "Professional Integrity and Physician-Assisted Death," *Hastings Center Report* 25 (May–June 1995): 8–17.

8. G. I. Benrubi, "Euthanasia—The Need for Procedural Safeguards," *New England Journal of Medicine* 326 (1992): 197–99.

9. W. Gaylin, L. R. Kass, E. D. Pellegrino, et al., "Doctors Must Not Kill," *Journal of the American Medical Association* 259 (1988): 2139–40.

10. New York Task Force on Life and the Law, *When Death Is Sought: Assisted Suicide and Euthanasia in the Medical Context,* 1994.

11. Steven H. Miles, "Physician-Assisted Suicide and the Profession's Gyrocompass," *Hastings Center Report* 25 (May–June 1995): 17–19.

12. Working Party to Review the British Medical Association's Guidance on Euthanasia, *The Euthanasia Report* (London: British Medical Association, 1988).

13. Council on Ethical and Judicial Affairs, AMA, "Physician Participation in Capital Punishment," *Journal of the American Medical Association* 270 (1993): 365–68.

14. R. Vance, "Medicine as Dependent Tradition: Historical and Ethical Reflections," *Perspectives in Biology and Medicine* 28 (1985): 282–302.

15. Y. Conwell and E. D. Caine, "Rational Suicide and the Right to Die: Reality and Myth," *New England Journal of Medicine* 325 (1991): 1100–03.

16. F. G. Miller, Timothy E. Quill, Howard Brody, J. C. Fletcher, Larry O. Gostin, and D. Meier, "Regulating Physician-Assisted Death," *New England Journal of Medicine* 331 (1994): 119–23.

17. K. M. Foley, "The Relationship of Pain and Symptom Management to Patient Requests for Physician-Assisted Suicide," *Journal of Pain and Symptom Management* 6 (1991): 289–97.

18. Daniel Callahan, "Regulating Physician-Assisted Death," letter, *New England Journal of Medicine* 331 (1994): 1656.

19. J. S. Cohen, S. D. Fihn, E. J. Boyko, A. R. Jonsen, and R. W. Wood, "Attitudes toward Assisted Suicide and Euthanasia among Physicians in Washington State," *New England Journal of Medicine* 331 (1994): 89–94.

20. J. G. Bachman, D. J. Doukas, R. L. Lichtenstein, and K. H. Alcser, "Assisted Suicide and Euthanasia in Michigan," letter, *New England Journal of Medicine* 331 (1994): 812–13.

21. D. J. Doukas, D. Waterhouse, D. W. Gorenflo, and J. Seid, "Attitudes and Behaviors on Physician-Assisted Death: A Study of Michigan Oncologists," *Journal of Clinical Oncology* 13 (1995): 1055–61.

22. J. Teno and J. Lynn, "Voluntary Active Euthanasia: The Individual Case and Public Policy," *Journal of the American Geriatrics Society* 39 (1991): 827–30.

23. Ira R. Byock, "The Euthanasia/Assisted Suicide Debate Matures," *American Journal of Hospice and Palliative Care* (March–April 1993): 8–11.

24. C. S. Cleeland, R. Gonin, A. K. Hatfield, et al., "Pain and Its Treatment in Outpatients with Metastatic Cancer," *New England Journal of Medicine* 330 (1994): 592–96.

25. Management of Cancer Pain Guideline Panel, *Management of Cancer Pain (Clinical Practice Guideline no. 9)* (Rockville, MD: Agency for Health Care Policy and Research, 1994).

26. I. Illich, *Medical Nemesis: The Expropriation of Health* (New York: Pantheon, 1976).

27. Howard Brody, *The Healer's Power* (New Haven: Yale University Press, 1992), pp. 221–37.

28. Howard Brody, "Assisted Death—a Compassionate Response to a Medical Failure," *New England Journal of Medicine* 327 (1992): 1384–88.

Part IV

Potentially Vulnerable Patients

7

PHYSICIAN-ASSISTED DEATH IN THE CONTEXT OF DISABILITY

Kristi L. Kirschner, M.D., Carol J. Gill, Ph.D.,
and Christine K. Cassel, M.D.

David Rivlin sustained a spinal cord injury at the age of twenty in a surfing accident. He had quadriplegia but maintained partial use of his right arm, and lived in his own home with assistance. In 1986, fifteen years after his spinal cord injury, Rivlin underwent surgery to remove a spinal cord aneurysm that was causing progressive neurological deterioration. Postoperatively, he had full paralysis of his four limbs and required a ventilator due to diaphragmatic paralysis. In May 1989 Rivlin petitioned the court to allow a physician to sedate him and remove his ventilator. The court concurred with his request, citing the right of the competent patient to refuse medical treatment—even life-sustaining treatment. He died on July 20, 1989, with the assistance of a hospice physician.[1-4]

Refusal of Life-Sustaining Treatment

David Rivlin's case appears to exemplify a prototypical case of a competent patient's right to refuse life-sustaining treatment. Judge Benjamin Cardozo articulated the autonomy-based premise in 1914 in the Schloendorff decision: "every human being of adult years and sound mind has a right to determine what shall be done with his own body . . ."[5] The President's Commission studying medical ethics in 1983 reiterated the principle that competent adults' rights extend to the right to refuse life-sustaining treatment if they so chose.[6] Arguments equating withdrawal of life-sustaining treatment with active euthanasia and assisted suicide were extensively discussed and largely discounted on the grounds that the removal of life-sustaining treat-

155

ment does not cause death but allows the natural dying process to proceed without artificial intervention.

Autonomy-based principles are intertwined with discussions of informed consent, which have been prominent since the 1960s. To give informed consent, patients need to understand the decision they are being asked to make, have information about the options available to them, know the risks and benefits of each option, and make decisions that are voluntary.[7] This model of decision making acknowledges that physicians are frequently not in the best position to make decisions in light of a person's unique values or cultural and religious background. Instead, by providing the medical facts, defining the treatment options, and articulating the medical risks and benefits associated with different treatments, physicians empower a patient to make his or her best decision. Applying this model, it could be argued that only David Rivlin could determine whether his quality of life with ventilator assistance was acceptable to him; he had lived it and experienced it for three years. He furthermore knew the consequences of removing the ventilator, and desired death.

No one doubts that Rivlin had the right to exercise control over his health decisions. He furthermore appeared to be making an informed decision. The state's interests in the preservation of life, protection of third parties, prevention of suicide, and promotion of the ethical integrity of medicine did not outweigh Rivlin's right to refuse medical treatment.[8] The judge in Rivlin's case did not believe there was a need or even an appropriate role for judicial involvement and reaffirmed Rivlin's right as a competent adult to refuse ventilatory support.

Some may question the possible role of depression in affecting Rivlin's decision-making capacity. Others would argue that if depression were indeed present, it was inevitable and based upon a realistic appraisal of his medical condition and life circumstances. In the current climate of high emotion and intense debate concerning the issues of physician-assisted suicide (PAS) and medical futility, David Rivlin's decision to be withdrawn from life-sustaining ventilation seems quite straightforward and noncontroversial.[9–14] But is it? The story of another man with quadriplegia who also used a ventilator may shed some further insight.

Larry McAfee was twenty-nine years old when he became quadriplegic from injuries incurred in a motorcycle crash.[15–17] From the beginning, McAfee required continuous ventilatory support. Like Rivlin, McAfee lived in nursing homes, as adequate funding to support him in his own home in the community was not offered in Georgia. In fact, he was transferred to a nursing home in Ohio for a time because Georgia did not have a nursing home capable of managing ventilator care. For seven months, he lived in a hospital intensive care unit. After four years, McAfee (like Rivlin) tired of institutional existence and developed the idea of having an "off" switch placed in the ventilator circuit that he could activate with his mouth. He petitioned the courts to have a physician supply him with adequate sedation to minimize his discomfort when he chose to activate the switch and disconnect the ventilator. The Georgia Supreme Court decided that McAfee had the right as a competent adult to refuse life-sustaining treatment and supported his decision based upon the severity of his disabling condition. They further held that "Mr. McAfee's right to be free from pain at the time the ventilator is disconnected is inseparable from his right to refuse medical treatment" and that sedation "in no way causes or accelerates death," thus indirectly absolving his physicians from a role in assisting in his death.[18]

Yet, after winning his court battle and having the necessary mechanisms in place to effect his death, McAfee ultimately chose not to exercise this right. Why? When his case came to public attention, there was an outpouring of assistance for McAfee, including a special arrangement from Georgia Medicaid. He was eventually able to move into a group home in the community with twenty-four-hour personal assistance.[19] Specialists in computer technology also worked with him to develop a system allowing the use of his skills as an engineer, and he was once again able to work. In short, when McAfee was presented with more options, he chose to live—despite the ongoing nature of his extensive disabling condition.

Rivlin, on the other hand, did not appear to have other viable options offered beyond his institutional existence. A closer examination of Rivlin's life circumstances reveals that prior to his neurological deterioration he had lived in his own home with assistance. He had returned to school, maintained an active social life, and had a couple of serious romantic relationships. After his surgery in 1986 when he required the use of a ventilator, Rivlin had financial coverage that would have allowed him to live in a nursing home, but not in his own home with twenty-four-hour assistance (the state was willing to provide $230 per day to maintain him in a nursing home but was unwilling to pay this amount for independent living).[2] Rivlin lived in the nursing home from 1986 to 1989 and found his world quite constricted. Without funds for adequate personal assistance, he no longer had realistic options of attending school, living in the community, or maintaining an active social life. When he felt that his life choices were limited to continued existence in the nursing home or death, Rivlin felt death was the preferable option. "Life is more than surviving," said Rivlin a few days before his death. "It's interacting with other people, it's having a family, it's having a career, it's having a wife. It's all of those things and I can't have them. . . . I've tried to figure out other ways but there is none."[1]

Both Rivlin and McAfee had extensive disabling conditions that required long-term ventilatory support to live. Given the choice of a life devoid of freedom in an institution versus death, they both felt death was preferable. Yet, when his options were expanded to include life in a group home with personal assistance services and potential for employment, Larry McAfee changed his mind. Both men wanted a level of self-determination that would allow them to pursue the life roles and goals that most people desire—the ability to live in their own home, the ability to pursue meaningful vocational and avocational goals, the ability to participate in society. We cannot be sure that Rivlin would have changed his mind had viable options been available to him, but his statements suggest that decisions about physician-assisted death for people with disabilities are not as simple as they seem. Understanding the barriers that blocked those options may shed further insight into the feasibility and limitations of exercising self-determination for people with extensive disabling conditions.

The Medical Model versus the Interactional Model of Disability

For both Rivlin and McAfee, some of the barriers were medical. A "cure" for spinal cord injury (as for many disabling conditions) is currently not possible. Disability may impose some intrinsic limitations or restriction of options. However, is it accurate to assume that these inherent consequences of disability account for the majority of restrictions a person with disability faces, or are they just one of many factors? A person with paraplegia, for example, may be unable to walk. This difficulty can be circumvented by the use of a wheelchair in a wheelchair-accessible environment. The problem of impaired mobility can therefore be characterized as a person's inability to walk or, alternatively, that person's need to have a wheelchair and an adapted environment (or perhaps most accurately, a combination of both).

In the medical model of disability, a person with a disability is sick and in need of care.[20] The disability is seen as a deficit—something to be cured, fixed, or prevented. In the interactional or minority group model of disability promoted by many disability activists and scholars, disability in and of itself is viewed as neutral. The consequences of disability—the handicaps—result from problematic interactions between the person and the environment.

In addition to medical and physical barriers, serious economic, social, public policy, and attitudinal barriers also exist. In the last half-century society has witnessed dramatic changes in the demographics and culture of disability. We have seen dramatic extensions in length of life for people with disabilities, chronic illnesses, and terminal conditions. It is estimated that thirty-five to forty-nine million Americans (one in seven) have a disabling condition (defined as an impairment that makes it difficult to perform at least one activity of daily living, or ADL).[21] The prevalence of disability also increases with aging. More than 70 percent of the elderly over age seventy-five are disabled; 40 percent are classified as severely disabled and require the assistance of another person for at least part of their ADLs.[22]

People with disabilities (as a group) also have lower incomes than nondisabled people, are largely unemployed, and are restricted in their choices of places to live. Approximately 70 percent of people with disabilities of working age (16–64) are unemployed compared with the unemployment rate of about 24 percent for nondisabled people (these numbers include the total percentage of the population unemployed for any reason, regardless of whether they are actively seeking employment).[21–22] Those who are employed make substantially less than their nondisabled counterparts. Though studies have documented ample evidence of desire to work, employment is prevented by such barriers as physical access problems, prejudice, cumbersome and often unreliable transportation systems, and loss of medical insurance (persons with a disability cannot be gainfully employed and remain on Medicare disability or Medicaid; they are often also unable to obtain other insurance secondary to "preexisting conditions").

Though the physical and economic barriers are substantial, the attitudinal barriers are even more insidious. For most of history, people with disabilities have been largely segregated and institutionalized. At times they have been considered cursed by God or bearers of a sign of moral weakness. They have been both pitied and feared. Our language surrounding disability reflects these attitudes—"invalid" (in-valid), "crippled," "defective," and "handicapped" all imply that one is abnormal or less than fully human. A 1991 Harris poll shows that while 92 percent of the population felt admiration for people with disabilities, 74 percent of those polled also felt pity and 47 percent expressed fear.[23] A number of studies have also shown that health care providers are not very effective at predicting the perceived quality of life of those people with extensive disabling conditions.[24–25] One study showed that 86 percent of those with quadriplegia judged their quality of life to be average to better than average, while only 17 percent of nondisabled health care providers believed this would be true if they had a high-level spinal cord injury.[25]

Traditionally, medical education has done little to dispel misperceptions and educate future physicians about issues related to disability medicine. It is reasonable to question whether physicians and other health care practitioners have enough knowledge of disability issues or the experience to allow accurate prognostication, adequate educaton about available resources, and facilitation of appropriate referrals for their patients with disabilities. Only 75 of the 125 U.S. medical schools have programs in physical medicine and rehabilitation (the field specializing in disability medicine), and only a few of these programs have required clerkships.[26] Few physicians in any specialty know much about independent living options, personal assistance services, augmentative technology, or disability rights. It is not surprising that patients may find their own feelings of despair tacitly and unconsciously validated by their health care providers, families, society at large, and the judicial system, as illustrated by another case.

Elizabeth Bouvia was a twenty-eight-year-old woman with cerebral palsy who on several occasions expressed the desire to die. She admitted herself to a public hospital in 1983 with the intention of "starving herself to death"—a position she later temporarily abandoned. In 1984, after she lost a substantial amount of weight, a nasogastric tube was placed. She petitioned the court for removal of the tube. In a written opinion, the Superior Court of California described Bouvia as follows:[27] "Since birth she has been afflicted with and suffered from severe cerebral palsy. She is quadriplegic . . . she is completely bedridden. Except for a few fingers of one hand and some slight head and facial movements, she is immobile. She is physically helpless and wholly unable to care for herself. She is totally dependent upon others for all her needs. These include feeding, washing, cleaning, toileting, turning, and helping her with eliminations and other bodily functions. She cannot stand or sit upright in bed or in a wheelchair. . . ."

Later in the opinion the court goes on to note that "in Elizabeth Bouvia's view, the quality of her life has been diminished to the point of hopelessness, uselessness, unenjoyability and frustration. She, as the patient, lying helplessly in bed, unable to care for herself, may consider her existence meaningless." The court concludes that "it is, therefore, immaterial that the removal of the nasogastric tube will hasten or cause Bouvia's eventual death."

One of the issues that faced the court was the question of whether Bouvia was suicidal, and, if so, whether that mattered. In a concurring opinion to the court decision, Justice Compton stated: "I have no doubt that Elizabeth Bouvia wants to die; and if she had the full use of even one hand, could probably find a way to end her life—in a word—commit suicide. In order to seek the assistance which she needs in ending her life by the only means she sees available—starvation—she has had to stultify her position before this court by disavowing her desire to end her life in such a fashion and proclaiming that she will eat all that she can physically tolerate. Even the majority opinion here must necessarily 'dance' around this issue."

"Afflicted, bedridden, helpless, dependent." Disability activists and people who knew Bouvia framed her story quite differently. Paraphrasing from editorial pieces written by activists at the time, a different picture emerges:[28–31] "Elizabeth Bouvia was a twenty-eight-year-old woman who also happened to have cerebral palsy. She had earned a college degree, lived in the community, and eventually married. During a relatively short period of time she left graduate school, lost a brother in a drowning accident, and had a miscarriage. Her husband left her. Due to a lack of financial resources, she was forced to live in public facilities when her father told her he could no longer care for her. She became quite depressed and even suicidal concerning her circumstances and perceived lack of options. She sought to die by starving herself."

Was Bouvia's disability the major factor in her desire to die or were her recent losses and hardships critical contributing factors? Was she a tragic woman whose cerebral palsy left her helpless and dependent or was she in reality an amazingly resourceful woman who had negotiated the many barriers of living with a disability quite successfully when a series of losses overwhelmed her and "burned her out"? Did Bouvia truly desire death or did she need support to deal with her depression and options that would allow her to rebuild her life and return to her own home in the community with some assistance?

"Disability burn-out," the term coined by the disability community to describe the fatigue and despair that results from continually fighting a system of barriers, is a real entity. "Disability only becomes a tragedy for me when society fails to provide the things we need to live our lives—job opportunities or barrier-free buildings, for example," reports one disability advocate. "It is not a tragedy that I use a wheelchair."[20] Others would argue that it is not society's responsibility to provide for the psychosocial needs of people with disabilities. Herein lies the crux of the argument concerning independence, autonomy, and self-determination.

Autonomy versus Self-Determination

Arguments about self-determination have been crucial to the disability rights movement. In common parlance, the terms *autonomy, inde-*

pendence, and *self-determination* are often used interchangeably. In the still evolving language and ideology of the disability civil rights movement, however, *self-determination* has emerged as the preferred term because autonomy conjures "bootstraps" images of rugged individualism. Understandably, people whose life options require the skillful selection and use of both personal and technical assistance may have little appreciation for an ethic that glorifies "doing it for yourself." In fact, some persons with disabilities critique the goal of self-sufficiency as rigid and nonprogressive. They argue that, however vigorously it may be denied, all human beings are vulnerable and need help, and that everyone would fare better under a value system that embraces cooperation and respectful interdependence.[32]

Likewise, disability advocates have sharply criticized Western concepts of dignity and quality of life as too mired in the dominant social values of autonomy and independence. They argue that society pressures people to feel unworthy or undignified if they rely on help to bathe and dress or use a catheter for bladder control. In the disability culture, on the other hand, such assistance is an accepted fact of daily living and carries no stigma. Given sufficient time and support for adjustment, persons with disabilities overwhelmingly report that their disability-related problems are an insignificant source of indignity compared to social barriers and devaluation. What matters to them, they say, is social respect and self-determination, and self-determination implies first and foremost that choices or options are available. The disability rights version of self-determination, then, emphasizes that the control or seat of decision making concerning one's life course lies within the individual, whether one is completely self-sufficient in the traditional sense or not.

The Apparent Irony of Self-Determination

All these observations appear to support arguments limiting physician-assisted dying, especially for people with disabilities. At the very least, they suggest a need for more stringent requirements for psychiatric evaluation and treatment and for the availability of social resources. Some would find these arguments, preventing disabled people from decisions they may make based on social discrimination and lack of resources for independent living, inherently paternalistic. Herein lies the apparent irony: although the disability rights movement has been based on the premise of self-determination, many disability rights advocates appear to limit self-determination about this most profound personal event—the end of life.

Disability rights activists who oppose sanctioning physician-assisted death assert, however, that singling out persons with incurable physical conditions for facilitated dying while opposing death wishes in "healthy" people is fundamentally discriminatory. Far from safeguarding their self-determination, many fear they will lose even more options as society gets accustomed to the idea. They cite recent cases of people with disabilities denied expensive health care or equipment by their insurers as well as what they believe are subtle but increasing pressures in health service settings to forgo aggressive life-saving measures.[33]

Rivlin, McAfee, and Bouvia were not terminally ill but had incurable disabilities. They all requested assistance from their health care providers in some form or other to facilitate their deaths. The critical question is: were these requests an expression of their ultimate autonomy to exercise control over their bodies and medical treatment or were their wishes to die a desire to escape the socially constructed part of disability—the pain of prejudice, economic deprivation, exclusion from the community, and unnecessarily restricted choices? If the latter scenario is a more accurate approximation of the truth, then their decisions are hardly acts of self-determination, but rather responses to coercive forces that should be opposed.

Conclusion

We have attempted to point out some of the potential pitfalls and latent complexities inherent in physician-assisted dying for people with disabilities, whether this assistance takes the form of abating life-sustaining treatment or enabling someone to commit suicide. We call for a more demanding standard in the assessment of self-determination and informed consent for everyone, but especially for persons with disabilities. We conclude with five points.

1. Self-determination requires a certain minimum level of empowerment and choice. The options available to a person with a disability may not meet this criterion. A forced choice is no choice at all.

2. To make an informed decision, individuals must have knowledge of the reasonable options available to them, as well as the risks and benefits of these options. They must not be coerced (overtly or covertly) to make any particular decision. Too often, especially in a society that is fearful and ambivalent about the place and worth of its disabled citizens, persons with disabilities have to deal with subtle as well as overt messages that stem from discrimination, represent misinformation, and reinforce their sense of despair.

3. Physicians are often inadequate providers of information regard-

ing all of the options that can improve life with a disability. In fact, physicians, nurses, and all health care providers would benefit from more knowledge and awareness of their limitations, fears, and perceptions in working with people with disabilities. Focusing on the disability when the real issues lie somewhere else may prevent us from offering adequate assessments, options, resources, and support services to patients with disabilities.

4. An assessment of another's quality of life may not be accurate and, in the case of disabilities, may in fact be more negative than the perception of the person who lives with the disability after a period of adjustment.

5. In a country that does not guarantee access to health care or adequate support for dignified assisted living to all its citizens, disempowered populations may be more vulnerable to the pressure to request PAS and other forms of physician assistance in dying. People with abridged choices due to social devaluation and economic oppression who are offered death as an option may be more inclined to choose this path than patients with a number of options available to them, and this may include people who are elderly, chronically ill, poor, and disabled. Disability advocates who oppose physician-assisted dying conclude that what may seem personal is in fact political and that the right to self-determination will be compromised, not expanded, by public policies and cultural values sanctioning death as reasonable for people with disabilities.

NOTES

We want to acknowledge Kathryn Montgomery Hunter, Ph.D., and Raymond H. Curry, M.D. for their assistance in reading prior drafts.

1. Margot Doughtery and S. R. Tessler, "Tiring of Life without Freedom, Quadriplegic David Rivlin Chooses to Die among Friends," *People* 32 (August 7, 1989): 56–58.

2. Paul K. Longmore, "To Live, to Die—Who Decides? The Strange Death of David Rivlin," *Western Journal of Medicine* 154 (May 1991): 615–16.

3. United Press International. "Man Disabled 18 Years Seeks Doctor to Cut Off Life Support," *Indianapolis Star,* July 7, 1989, p. A-11.

4. Paul K. Longmore, "Disabled Need Access to Life—Not Death," *Detroit News,* July 18, 1989, p. 11A.

5. *Schloendorff v. Society of New York Hospital,* 211 N.Y. 125, 105 N.E. 92,93 (1914).

6. President's Commission for the Study of Ethical Problems in Medicine and

Biomedical and Behavioral Research, *Deciding to Forego Life-Sustaining Treatment: A Report of the Ethical, Medical, and Legal Issues in Treatment Decisions* (Washington, D.C.: Government Printing Office, 1983).

7. President's Commission for the Study of Ethical Problems in Medicine and Biomedical and Behavioral Research, *Making Health Care Decisions: A Report on the Ethical and Legal Implications of Informed Consent in the Patient-Practitioner Relationship*, vol. 1 (Washington, D.C.: Government Printing Office, 1982).

8. *Bartling v. Superior Court*, 163 Cal.App.3d 186, 209 Cal. Rptr. 220 (1984).

9. Paul Cotton, "Medicine's Position Is Both Pivotal and Precarious in Assisted Suicide Debate," *JAMA* 273 (1995): 363–64.

10. Don Colburn, "Assisted Suicide Bill Passes: Oregon Law Puts State at the Center of Ethical Debate," *Washington Post Health*, November 15, 1994, p. 9.

11. Timothy E. Quill, Christine K. Cassel, and Diane E. Meier, "Care of the Hopelessly Ill: Proposed Criteria for Physician-Assisted Suicide," *New England Journal of Medicine* 327 (1992): 1380–84.

12. Report of the Task Force on Physician-Assisted Suicide of the Society for Health and Human Values, "Physician-Assisted Suicide: Toward a Comprehensive Understanding," *Academic Medicine* 70 (1995): 583–90.

13. Steven H. Miles, "Physician-Assisted Suicide and the Profession's Gyrocompass," *Hastings Center Report* 25 (1995): 17–19.

14. Bethany Spielman, "Bargaining about Futility," *Journal of Law Medicine and Ethics* 23 (1995): 136–42.

15. Joseph P. Shapiro and Larry McAfee, "Invisible Man," *U.S. News and World Report*, February 19, 1990, pp. 59–60.

16. Paul K. Longmore, "The Shameful Treatment of Larry McAfee," *Atlanta Journal-Constitution*, September 10, 1989, pp. B1, 3.

17. Stanley S. Herr, Barry A. Bostrom, and Rebecca S. Barton, "No Place to Go: Refusal of Life-Sustaining Treatment by Competent Persons with Physical Disabilities," *Issues in Law and Medicine* 8 (1992): 3–36.

18. *State v. McAfee*, 385 S.E. 2d 651 (S.C. Ga. 1989).

19. Associated Press, "Right-to-Die Litigant Who Chose to Live," *Chicago Tribune*, October 4, 1995, p. 11.

20. Joseph P. Shapiro, *No Pity: People with Disabilities Forging a New Civil Rights Movement* (New York: Times Books, 1993).

21. John M. McNeil, *Americans with Disabilities, 1991–1992* (Washington, D.C.: U.S. Department of Commerce, Bureau of the Census, 1993), Current Population Reports, series P70, no.33.

22. Information from the National Association of Rehabilitation Facilities Research and Information Center, August 9–11, 1990.

23. The ICD Survey of Disabled Americans, Louis Harris and Associates, Inc., New York, March 1986.

24. John R. Bach and Margaret C. Tilton, "Life Satisfaction and Well-being Measures in Ventilator Assisted Individuals with Traumatic Tetraplegia," *Archives of Physical Medicine and Rehabilitation* 75 (1994): 626–32.

25. Kenneth A. Gerhart, Jane Koziol-McLain, Steven R. Lowenstein, and Gale G. Whiteneck, "Quality of Life Following Spinal Cord Injury: Knowledge and

Attitudes of Emergency Care Providers," *Annals of Emergency Medicine* 23 (April–June 1994): 807–12.

26. Richard S. Materson, "The Scrooge–Van Winkle Time Machine: Suppose We Awakened Tomorrow and There Were No More Physiatrists," *Archives of Physical Medicine and Rehabilitation* 76 (1995): 12.

27. *Bouvia v. Glenchur*, 225 Cal Rptr 297 (C.A. 2nd Dis., issued 6/5/86).

28. Diane Coleman, "Withdrawing Life-Sustaining Treatment from People with Severe Disabilities Who Request It: Equal Protection Considerations," *Issues in Law and Medicine* 8 (1992): 37–53.

29. Harlan Hahn, "Can Physical Disability Make a Life Not Worth Living?" *Los Angeles Times*, December 9, 1983, p. II7.

30. Carol Gill, "When Society Gives Up on the Disabled," *Los Angeles Herald Examiner*, May 5, 1986.

31. Paul K. Longmore, "Urging the Handicapped to Die: Bouvia Decision Is Victory for Bigotry, Not Self-Determination," *Los Angeles Times*, April 25, 1986, II7.

32. Paul K. Longmore, "The Second Phase: From Disability Rights to Disability Culture," *Disability Rag and Resource* 16 (1995): 4–11.

33. R. Powell, "Cost, Benefits and Quality of Life: Rationale or Rationing?" *Disability Rag and Resource* 15 (1994): 24–27.

8

PHYSICIAN-ASSISTED SUICIDE, ABORTION, AND TREATMENT REFUSAL
USING GENDER TO ANALYZE THE DIFFERENCE

Susan M. Wolf, J.D.

The debate on whether to legitimate physician-assisted suicide and whether the federal Constitution invalidates state prohibitions on the practice proceeds for the most part as if the patient's gender were irrelevant.[1] But the arguments for recognizing a constitutional right to be free to obtain assisted suicide[2] largely build on rights to abortion and the termination of life-sustaining treatment.[3] Indeed, the Ninth Circuit, in deciding that the Fourteenth Amendment protected a right to be free to obtain assisted suicide, stated, "*Casey* . . . and *Cruzan* . . . are fully persuasive, and leave little doubt as to the proper result."[4]

We will see in the 1996–1997 term if the Supreme Court accepts this assertion. But whether it does or not, this reasoning makes ignoring gender peculiar. Abortion analysis clearly requires attention to gender; indeed, numerous scholars have claimed that abortion is fundamentally an issue of gender equality.[5] And there is a growing literature, to which I have contributed, arguing that termination of treatment requires attention to gender as well,[6] a step that many empirical studies have already taken.[7] Thus it is odd to proceed as if gender suddenly becomes irrelevant in analyzing assisted suicide.

Indeed, I have argued elsewhere at length that gender is quite relevant.[8] There I point out that the cases central to the U.S. debate mostly feature women patients. Moreover, health characteristics that may increase vulnerability to assisted suicide as well as euthanasia (depression, inadequate pain relief, lack of health insurance, and difficulty obtaining satisfactory health care) differentially affect women. Suicide

167

statistics also show a clear gender effect, with women attempting suicide more often than men. These facts raise the question of whether women would more often seek assistance or do so for different reasons and would die in greater numbers than men if assisted suicide were legitimated. In addition, our culture partakes of traditions that have long revered women's self-sacrifice. Indeed, in a society and health care system marred by persisting sexism and gender inequities, it would be surprising to find assisted suicide unaffected.

In this chapter I take on another piece of the puzzle. I examine the claim that rights to abortion and termination of treatment ground a constitutional right to be free to obtain assisted suicide.[9] Specifically I analyze the assertion that the constitutionally protected liberty interest in abortion and termination of treatment embraces a protected interest in assisted suicide, and that abortion and treatment refusal case law similarly shows that countervailing state interests fail to justify a ban. I argue that one cannot sort out the relationships among abortion, termination of treatment, and assisted suicide without attending to gender.[10] Yet paying attention to gender reveals critical distinctions. It shows that protected interests in abortion and treatment refusal fail to ground a protected interest in assisted suicide. It further shows that even if there were a protected interest in assisted suicide, the state would have stronger countervailing interests in preventing this practice than abortion or treatment refusal and may well be able to justify a ban.

Several caveats apply. First, this is not an argument that women (or the wider group I discuss in the conclusion) have no constitutional right to be free to obtain assisted suicide, while others do. It is an argument that because abortion is uniquely a right of women and because the right of all to refuse treatment rests on an interest of heightened importance to women—an interest in being free of unwanted bodily invasion—attention to gender reveals the true contours of those rights. Moreover, because women tend to be among the many who are especially vulnerable in the U.S. health care system and broader society, attention to gender also illuminates countervailing state interests not uniquely associated with women.

Second, this analysis focuses on claimed rights to seek assisted suicide rather than addressing both assisted suicide and euthanasia.[11] The recent constitutional litigation concerns a claimed right only to assisted suicide,[12] and advocacy for legalization in the United States has centered increasingly on assisted suicide rather than both.[13] These trends reflect the fact that claims of personal liberty are stronger and risks of mistake and abuse weaker when an individual seeks only help in a fatal act that he or she will ultimately perform. Thus even the Dutch, who have permitted both assisted suicide and euthanasia and have found the latter practice to predominate,[14] are now starting to encourage assisted suicide instead, because of the greater assurance of individual choice.[15] Thus focusing on assisted suicide in isolation from euthanasia favors those who seek to legitimate the practice, and makes more difficult arguments against it.

Yet there are many, including myself, who regard the isolation as artificial.[16] Certainly there is a distinction between the two, hinging on who performs the final fatal act, the patient or the physician.[17]

However, advocates of euthanasia themselves have often claimed that this distinction makes no real difference.[18] Moreover, some have argued that legitimating assisted suicide but not euthanasia would discriminate against patients who lack the physical capacity to take pills or otherwise kill themselves.[19] And certainly in the termination of treatment area, the courts from the start have found that rights to forgo treatment are not limited to patients contemporaneously and competently deciding for themselves.[20] Finally, many analysts have claimed that allowing assisted suicide would lead to euthanasia, even if initially only the former practice were legalized.[21]

In this chapter I nonetheless accept the more difficult challenge for an opponent of both practices.[22] I remain focused on assisted suicide, challenging the claim of a right to be free to obtain that alone rather than claims of a right to both. Yet in the real-world debate this severing of assisted suicide from euthanasia deserves to be challenged. It is essential to ask whether the supposed right to assisted suicide can be contained. If it leads logically to a broader right to euthanasia or practically to wider physician action including euthanasia, then euthanasia becomes an inevitable part of any argument over a claimed liberty interest in being free to obtain assisted suicide and countervailing state interests in prohibiting the practice. Lastly, it is important to be clear about the limits of this argument. I consider only the claim that Fourteenth Amendment abortion and treatment refusal jurisprudence establishes a constitutional right to be free to obtain assisted suicide, the claim accepted by the Ninth Circuit in *Compassion in Dying*. I do not consider other possible constitutional bases or arguments, such as the equal protection rationale embraced by the Second Circuit in *Quill*.[23] Moreover, any constitutional argument has limits: even if assisted suicide enjoys no constitutional protection, the states could still legitimate it through political processes. Lack of constitutional protection only means the Constitution fails to preempt that political struggle by prohibiting a ban. Indeed, the question of whether states should ban or legitimate assisted suicide is a difficult question on which reasonable people may disagree. But I hope to show that the question of whether the Fourteenth Amendment deprives states of this choice by prohibiting a ban—given that the Constitution says nothing about assisted suicide and most states have traditionally criminalized it—is a less vexing matter.

Is There a Protected Liberty Interest?

Case law and commentary have suggested that a right to be free to obtain assisted suicide is safeguarded by the Fourteenth Amendment's protection of liberty as a matter of substantive due process. They have asserted that the Supreme Court's construction of the liberty guarantee in the *Cruzan*[24] termination of treatment case and the *Casey*[25] abortion case would protect assisted suicide as well.[26] Yet foregrounding gender shows that *Cruzan* and *Casey* concern a right to be free of the bodily invasions of unwanted treatment and pregnancy. A right to be free of such bodily invasion, something of special importance to women, does not establish a right to be able to obtain an invasion for the purpose of ending one's life.

Moreover, *Cruzan* and *Casey* establish a rights-bearer's entitlement to live free. This experience of freedom, bound up with the decisional authority to say no, is particularly fundamental to women's flourishing. But neither case establishes a rights-bearer's entitlement to surrender freedom irrevocably through death.

Third, to the extent the Constitution's protection of the abortion decision is properly understood at least in part as a protection of gender equality, assisted suicide finds no support. The literature offers an occasional suggestion that banning assisted suicide may disadvantage women, thus implying a claim of gender equality.[27] However, I argue that women's equality, which indeed supports rights to abortion and treatment refusal, cuts the other way when considering assisted suicide. A long history of valorizing women's self-sacrifice and encouraging women's deaths makes legitimating assisted suicide a fatal threat to women's equality.

Refusing Invasion versus Being Free to Obtain It

Determining whether *Cruzan* and *Casey* ground a liberty interest that encompasses assisted suicide forces careful examination of the kind of liberty interest those cases recognize. *Cruzan* clearly acknowledges that the liberty interest a competent patient would have is a right to be free of bodily invasion. Despite more sweeping subsequent language in *Casey*, it too at root recognizes a right to be free of another invasion, unwanted pregnancy.

Cruzan, of course, recognizes a liberty interest only in dicta. The Supreme Court ruled that Missouri had infringed no constitutional right of the incompetent patient in question; the state could constitutionally require "clear and convincing" evidence of her wishes while formerly competent before permitting her guardians to forgo life-sustaining treatment. Yet Chief Justice Rehnquist, writing for the Court, conceded, "The principle that a competent person has a constitutionally protected liberty interest in refusing unwanted medical treatment may be inferred from our prior decisions."[28] He reviewed Supreme Court cases finding a liberty interest to decline vaccination, "'forcible injection of medication,'" and bodily searches and seizures.[29] Over and over, he framed the protected interest as an interest in refusing treatment. He even clarified that it was "the forced administration of . . . treatment" that implicated the interest.[30] Justice Rehnquist concluded that "for purposes of this case, we assume that the . . . Constitution would grant a competent person a constitutionally protected right to refuse lifesaving hydration and nutrition."[31]

This construction of the protected interest as a right to exclude something from the body is even more explicit in Justice O'Connor's concurrence: "[T]he liberty interest in refusing medical treatment flows from decisions involving the State's invasions into the body. . . . Because our notions of liberty are inextricably entwined with our idea of physical freedom and self-determination, the Court has often deemed state incursions into the body repugnant to the . . . Due Process Clause."[32] She emphasized the physical "intrusion and restraint" involved in forcible treatment.[33]

Justice Brennan, writing in dissent joined by Justices Marshall and Blackmun, insisted on a "fundamental right to be free of unwanted" treatment.[34] He asserted that "[t]he right to be free from [unwanted] medical attention . . . is deeply rooted in this Nation's traditions" and cited the "'inviolability of the person.'"[35] He framed the "right to be free from unwanted medical attention" as "a right to evaluate the . . . treatment . . . and to make a personal decision whether to subject oneself to the intrusion."[36]

Justice Stevens in dissent similarly emphasized that what was at stake was "[h]ighly invasive treatment."[37] His opinion includes broader language about "the liberty to make . . . choices constitutive of private life,"[38] and asserts that "[c]hoices about death touch the core of liberty."[39] But this is married to language explicating "rights pertaining to bodily integrity" and emphasizing the right to be free from "physically invasive" procedures.[40]

Two years after *Cruzan* the Court again construed the Constitution's liberty guarantee, this time in the abortion context. Justices O'Connor, Kennedy, and Souter, forming the governing plurality in *Casey,* con-

firmed that women have a liberty interest in deciding whether to
terminate a pregnancy. However, they went on to reject *Roe*'s trimester
formulation and revise the test for determining when state interests
overcome the liberty interest. In parts of their opinion, they cast the woman's protected interest as an interest in choice: "These matters, involving the most intimate and personal choices a person may make in
a lifetime, choices central to personal dignity and autonomy, are central to the liberty protected by the Fourteenth Amendment. At the heart
of liberty is the right to define one's own concept of existence. . . ."[41]
These are the portions that some commentators now claim support a
liberty interest in assisted suicide. They read Justice O'Connor, in
particular, who emphasized bodily invasion in *Cruzan,* as now abandoning that idea in favor of a much broader understanding of liberty.[42]

Yet a more careful reading of *Casey* shows that the plurality is not
abandoning the bodily invasion idea at all. Rather they clarify—in a
portion of the opinion joined by two other justices, and so representing
a controlling majority view—that the liberty interest at stake in the
abortion cases "stands at the intersection of two lines of decisions."[43]
The first line concerns procreation. These cases concerning the right to
prevent or terminate pregnancy are based on "the liberty relating to
intimate relationships, the family, and decisions about whether . . . to
beget or bear a child."[44] Here the language of "choice" dominates.
Indeed, it echoes the shift in common parlance from discussing a right
to abortion to discussing a right to choice.

But it is the other line of cases that touches on end-of-life issues. Here
liberty is a matter of "personal autonomy and bodily integrity," growing out of "cases recognizing limits on governmental power to mandate
medical treatment."[45] Far from turning away from the *Cruzan* definition of liberty, the plurality here cites the case.[46]

Thus *Cruzan* continues to stand for the proposition that there is a
protected liberty interest in rejecting invasive treatment, even when the
predicted consequence is death. However, at the beginning of life, in
what the plurality calls the "unique" circumstances of abortion,[47] the
liberty interest is founded in part on what appear to be broader notions
of "choice."

What does this mean for analysis of assisted suicide? First we must
ask which of the two lines of cases on liberty is most relevant. The
plurality has not merged the two lines together; they are careful to
distinguish them. Moreover, they distinguish them not just abstractly,
but by focusing in *Cruzan* on what is really at issue in facing the end
of life and in *Casey* in facing the beginning. Clearly assisted suicide is
closer to termination of treatment than abortion. The first two are end-
of-life issues concerning a single individual's dominion over his or her

own body with no question of another fetal being.[48] Thus liberty as a right to be free of bodily invasion is most germane.

Second, the plurality strongly suggests that even in the abortion domain, the liberty interest is not just a free-floating interest in "choice." Instead, it involves a choice to get something out of one's body. Only this understanding makes sense of the plurality's assertion that the abortion right sits at the intersection of *two* lines of cases, those on procreative choice and those on refusing bodily invasion. If abortion were just about "choice," the second line of cases would be irrelevant. And abortion is indeed about a right to be free of unwanted invasion, the invasion of pregnancy. The state cannot compel a women to tolerate that invasion.

Thus even the abortion right embraces an understanding of liberty as the right to be free of unwanted bodily invasion. Those who quote the "choice" language in *Casey* out of context capture only part of the plurality's analysis. *Casey* reaffirms rather than erases *Cruzan*'s definition of liberty.

That definition clearly embraces the right to be free of unwanted bodily invasion. But it is not at all clear that it covers a right to be free to obtain bodily invasion for the purpose of ending your own life. This is not an artificial distinction. Removing an unwanted fetus from the body restores the status quo ante (not being pregnant) and allows a woman to continue her life plan before it was interrupted by unwanted pregnancy. Removing unwanted life-sustaining treatment also restores the status quo ante (life with a disability or illness) and allows a person to continue what may be a dying process. But assisted suicide removes nothing from the body[49] and restores no status quo ante. It intervenes to change the life course radically.[50]

There is a potential for confusion here. Certainly both abortion and treatment refusal can require a second bodily invasion—the doctor may have to enter the body to remove the fetus or the feeding tube. This is no surprise. The body is complex and removing something may require skillful entry and exit, as well as control of associated symptoms. Yet the fact that abortion and treatment refusal may require invasion does not alter the point of all this activity—removal of something from the body.[51] This is not the case in assisted suicide. No primary invasion is being removed when the physician supplies the means of bodily invasion for suicide.

Distinguishing between removal of bodily invasion and the demand for it accords with precedent. *Cruzan* in particular emphasizes that the traditional core of liberty in this country is a right to keep the government out of one's body. The Constitution protects this in more than one place, including in the search and seizure restrictions of the Fourth

Amendment as well as the Due Process Clause's protection of liberty in the Fourteenth. It has ancient roots in Anglo-American law, in the common law right to be free of unconsented invasion, in penal codes' prohibitions on battery, and in state constitutional provisions. It thus clearly meets the Court's test for substantive due process protection: it is rooted in our traditions and is truly "fundamental" to "the concept of ordered liberty."[52]

It is especially fundamental for women. Women live at risk of unwanted bodily invasion. That invasion comes in many forms: incest and sexual abuse of girls, unwanted impregnation and pregnancy in women of reproductive age, rape of women of all ages. Drucilla Cornell has argued that critical to a woman's sense of self is the confidence that she can keep others out of her body.[53] Without this, a woman's psychological sense of boundaries and basic sense of physical security are threatened. Indeed, the power of unwanted bodily invasion is well known. It is a common means of terrorizing women in domestic violence, brutalizing them in torture, and committing aggression against them in war.[54] Men, too, can be threatened by rape and other forms of unwanted invasion. But the problem is more widespread for women, the need to define who can gain access to the body through intercourse is inescapable, and the threat of unwanted invasion through pregnancy is unique to women. Thus for women the right to exclude unwanted bodily invasion is absolutely fundamental.

None of the same can be said of the supposed right to be free to obtain bodily invasion to kill oneself. Indeed, suicide was traditionally prohibited.[55] Though the states have decriminalized it,[56] that does not create a right to suicide. In fact, a person attempting suicide may not only be stopped, he or she may be committed to a mental health facility for evaluation.[57] And the decriminalization of suicide itself has not affected state prohibitions on assisting a suicide. Assisting a suicide remains criminal in most states.[58] As the majority opinion of the Second Circuit finds in *Quill,* the supposed right to assisted suicide is not "implicit in our understanding of ordered liberty," nor was it "ever . . . recognized in any state."[59] Assisted suicide therefore fails the test for substantive due process protection.

The acknowledgment in *Cruzan* and *Casey* of a protected liberty interest in being free of state-compelled bodily invasion thus cannot accomplish what advocates of assisted suicide wish. It cannot ground a right to be free to obtain bodily invasion to kill oneself.[60] Lifting *Casey*'s procreative "choice" language out of context does not do the trick. Assisted suicide is neither procreative choice nor refusal of governmentally compelled bodily invasion, and cannot be rooted in the ancient right to exclude the government from one's body.

The Interest in Living Free versus in Ending Life and Freedom

Even the parts of *Casey* and *Cruzan* that emphasize the decisional freedom aspect of liberty focus on the interest in continuing with one's life unencumbered rather than any interest in ending one's life altogether. Advocates of assisted suicide have quoted the governing plurality's statement in *Casey* that "At the heart of liberty is the right to define one's own concept of existence, of meaning, of the universe, and of the mystery of human life."[61] But this statement follows a list of personal decisions protected by the Constitution, and that list includes nothing resembling assisted suicide. Instead, it enumerates "marriage, procreation, contraception, family relationships, child rearing, and education." "Our precedents 'have respected the private realm of family life'. . . ." "These matters . . . are central to the liberty protected by the Fourteenth Amendment."[62] The plurality emphasizes that the choice about procreation made in electing abortion is a protected liberty interest because the state cannot force upon a woman a certain role and place in society. Instead, a woman must be free to choose these herself.[63] The opinion recognizes the special stake of women in being able to reject an unwanted pregnancy: "The ability of women to participate equally in the economic and social life of the Nation has been facilitated by their ability to control their reproductive lives."[64] Indeed, the opinion refers to "the *urgent* claims of the woman to retain the ultimate control over her destiny and body, claims implicit in the meaning of liberty."[65]

This is a concept of liberty as the right to live unencumbered by unwanted pregnancy in order to carve out a destiny other than mother of that child-to-be. There is no support here for a concept of liberty as the right to forfeit one's liberty permanently by purposefully ending one's life. This reflects a traditional distinction drawn in understanding the role of the liberal state in promoting liberty. John Stuart Mill, in particular, has argued that the liberal state properly supports individual freedom and enforces freely made choices but cannot properly support and enforce choices made to surrender freedom irrevocably, as by selling oneself into slavery.[66] Thus the liberty interest recognized by *Casey* does not protect every conceivable choice. It protects the choice to say no and go on from there unencumbered. It offers no protection to choices whose goal is to encumber one's life radically, that is, to end it and thereby end choice irrevocably.

One response might be that *Casey* fails to consider liberty at the end of life because it is about something else, abortion. But *Casey* cites *Cruzan*, as noted above. And it does so in explicating liberty "as a rule . . . of personal autonomy and bodily integrity, with doctrinal affinity to cases recognizing limits on governmental power to mandate medical treatment or bar its rejection."[67] Thus *Casey* frames the liberty interest protected by *Cruzan* as another example of the right to live unencumbered, to make certain choices free of government mandate. There is no hint that the interest protects a choice to end life and autonomy by assisted suicide.

Of course, exercise of the right that *Cruzan* indicates is protected, the right to refuse life-sustaining treatment, will often (though not always) eventuate in death. But *Cruzan* itself derives that right from cases recognizing a liberty interest in refusing unwanted treatments such as vaccination and antipsychotic drugs.[68] The liberty interest that *Cruzan* recognizes is an interest not in choosing death but in refusing treatment.[69] Indeed, the Court grounds its opinion in part in a long line of judicial decisions beginning with *Quinlan* that find a right to be free of unwanted bodily invasion even when the likely consequence is death, rather than finding a right to death itself.[70] The Court clearly distinguishes the state's obligation to respect refusal of life-sustaining treatment from the state's traditional and proper opposition to assisted suicide.[71] Thus the opinion acknowledges the state's "interest in the protection and preservation of human life" and indicates that one of the ways states demonstrate this commitment is by "imposing criminal penalties on one who assists another to commit suicide."[72]

Here again gender helps distinguish the protected zone of liberty from what remains outside of it. As noted above, the plurality's opinion in *Casey* recognizes that a woman must be permitted by the state to say no to unwanted pregnancy in order to realize her life goals and define her own role in society. Indeed, women must be able to refuse a whole roster of bodily invasions in order to live freely and flourish. These include unwanted pregnancy, incest, and unwanted intercourse. It would be hard to dispute that the ability to say no to these is fundamental to women's liberty and flourishing. The fact that women often suffer bodily invasion despite saying no makes this interest all the more fundamental.

The special importance to women of being able to refuse unwanted bodily invasion carries over into the domain of life-sustaining treatment. There, too, Miles and August have argued that women's no is often overridden. In examining state appellate decisions in cases concerning life-sustaining treatment, they found that courts tended to dismiss now-incompetent women's expressions of treatment preferences while previously competent. Courts saw men's prior remarks as rational but women's as "unreflective, emotional, or immature"; "some courts simply . . . [did] not recognize women's views"; a higher evidentiary standard was applied in women's cases; and while men's treatment refusals were seen as resistance to medical assault, women were seen as needing treatment to avoid medical neglect.[73] Thus a man's no had more weight than a woman's.

Women have a potent interest in being able to refuse the bodily invasions of unwanted treatment, pregnancy, intercourse, and other penetrative assault. The difficulty women have in getting others to honor their refusals only heightens that interest. What does that tell us, then, about women's interest in being free to obtain assistance with suicide? Very little, I would submit. The interest in living free of unwanted encumbrance bears little relation to the claimed interest in getting help to end one's life. Women need the freedom to fend off unwanted invasions of all sorts, sexual, violent, and medical. But the claimed right to be free to obtain assisted suicide seeks something opposite, a physician who will provide invasive drugs or other means to ensure a fatal suicide. The demand for assisted suicide is a demand for a third party's involvement in purposefully ending a woman's life. That is something women already have in abundance and most people decry. Women are differentially the victims of fatal domestic violence.[74] Moreover, as noted above, women already attempt suicide substantially more often than men, though they succeed less often.[75] It is hardly clear that liberty is advanced by ensuring women's attempts are more uniformly successful.[76]

Promoting Gender Equality versus Ensuring the Deaths of Women

The governing plurality's language in *Casey* about the importance of protecting the abortion option to secure women's "ability . . . to participate equally in . . . economic and social life"[77] echoes extensive commentary suggesting that the abortion right is fundamentally a matter of gender equality.[78] Unless women can control their reproductive lives, they are profoundly hampered in competing with men in the workplace, accepting equal public responsibilities, and realizing their own personal goals.

A comparable argument can be made about the ability to refuse unwanted medical treatment. Women labor under a special burden in trying to control their treatment and establish relationships with medical professionals that are as respectful and satisfactory as men's. The long history of physician paternalism is particularly acute in the case of women patients.[79] Indeed, the American Medical Association's Council on Ethical and Judicial Affairs issued a report in 1991 on gender disparities in health care. The report noted that women receive more care than men, even for the same illness, but the care is generally worse. The report cites numerous studies documenting women's greater difficulties in establishing satisfactory physician-patient relationships and receiving good care.[80]

All of this would suggest that women might have a difficult time ensuring that the use of life-sustaining treatment conforms with their wishes. As noted above, Miles and August indeed report this in the litigated appellate cases they studied. The authors found that women's choices were more often belittled and disregarded than men's, so that it was more difficult for women to forgo unwanted life-sustaining treatment.[81]

This means that recognizing a constitutionally protected interest in forgoing life-sustaining treatment, one that cannot be overridden by state courts or legislatures and that even in clinical settings commands the respect of a constitutional right, will help advance gender equity. Certainly abortion, as a procedure only women choose, is more starkly a matter of women's equality. But given the baseline difficulties women may face in forgoing treatment, constitutional protection is likely to advance gender equality there, too.

In addition, if women must be able to refuse unwanted bodily invasions generally in order to achieve a sense of personal boundaries, intactness, and physical security, then protecting the right to refuse unwanted medical invasions is especially important to women. The feeling of boundedness and security that most men may achieve with little effort, women may find far more effortful and problematic. Thus protecting the right to refuse unwanted bodily invasions is indeed a matter of gender equity.

What does all of this mean for the claimed right to be free to obtain assisted suicide? Clearly, securing assistance in suicide has little to do with women's need to refuse unwanted bodily invasion and so secure their boundaries. Indeed, when the physician assists by prescribing a lethal medication, for instance, he or she is offering the fatal instrument of bodily invasion. So this portion of the gender equity argument applies to abortion and treatment refusal but fails to apply to assisted suicide.

Moreover, by deliberately offering a woman the means of her own death, the physician is fitting into a long history of socially encouraging women's suicides. I have summarized the history elsewhere.[82] Suicide in Greek tragedy is "a woman's solution," the way wives join their husbands in death.[83] Societal gender roles bless women's suicides through history. "By the mid-nineteenth century characterizations of women's suicides meshed with the ideology . . . of 'True Womanhood. . . .'"[84] Thus "virtue for women lies in self-sacrifice."[85] The physician who offers a woman the means to kill herself may be reinforcing not disrupting a history of fatal gender inequity.

What about the other portion of the argument pertaining to treatment refusal, that constitutional recognition can help correct a tendency to denigrate women's choices? One might argue that this does apply to assisted suicide, by taking the Miles and August analysis of treatment refusal and extending it to assisted suicide. In other words, one might speculate that women's requests for assistance would be differentially ignored.[86]

However, elsewhere I have offered numerous reasons to expect that women would request assisted suicide at higher rates than men and that their requests would be differentially granted.[87] First, the fact that women attempt suicide more often than men[88] suggests that women might more often seek physician assistance simply as part of the sequence of actions that constitute the attempt. Women might also seek physician assistance as a search for reassurance, symptomatic relief, relationship, or some other kind of help rather than a striving to die. Indeed, the fact that women more often attempt suicide but less often succeed may reflect more than a male tendency to use firearms; it may mean that many women wish not to "succeed" so much as change their circumstances, and attempting suicide is one way to do that.[89] If so, then the predominance of women among those taking steps toward suicide may predict more women asking their physicians for assistance.

The response among physicians may also be quite different from the dismissal Miles and August find among judges. Those authors analyze that dismissal to be part of broader societal patterns of sexism, including a tendency to regard women as more emotional and less rational than men, to accord women's preferences less weight, to denigrate their agency, and to infantilize them as beings in need of protection. But societal sexism may make physicians more, not less, willing to assist suicide for a woman patient. In a society that unfortunately still tends to regard women's lives as less valuable than men's and that particularly devalues older women's lives, physicians may be more ready to support a woman patient's judgment that life is no longer worth living. The long cultural history of regarding women's self-sacrificing behavior as feminine and virtuous further supports this speculation.[90]

Finally, the gender disparities that still plague health care may differentially drive women to seek assisted suicide. Women are more likely to receive inadequate pain relief[91] and more commonly suffer from depression.[92] Both depression and inadequately controlled pain are thought to place patients at risk for seeking assisted suicide or euthanasia.[93] Women are also differentially at risk because of difficulties obtaining good care to cope with serious illness, pain, and other symptoms. The AMA report noted above on gender disparities suggests that women face greater barriers to getting good care generally. And women more often rely on government entitlement programs, with older women in particular less likely than older men to have private health insurance.[94] Women also tend to make less money than men.[95]

Thus there is ample reason to expect that women may more often seek assisted suicide and that physicians may more frequently acquiesce. And aside from sheer frequency issues, women's requests for assistance and physicians' acquiescence may often be a product of background gender disparities and sexism. Thus even if the numbers were no different, there would be cause for concern.

Against this background, it is difficult to argue that constitutional protection for assisted suicide would advance gender equity. Indeed, given the fact that more women than men attempt suicide, constitutional protection may simply ensure that more women die. And many of those women will surely be driven in part by background gender inequalities. Protecting assisted suicide would make those inequalities fatal.

Of course, some of the gender inequalities may also apply to forgoing treatment. Assigning lesser value to women's lives and valorizing female self-sacrifice, plus the greater barriers to women's access to good care and health care coverage, might make women more ready to throw in the towel and refuse treatment and might make physicians more ready to go along with that choice. But a gender equality analysis of forgoing treatment cannot lose sight of the fundamental importance to women of being able to refuse bodily invasion. Background gender inequities that may influence individuals' decisions are a serious problem and should be addressed. However, the basic freedom to exclude others from one's body cannot be abridged.

That basic freedom plays no part when it comes to assisted suicide. Thus the gender inequities that will be made fatal by constitutional protection for assisted suicide dominate the analysis. The important goal of gender equity militates against protecting assisted suicide, even as that goal supports constitutional protection for abortion and treatment refusal.

What Are the Countervailing State Interests?

Even if the courts find a protected liberty interest in assisted suicide, they must then proceed to analyze the countervailing state interests. I argue that the state interests are greater than in the case of abortion or treatment refusal. First, the state has a stronger interest in protecting the lives of born persons than fetuses, whose status is contested. Moreover, the state's related interest in preventing suicide is directly implicated by assisted suicide but not by efforts to be free of unwanted bodily invasion through treatment refusal.

Second, the state interest in protecting the integrity of the medical profession, combined with the profession's acknowledged history of sexism, supports facilitating physician aid in abortion (where physician involvement generally remains necessary) and aid in forgoing treatment (where the same is true). That state interest does not support facilitating assisted suicide. Physician involvement is not necessary for suicide, and the dangers in permitting physicians to act on persisting professional sexism and stereotypes are substantial. Error and abuse are predictable, and their burden will fall most heavily on those historically ill-served by the health care system, including women.

Third, the state has an interest in preventing fatal practices that will be applied inequitably to jeopardize the lives of women, not to mention the elderly, the disabled, and others whose lives tend to be disvalued. This interest is weightier than in the case of abortion. Abortion, too, may be urged upon those who are disvalued or whose reproduction is disvalued, but abortion is not intentionally fatal to the woman herself and the woman's interest in being free of unwanted pregnancy is strong. In the case of treatment refusal, again the disvalued may feel more pressure to forgo life-sustaining treatment. But treatment refusal, too, is not about intentionally helping to bring on the death of a patient, and the patient's interest in being free of unwanted treatment is also strong.

Thus abortion and treatment refusal jurisprudence not only fails to establish a protected liberty interest in assisted suicide, but also fails to indicate that such a liberty interest would prevail over countervailing state interests. Indeed, the *Compassion in Dying* court concedes that the countervailing state interests are strong enough to justify extensive regulation of assisted suicide, even for patients who are terminal and competent.[96] What the court refuses to permit is a ban.

The precise test that courts should use to analyze a ban on assisted suicide is controversial, hinging in part on whether the ban is challenged "on its face" (in which case, at least two different tests have been put forward) or "as applied" to terminal, competent patients (in which case the ban remains as to all other patients).[97] The point of this chapter, however, is to show that abortion and treatment refusal case law fails to settle the assisted suicide constitutional question. The Supreme Court has had no opportunity to consider a ban in the termination of treatment context, because *Cruzan* did not raise the question. *Casey,* too, merely considered whether challenged regulations imposed an "undue burden" on the abortion right, not whether a ban was sustainable. Thus neither case undermines an assisted suicide ban. Moreover, the Court's tolerance since *Roe v. Wade* for a state ban on abortion after fetal viability (except when the woman's health or life is endangered) supports the likelihood that states can justify an assisted suicide ban. As I argue in the next section, state interests in protecting the actual lives of born persons are greater than state interests in protecting the potential lives of fetuses. And traditional state interests in protecting life and preventing suicide persist even when people are at their most vulnerable: sick or disabled at the end of life, and for whatever reason (including poor pain relief, inadequate medical care, or psychological distress) seeking assistance with suicide.

Protecting the Lives of Persons versus Potential Persons; Preventing Suicide versus Honoring Treatment Refusal

Some commentators suggest that the state has a greater interest in opposing abortion than assisted suicide because the state has an acknowledged interest in potential fetal life but little interest in preventing assisted suicide, at least among competent adults.[98] Yet this misunderstands the comparison. In the abortion cases, the entity being protected has no agreed moral status, and the Supreme Court's abortion decisions have never held the fetus to be a person. However, in cases of assisted suicide, the being whose life is at stake is incontrovertibly a person.[99] And traditionally the state has had a clear interest in protecting persons' lives.[100] Thus it would seem that the state has a stronger interest in protecting life in the assisted suicide case than the abortion case. Even after fetal viability, the state interest in protecting potential life fails when it conflicts with the woman's life and health. This suggests that the Constitution protects the lives of born persons to a greater extent than the lives of merely potential persons. If the state interest in potential life can justify a ban on abortion after viability (at least when the woman's health or life is not in danger), then the state interest in actual life is even more likely to permit a ban.

Related to the state interest in protecting life is the more specific state interest in preventing suicide. The latter interest is directly implicated in the case of assisted suicide. However, *Compassion in Dying* maintains that the state interests both in preventing suicide and in protecting life are weak at the end of life. "While the state has a legitimate interest in preventing suicides in general, that interest, like the state's interest in preserving life, is substantially diminished in the case of terminally ill, competent adults who wish to die."[101] This is too glib. *Cruzan* shows that the state interest remains strong in end-of-life cases; Missouri's interest defeated the authority of Nancy Cruzan's parents to discontinue artificial nutrition, though their daughter was in a persistent vegetative state. And Chief Justice Rehnquist's opinion acknowledged that most states criminalize assisted suicide in an exercise of their interest in protecting life.[102] Thus the state interests at the end of life are not confined to protecting noncognitive patients such as Cruzan. And those countervailing interests apply even when a person competently elects suicide: "We do not think a State is required to remain neutral in the face of an informed and voluntary decision by a physically able adult to starve to death."[103]

Moreover, Chief Justice Rehnquist's focus on the state interest in banning assisted suicide rather than suicide itself reflects the fact that even if individuals may kill themselves, the state has a strong interest in preventing citizens from becoming involved in intentionally bringing on the deaths of each other, whether directly or by assisting suicide. Thus *Compassion in Dying* misses the boat in saying that "[w]hen patients . . . do not wish to pursue life, the state's interest in forcing them to remain alive is clearly less compelling."[104] Blocking a competent, terminal patient's suicide (which no state now does) might be "forcing them to remain alive"; blocking third-party assistance is not.

The dangers of third-party assistance with suicide are substantial. *Compassion in Dying* acknowledges that "[a] state may properly assert an interest in prohibiting . . . assistance . . . on the grounds that allowing others to help may increase the incidence, undercut society's commitment to the sanctity of life, and, adversely affect the person providing assistance."[105] A third party's involvement may also lead to pressure, subtle or blatant, on the patient. These concerns are particularly acute in the case of women. Their large number of unsuccessful suicide attempts (compared to men's) may be rendered fatally successful by third-party assistance, even if those attempts were motivated more by a desire to change circumstances than to die. Moreover, women may be encouraged to undervalue their own lives and engage in self-sacrificing behavior. Indeed, a three-judge panel of the Ninth Circuit in *Compassion in Dying*, writing prior to the *en banc* consideration, found a state interest in protecting the elderly, the infirm, the poor, minorities, and the disabled from similar pressure. The panel noted that undertreated pain, lesser resources, and societal discrimination rendered these populations vulnerable to third-party pressure, especially from a physician.[106]

The Ninth Circuit *en banc* dismissed these concerns, but the court's reasoning does not bear scrutiny. The court asserts that the state interest in preventing third-party involvement diminishes with the interest in preventing suicide itself.[107] But this simply ignores the separate dangers of third-party action. Second, the court expresses completely unsupported faith that physicians will prevent such harms,[108] ignoring the fact that physicians are human and subject to the same biases as the broader culture.[109] Lastly, the court rejects the notion that those "who have historically received the least adequate health care" will now be urged to assisted suicide and will be vulnerable to that urging.[110] But there is nothing implausible in the notion that this population will be encouraged to take the least expensive and demanding health care option.[111] And someone who is terminally ill, who may have uncontrolled pain or other symptoms, may be quite vulnerable to such urging.

Finally, one cannot judge the state interest by focusing only on competent, terminal patients. There is good reason to expect any practice authorized for that population to slip outside those boundaries. The Dutch practice has already done so, extending to the incompetent, those without physical illness, and children.[112] And the fact that *Compassion in Dying* and many advocates of assisted suicide assert no real difference between that and termination of treatment suggests that the numerous court decisions extending rights to forgo treatment to the incompetent and nonterminal would ground a similar extension of any right to assisted suicide. Thus state interests are strong in protecting life and preventing suicide among the competent and terminal, as well as others.[113]

The Necessity of Physician Involvement versus Inadequate Justification for Its Dangers

The state's countervailing interests pertaining to physicians are often narrowly framed as protecting the integrity of the medical profession.[114] However, physicians wield life-and-death powers in abortion, termination of treatment, and assisted suicide. State interests in protecting life extend to protecting patients from inappropriate, fatal physician behavior, not just protecting the integrity of the medical profession itself.

Obviously there is a potential for inappropriate, fatal physician behavior, including mistake and abuse, in performing all three practices. But in the case of abortion and termination of life-sustaining treatment this risk must be balanced against the general necessity of physician involvement.[115] Thus prohibiting physicians from performing abortions would certainly create enormous barriers for women who wish to end unwanted pregnancies. And prohibiting physicians from terminating treatment already begun would make it extremely difficult for patients to stop treatment themselves. The patient on a ventilator, for instance, would be hard-pressed to extubate herself, could not be expected to manage the respirator machinery, and would in most cases lack the expertise to direct her own "terminal weaning."

Yet suicide is an act that does not require a physician. Many people kill themselves each year with no physician help at all. And even those who prefer to use drugs, the one modality largely controlled by physicians, can get instructions from books and newsletters and often can get the drugs without a physician knowingly assisting suicide. It is understandable that people may wish the easier access to drugs and expert instruction that would follow legitimation of physicians' assisting suicide. But that comes at a price, the risks that go with physician involvement.

In abortion and terminating treatment, those risks are unavoidable, as physicians must generally be involved. But that is not so with suicide. Physicians need not be involved. And there are good reasons to keep them out of the business. I and others have written elsewhere about the transformation in the physician's role, medical ethics, and medical education that will be wrought by authorizing physicians to violate the ancient Hippocratic injunction to "give no deadly drug, even if asked."[116] The fact that some physicians have apparently been doing it and that some evidently approve, as the court notes in *Compassion in Dying*,[117] does not alter the fact that officially allowing all physicians to deliberately take their patients' lives would be a substantial change in physicians' authority and role. And permitting physicians to take deliberate steps to bring about the deaths of patients poses special problems for women. It allows background gender inequities, continuing societal sexism, and the particular gender dynamics that remain problematic in physician-patient relationships[118] to result in women's deaths.

State Interests in Blocking Physicians from Intentionally Seeking the Deaths of Their Patients, Given Gender Inequities

A fatal practice likely to show significant gender inequities should be a candidate for state prohibition. The state has a recognized interest in protecting the lives of the vulnerable. Here the vulnerability is particularly objectionable because it stems from a history of discrimination, as I suggested in analyzing how patterns of inadequate pain relief, depression, unsatisfactory physician-patient relationships, lack of private insurance, historical valorization of women's self-sacrifice, and continuing sexism may leave women more at risk than men for assisted suicide.

This argument is not grounded merely on the expectation that women may numerically predominate if assisted suicide is legitimated.[119] It is also grounded on the above analysis of why women may seek assisted suicide and why physicians may accede.[120] It rests on the persistence of inequity and sexism in both cases. And though I focus here on gender inequity, broader arguments could be offered about the state interest in avoiding other patterns of fatal inequity based on the persistence of prejudice against the elderly, disabled, and others historically disvalued. One might assert, of course, that the same sort of gender argument could support state interests in banning abortion or termination of treatment. In other words, one could claim that women without the resources to raise a child will differentially seek abortion, or that the difficulties women have in getting good medical care and in marshaling the resources to cope with serious illness will differentially motivate women to forgo treatment. But neither abortion nor honoring treatment refusal is fundamentally about deliberately seeking the deaths of women, whether directly (as through euthanasia) or by helping them kill themselves. Thus the countervailing state interest is strongest in the case of assisted suicide. And the individual liberty interest against which the state's is counterposed is weakest, neither the interest in being free of unwanted bodily invasion nor the interest in personal choice about reproduction and the family. Indeed, I have claimed above that assisted suicide implicates no constitutional liberty interest at all.

Conclusion: Reunderstanding Gender

Because my analysis focuses on gender, it might be misconstrued as applying only to women, as I suggested above. But gender is important here because it shows that abortion and treatment refusal case law, properly understood, provides no reason to conclude that the Fourteenth Amendment's liberty guarantee protects an interest in being free to obtain assisted suicide. This is a conclusion that applies to all, not simply women. It is in the nature of abortion and treatment refusal that each involves getting something out of the body. I have argued that this is particularly important to women, because women historically have been subordinated by being subjected to unwanted bodily invasion and loss of control over their bodies. But they are not alone. Chattel slavery, for example, involved radical loss of control over the body, rape, and other unwanted bodily invasions as a means of subjugation. Male-on-male rape is another instance of unwanted bodily invasion used as a means of subordination. To look at the liberty interest protected by *Cruzan* and *Casey* purely as decisional control and thus to forget that these cases involve physical control of the body is to view the Fourteenth Amendment from the standpoint of someone who has not been subordinated by physical domination.[121] In that sense, it is to take the view of the subordinator. Yet the Fourteenth Amendment is an anti-slavery amendment. It is precisely about protection for those who have been subordinated and robbed of physical control.

Gender also is important for what it reveals about the state's countervailing interests. It forces attention to the state interests in protecting those ill-served by the health care system and those for whom a regime of assisted suicide would pose a danger. Here, too, women are not alone. People of color also have a long history of being ill-served by the U.S. health care system.[122] Individuals lacking health insurance and those who are poor and dependent on government entitlement programs are vulnerable as well to being offered assisted suicide long before they are offered adequate care for serious illness, much less good palliative care, pain relief, and hospice care.

Thus a gender analysis brings to the fore problems that are not confined to women. Many are problems shared by others who have historically been subordinated. It is consequently no accident that California polls show support for legalizing assisted suicide to be strongest among affluent white males, while people of color, the aged, and women are more skeptical.[123] And many of the arguments I make above could be restated to focus on race, age, disability, or lack of medical insurance.

Broadening my argument to embrace other characteristics histori-cally used to stigmatize and subordinate people reveals a deeper dy-namic. Gender, like these other characteristics, has been *made* to matter. It has been socially constructed as important and a way of distributing power.[124] Indeed, its very meaning is socially constructed, with a contested relationship to biological sex.[125]

This means that my gender argument is not just about biological females. It reaches others to whom the traits of the subordinated gen-der are attributed, all who are "feminized."[126] In the assisted suicide debate, that is a much larger group than biological women. It includes others threatened with loss of bodily integrity, whose authority over their own lives is at risk, and whose subordinated social position makes it more likely they will be offered death than the resources to cope with serious disease.

Reunderstanding gender thus shows the argument's full reach. The rights analysis advanced to legitimate assisted suicide fails not just for women but also for the larger group. It assumes a rights-bearer with no history of being disadvantaged, encouraged to exit, and even put to death. The analysis of countervailing state interests similarly ignores the context and the history. It thus erases the state interest in shielding those whom our country's history of inequity renders more vulnerable to death through assisted suicide.

After all, ours is a nation born of inequity, whose founding document excluded people by race and gender from basic democratic participation.[127] It is a nation that continues to see people disadvantaged on the basis of race and gender as well as class. Assisted suicide does not sit outside that history. It does not float in space with no context. Advocates for legitimation may plead the rights of abstract rights-bearers, people without race, gender, or class. But such people do not exist.

In the real world, assisted suicide will be administered by flawed physicians to flawed patients. Unlike abortion, it will prove fatal to the person who requests it. Unlike termination of treatment, it will legitimate physicians' involvement in deliberately bringing about the deaths of their patients.

We live in a profoundly imperfect nation in hard times. Only recently and ambivalently has this country begun to deal with the legacies of slavery and denying fundamental rights to women. And this remains the only industrialized nation with a hefty portion of its population lacking health care coverage.[128] In this real context, assisted suicide will unavoidably be a fatal instrument of inequity.

Whether a state should nonetheless legitimate the practice should be a matter of the most serious debate. It requires a process of democratic deliberation that includes those citizens who will actually suffer from the inequity. I have argued that nothing in the abortion or treatment refusal cases relieves citizens of this momentous decision by constitutionally prohibiting a ban. *Casey* and *Cruzan* assign the fate of assisted suicide not to the Court but to the citizenry. Let those who struggle to refuse unwanted bodily invasion, to exert control over their lives, and to secure good health care be persuaded.

NOTES

Thanks to Arthur Caplan, Jim Chen, Rebecca Dresser, Dan Farber, Phil Frickey, Jeff Kahn, and Dorothy Roberts for insightful comments on prior drafts; to Robert Burt, Sam Gorovitz, and the University of Minnesota Law School Faculty Workshop for thought-provoking reactions to earlier work in this vein; to David Weissbrodt as well as the University of Minnesota Law Library for help with sources; and to Laurie Nesseth of the University of Minnesota Law School for able research assistance. This work was supported by the University of Minnesota Law School's Fesler Research Fellowship, a University of Minnesota Faculty Summer Research Fellowship, and a McKnight Summer Fellowship.

1. Indeed, Seth Kreimer asserts, "the concerns of women's equality that are implicated by abortion are absent from the arguments for assisted suicide or euthanasia." Seth F. Kreimer, "Does Pro-Choice Mean Pro-Kevorkian? An Essay

on *Roe, Casey,* and the Right to Die," *American University Law Review* 44 (1995): 803–54, 810. He goes on to consider gender briefly in a footnote. See id. at 850 n.170.

The few analyses in the scholarly literature that do pay serious attention to gender include Jocelyn Downie and Susan Sherwin, "A Feminist Exploration of Issues around Assisted Death," *St. Louis University Public Law Review,* forthcoming; Susan M. Wolf, "Gender, Feminism, and Death: Physician-Assisted Suicide and Euthanasia," in Susan M. Wolf, ed., *Feminism and Bioethics: Beyond Reproduction* (New York: Oxford University Press, 1996), pp. 282–317; Leslie Bender, "A Feminist Analysis of Physician-Assisted Dying and Voluntary Active Euthanasia," *Tennessee Law Review* 59 (1992): 519–46. Analyses in the press that do the same include B. D. Colen, "Gender Question in Assisted Suicides," *Newsday,* November 25, 1992, p. 17; Ellen Goodman, "Act Now to Stop Dr. Death," *Atlanta Journal and Constitution,* May 27, 1992, p. A11.

The case law on the constitutional status of assisted suicide, which ignores the significance of gender, includes *Quill v. Vacco,* 80 F.3d 716 (2d Cir. 1996) *cert. granted,* 65 U.S.L.W. 3254 (Oct. 1, 1996) (No. 95-1858); *Compassion in Dying v. Washington,* 79 F.3d 790 (9th Cir.) (en banc), *cert. granted sub nom. Washington v. Glucksberg,* 65 U.S.L.W. 3254 (Oct. 1, 1996) (No. 96-110); *People v. Kevorkian,* 527 N.W.2d 714 (Mich. 1994).

2. By "assisted suicide" I mean physician-assisted suicide throughout this chapter, setting aside for now questions of assistance by family members and other nonphysicians. This is because the U.S. litigation concerning a claimed constitutional right to assisted suicide concerns exclusively physician-assisted suicide so far. See *Quill,* 80 F.3d 716; *Compassion in Dying,* 79 F.3d 790. Even Jack Kevorkian, though he has been stripped of his medical license in Michigan, continues to argue that he acts as a physician striving to relieve his patients' suffering when he assists in suicide. See Jack Lessenberry, "In Latest Suicide Trial, Kevorkian Asserts 'Duty as a Doctor,'" *New York Times,* May 4, 1996, sec. 1, p. 10.

3. Both *Quill* and *Compassion in Dying* build on abortion and treatment refusal rights. The commentary doing so is extensive, including Robert M. Kline, "The Right to Assisted Suicide in Washington and Oregon: The Courts Won't Allow a Northwest Passage," *Boston University Public Interest Law Journal* 5 (1996): 213–37; Sylvia A. Law, "Physician-Assisted Death: An Essay on Constitutional Rights and Remedies," *Maryland Law Review* 55 (1996): 292–342, 301–307; Kathryn L. Tucker and David J. Burman, "Physician Aid in Dying: A Humane Option, a Constitutionally Protected Choice," *Seattle University Law Review* 18 (1995): 495–508; John A. Powell and Adam S. Cohen, "The Right to Die," *Issues in Law and Medicine* 10 (Fall 1994): 169–82; Robert A. Sedler, "Constitutional Challenges to Bans on 'Assisted Suicide': The View from Without and Within," *Hastings Constitutional Law Quarterly* 21 (1994): 777–97; Ronald Dworkin, *Life's Dominion: An Argument about Abortion, Euthanasia and Individual Freedom* (New York: Alfred A. Knopf, 1993); Brian C. Goebel, Note, "Who Decides If There Is 'Triumph in the Ultimate Agony'? Constitutional Theory and the Emerging Right to Die with Dignity," *William and Mary Law Review* 37

(1996): 827–901; Jonathan R. MacBride, Comment, "A Death without Dignity: How the Lower Courts Have Refused to Recognize That the Right of Privacy and the Fourteenth Amendment Liberty Interest Protect an Individual's Choice of Physician-Assisted Suicide," *Temple Law Review* 68 (1995): 755–810; Steven J. Wolhandler, Note, "Voluntary Active Euthanasia for the Terminally Ill and the Constitutional Right to Privacy," *Cornell Law Review* 69 (1984): 363–83.

However, commentators rejecting the notion that abortion or treatment refusal jurisprudence successfully grounds a right to assisted suicide include New York State Task Force on Life and the Law, *When Death Is Sought: Assisted Suicide and Euthanasia in the Medical Context,* New York, May 1994, pp. 67–75 [hereinafter New York State Task Force]; Yale Kamisar, "Against Physician-Assisted Suicide—Even a Very Limited Form," *University of Detroit Mercy Law Review* 72 (1995): 735–69; Kreimer, "Does Pro-Choice Mean Pro-Kevorkian?"; Alexander Morgan Capron, "Easing the Passing," *Hastings Center Report* 24 (July–August 1994): 25–26; Thomas J. Marzen, "'Out, Out Brief Candle': Constitutionally Prescribed Suicide for the Terminally Ill," *Hastings Constitutional Law Quarterly* 21 (1994): 799–826; Willard C. Shih, Note, "Assisted Suicide, the Due Process Clause and 'Fidelity in Translation,'" *Fordham Law Review* 63 (1995): 1245–82.

Note that one might try to ground a Fourteenth Amendment right to be free to obtain assisted suicide not in abortion or treatment refusal jurisprudence but in case law concerning substantive due process rights that do not involve bodily invasion, such as the right to marry. See *Loving v. Virginia,* 388 U.S. 1 (1967). However, this chapter focuses on the assertion that abortion and treatment refusal jurisprudence is an adequate basis for finding constitutional protection, the assertion accepted in *Compassion in Dying.*

4. 79 F.3d at 813 (citations omitted).

5. See, e.g., Cass R. Sunstein, *The Partial Constitution* (Cambridge, Mass.: Harvard University Press, 1993), pp. 270–85; Laurence H. Tribe, *Abortion: The Clash of Absolutes* (New York: Norton, 1990), p. 105; Ruth Bader Ginsburg, "Some Thoughts on Autonomy and Equality in Relation to *Roe v. Wade*," *North Carolina Law Review* 63 (1985): 375–86, 377–86; Sylvia A. Law, "Rethinking Sex and the Constitution," *University of Pennsylvania Law Review* 132 (1984): 955–1040, 1013–28; Kenneth L. Karst, "The Supreme Court 1976 Term—Forward: Equal Citizenship under the Fourteenth Amendment," *Harvard Law Review* 91 (1977): 1–294, 57–59.

6. See, e.g., Wolf, "Gender, Feminism, and Death," p. 308; Steven H. Miles and Allison August, "Courts, Gender and 'The Right to Die,'" *Law, Medicine and Health Care* 18 (1990): 85–95.

7. See, e.g., Lawrence J. Schneiderman et al., "Attitudes of Seriously Ill Patients toward Treatment That Involves High Cost and Burdens on Others," *Journal of Clinical Ethics* 5 (1994): 109–12.

8. Wolf, "Gender, Feminism, and Death."

9. Throughout this chapter I frame the right at issue as a right to be free to obtain assisted suicide rather than as a right to assisted suicide. In doing this, I am bowing to the claim frequently made by proponents of assisted suicide, that they seek only a negative liberty, not a positive entitlement. However, this claim deserves careful

scrutiny. If assisted suicide is such a valuable practice, why should the poor and those lacking health insurance not be entitled to it? Cf. *Harris v. McRae*, 448 U.S. 297, 316–17 (1980) (upholding denial of abortion funding for poor women).

10. Strictly speaking, this chapter analyzes both gender and biological sex, in that I address both the biological fact that women are subject to unwanted pregnancy and the social fact that those who are gendered female or "feminized" (see my conclusion) are subject to subordination through an array of bodily invasions and unsatisfactory interactions with the health care system. A longer and more detailed treatment of this topic would disaggregate sex and gender. However, I rely on "gender" as the primary rubric here because my argument focuses on the significance of being vulnerable to subordination through various sorts of bodily invasion and of having a negative history with the health care system. As I explain in my conclusion, these are not concerns confined to biological females.

11. By "euthanasia" I mean active euthanasia only. I avoid the older use of the term to include termination of life-sustaining treatment because it is confusing. Law and ethics treat the two practices so differently that embracing them under the same rubric thwarts clear debate.

12. See *Quill*, 80 F.3d 716, 730–31; *Compassion in Dying*, 79 F.3d 790.

13. See, e.g., Charles H. Baron et al., "A Model State Act to Authorize and Regulate Physician-Assisted Suicide," *Harvard Journal on Legislation* 33 (1996): 1–34, 9–10; Timothy E. Quill, Christine K. Cassel, and Diane E. Meier, "Care of the Hopelessly Ill: Proposed Clinical Criteria for Physician-Assisted Suicide," *New England Journal of Medicine* 327 (1992): 1380–84; Robert F. Weir, "The Morality of Physician-Assisted Suicide," *Law, Medicine and Health Care* 20 (1992): 116–26; Sidney H. Wanzer et al., "The Physician's Responsibility toward Hopelessly Ill Patients: A Second Look," *New England Journal of Medicine* 320 (1989): 844–49, 847–49.

14. See Paul J. van der Maas et al., "Euthanasia and Other Medical Decisions concerning the End of Life," *Lancet* 338 (1991): 669–74, 671.

15. See Marlise Simons, "Dutch Doctors to Tighten Rules on Mercy Killings: Patient Would Administer Drug," *New York Times*, September 11, 1995, p. A3.

16. See, e.g., New York State Task Force on Life and the Law, pp. 82–85, 141–45; Yale Kamisar, "Are Laws against Assisted Suicide Unconstitutional?" *Hastings Center Report* 23 (May–June 1993): 32–41, 35–36. Even the majority in *Compassion in Dying* conceded that "it may be difficult to make a principled distinction between" assisted suicide and euthanasia. 79 F.3d at 831.

17. For general discussion of the distinction, see New York State Task Force on Life and the Law, pp. 82–85. One can also distinguish among voluntary, involuntary, and nonvoluntary euthanasia, based on whether the patient has competently requested euthanasia, refused it, or said nothing. Ibid., p. 1.

The majority in *Compassion in Dying* confuses these well-accepted distinctions by saying, "We define euthanasia as the act . . . of painlessly putting to death persons suffering from . . . disease, . . . but *not* at the person's request." 79 F.3d at 832 n.120 (emphasis in the original). Thus they arbitrarily exclude voluntary euthanasia from the category of "euthanasia." They engage in similarly unjustified semantics in saying, "[W]e are doubtful that deaths resulting from terminally ill patients taking medication prescribed by their doctors should be classified as 'suicide.'" 79 F.3d at 824. Their argument is that assisted suicide is merely hastening a dying process already under way. But that assumes "assisted suicide" applies only to terminally ill patients (which it does not) and that it simply accelerates a preexisting physiological process, such as renal failure. But assisted suicide introduces a whole new physiological process: response to the drug or other modality used. The majority's verbal acrobatics are therefore unpersuasive.

18. See, e.g., Glenn C. Graber and J. Chassman, "Assisted Suicide Is Not Voluntary Euthanasia, but It's Awfully Close," *Journal of the American Geriatrics Society* 41 (1993): 88–89; Dan W. Brock, "Voluntary Active Euthanasia," *Hastings Center Report* 22 (March–April 1992): 10–22, 10; Eric H. Loewy, "Healing and Killing, Harming and Not Harming," *Journal of Clinical Ethics* 3 (1992): 30.

19. See, e.g., Franklin G. Miller et al., "Regulating Physician-Assisted Death," *New England Journal of Medicine* 331 (1994): 119–23, 120; Sedler, "Constitutional Challenges to Bans on 'Assisted Suicide,'" pp. 791–95; *Rodriguez v. British Columbia,* 107 D.L.R.4th 342, 363, 415 (Can. 1993) (Lamer, C. J. C., and MacLachlin, J., dissenting). Cf. *Compassion in Dying,* 79 F.3d at 831–32 (physician administration of drugs may be necessary when the patient is unable to self-administer).

20. See *In re Quinlan,* 355 A.2d 647 (N.J.), *cert. denied,* 429 U.S. 922 (1976).

21. See, e.g., New York State Task Force, p. 145.

22. My opposition has been articulated in a number of publications, including Susan M. Wolf, "Pediatric Euthanasia and Assisted Suicide," in Linda L. Emanuel, ed., *Assisted Death: Balancing Considerations regarding Physician-Assisted Suicide and Euthanasia in the USA,* forthcoming; "Gender, Feminism, and Death"; "*Final Exit*: The End of Argument," *Hastings Center Report* 22 (January–February 1992): 30–33; and "Holding the Line on Euthanasia," *Hastings Center Report* 19 (January–February 1989): supp. 13–15.

23. This chapter focuses on the claim that the Fourteenth Amendment's protection of liberty reaches assisted suicide, the central holding in *Compassion in Dying.* Outside the scope of this chapter are other claimed constitutional protections for assisted suicide, such as the Equal Protection Clause relied on in *Quill* and the First Amendment protection advocated by Ronald Dworkin. See Dworkin, *Life's Dominion.* I take the liberty claim as my focus because the case law and commentary to date have for the most part seen that as the leading argument for constitutional protection of assisted suicide. See generally Kreimer, "Does Pro-Choice Mean Pro-Kevorkian?"

24. *Cruzan v. Director, Mo. Dep't of Health,* 497 U.S. 261 (1990).

25. *Planned Parenthood v. Casey,* 505 U.S. 833 (1992).

26. See, e.g., *Compassion in Dying,* 79 F.3d at 799–816; citations in n. 3 above, esp. Kline, "The Right to Assisted Suicide in Washington and Oregon"; Law, "Physician-Assisted Death"; Goebel, Note, "Who Decides If There Is 'Triumph in the Ultimate Agony?'"; Tucker and Burman, "Physician Aid in Dying"; MacBride, Comment, "A Death without Dignity."

27. See Kreimer, "Does Pro-Choice Mean Pro-Kevorkian?" p. 850 n.170.

28. 497 U.S. at 278.

29. 497 U.S. at 278 (citations omitted). He also cited two cases implicating a traditional liberty interest to be free of bodily incarceration for medical treatment. 497 U.S. at 278–79.

30. 497 U.S. at 279.

31. 497 U.S. at 279.

32. 497 U.S. at 287 (O'Connor, J., concurring) (citations omitted).

33. See 497 U.S. at 288. I omit discussion of Justice Scalia's concurrence because he rejected the very notion that a constitutionally protected interest was implicated in the case.

34. 497 U.S. at 302 (Brennan, J., dissenting).

35. 497 U.S. at 305 (Brennan, J., dissenting) (citations omitted).

36. 497 U.S. at 309 (Brennan, J., dissenting).

37. 497 U.S. at 339 (Stevens, J., dissenting).

38. 497 U.S. at 341 (Stevens, J., dissenting) (citation omitted).

39. 497 U.S. at 343 (Stevens, J., dissenting).

40. 497 U.S. at 342 (Stevens, J., dissenting) (citation omitted).

41. 505 U.S. at 851.

42. Justice Souter was not yet sitting on the Court when *Cruzan* was decided, and Justice Kennedy joined the Chief Justice's opinion for the Court. As noted above, Justice O'Connor wrote a separate concurrence.

43. 505 U.S. at 857.

44. 505 U.S. at 857.

45. 505 U.S. at 857.

46. They do so again, thus reinforcing my point, in saying that "state regulation with respect to the child a woman is carrying" is especially deserving of constitutional scrutiny because "the state has touched not only upon the private sphere of the family but upon . . . bodily integrity. . . . Cf. *Cruzan. . . .*" 505 U.S. at 896.

47. 505 U.S. at 852.

48. The Court has not yet decided a case involving termination of treatment (or, of course, assisted suicide) for a pregnant woman. For such a case, see *In re A.C.,* 573 A.2d 1235 (D.C. 1990) (en banc).

49. One might claim that assisted suicide removes pain or suffering from the body. But that is figurative, not literal removal of a discrete entity such as a tube or fetus. Pain and suffering are not actual, removable things lodged in the body but phenomena or states the person experiences.

50. I am grateful to Phil Frickey for suggesting this line of argument.

51. Justice Blackmun's concurrence in *Casey* seems to recognize that a right to seek abortion may entail a right to seek bodily invasion for the purpose of removing the fetus. See 505 U.S. at 927 n.3 (Blackmun, J., concurring). Unfortunately, his language is unnecessarily broad and seems to suggest that a constitutional right to refuse bodily invasion (as in treatment) is paralleled by a right to obtain invasion (or treatment). He loses sight here of the difference between what I am calling the primary and secondary bodily invasions.

52. The quoted language is from *Palko v. Connecticut,* 302 U.S. 319, 325 (1937). For a general statement of the standard, which the Justices have often

articulated, see the Court's controversial opinion in *Bowers v. Hardwick,* 478 U.S. 186, 191–92 (1986).

53. See Drucilla Cornell, *The Imaginary Domain: Abortion, Pornography and Sexual Harassment* (New York: Routledge, 1995), pp. 46–52, and *Transformations: Recollective Imagination and Sexual Difference* (New York: Routledge, 1993), p. 144. For extended discussion of the significance of bodily invasion to women, see Robin West, "Jurisprudence and Gender," *University of Chicago Law Review* 55 (1988): 1–72.

54. On domestic violence see, e.g., Catherine F. Klein and Leslye E. Orloff, "Providing Legal Protection for Battered Women: An Analysis of State Statutes and Case Law," *Hofstra Law Review* 21 (1993): 801–1189, 857–58. The plurality opinion in *Casey* notes the frequency of sexual assault in domestic violence against women. See 505 U.S. at 889, 891. On torture see, e.g., Ximena Bunster-Burotto, "Surviving beyond Fear: Women and Torture in Latin America," in Miranda Davies, ed., *Women and Violence* (Atlantic Highlands, N.J.: Zed Books, 1994), pp. 156–76. On war see, e.g., Amnesty International, *Human Rights Are Women's Right,* New York, 1995, pp. 18–22.

55. Justice Scalia recites the history in his *Cruzan* concurrence: "At common law in England, a suicide . . . was criminally liable." 497 U.S. at 294 (Scalia, J., concurring) (citations omitted). At least some of the American colonies adopted this approach. See Thomas J. Marzen et al., "Suicide: A Constitutional Right?" *Duquesne Law Review* 24 (1985): 1–242, 64–68.

56. See Marzen et al., "Suicide," p. 98. Justice Scalia explains: "Although the States abolished the penalties imposed by the common law (i.e., forfeiture and ignominious burial), they did so to spare the innocent family and not to legitimize the act." 497 U.S. at 294 (Scalia, J., concurring).

57. See *Compassion in Dying,* 79 F.3d at 820 & n. 83; *People v. Kevorkian,* 527 N.W.2d at 732 & nn.55, 56. "At common law, even a private person's use of force to prevent suicide was privileged." 497 U.S. at 298 (Scalia, J., concurring) (citations omitted). State law typically permits at least temporary commitment for mental health evaluation when a person attempts suicide and is suspected of being mentally ill. See, e.g., Kate E. Bloch, Note, "The Role of Law in Suicide Prevention: Beyond Civil Commitment—A Bystander Duty to Report Suicide Threats," *Stanford Law Review* 39 (1987): 929–53, 933–35.

58. See *Cruzan,* 497 U.S. at 280 & n.8; Alan Meisel, *The Right to Die,* 2d ed. (New York: Wiley, 1995), vol. 2, p. 478; Antonios P. Tsarouhas, "The Case against Legal Assisted Suicide," *Ohio Northern University Law Review* 20 (1994): 793–814, 795–96 (citing prohibitions in statute, case law, and the Model Penal Code). Assisted suicide has long been criminal. "Case law at the time of the adoption of the Fourteenth Amendment generally held that assisting suicide was a criminal offence." 497 U.S. at 294 (Scalia, J., concurring) (citing, *inter alia,* Marzen et al., "Suicide," p. 76). See also Marzen et al., "Suicide," p. 98.

Judge Calabresi's concurrence in *Quill* questions the continued vitality of New York's prohibition on assisted suicide. 80 F.3d at 732–35. However, he does so in part by construing case law authorizing physicians' termination of unwanted treatment as eroding the basis for prohibiting assisted suicide. Though the distinction between assisted suicide and terminating treatment has certainly been questioned, this chapter argues there are significant differences, as most of the Justices' opinions in *Cruzan* acknowledged. Judge Calabresi also questions whether there is any reason to criminalize assisted suicide once suicide itself has been decriminalized. Yet the reasons for decriminalizing suicide—avoiding cruelty to the surviving family, recognition that many suicides are the product of mental illness, and the like—do nothing to undermine the state's interest in preventing citizens from killing others or from participating in the intentional taking of life.

59. 80 F.3d at 724–25 (citations omitted).

60. The Michigan Supreme Court concluded as much in *People v. Kevorkian*, focusing on *Cruzan*:

> The right to refuse medical treatment meets the "ordered liberty" and the "historical underpinnings" tests [for constitutional protection] because it is rooted in the common-law doctrine of informed consent, which embodies the notion of bodily integrity. A person may refuse life-sustaining medical treatment because the treatment itself is a violation of bodily integrity. Suicide enjoys no such foundational support, however. When one acts to end one's life, it is the intrusion of the lethal agent that violates bodily integrity.

527 N.W.2d at 732 n.59.

61. 505 U.S. at 851, quoted, for example, by Dworkin, *Life's Dominion*, p. 171.

62. 505 U.S. at 851 (citations omitted).

63. See 505 U.S. at 852.

64. 505 U.S. at 856 (citation omitted).

65. 505 U.S. at 869 (emphasis added).

66. See John Stuart Mill, "On Liberty," in Marshall Cohen, ed., *The Philosophy of John Stuart Mill: Ethical, Political and Religious* (New York: Random House, 1961), pp. 185–319, 304. Certainly there are differences between selling oneself into slavery and assisted suicide, a prominent one being that the slave continues to live and may later change her mind about the enslavement; the liberal state cannot then properly enforce the agreement against her. But that is not the only argument for Mill's position. Even if she cannot change her mind (because she loses cognitive capacity, or hypothetically agreed to be both enslaved and lobotomized, or agreed to be enslaved and then killed), it is improper for a liberal state to support agreements whose purpose is to eradicate freedom irrevocably. Such agreements create relationships (such as master-slave) and hence institutions (such as slavery) whose goal is to eradicate freedom. A state committed to individual freedom cannot properly support relationships and institutions whose purpose is to deliver individuals into a circumstance in which they can no longer exercise freedom. Yet that is the purpose of assisted suicide: to secure death, the end of freedom.

This does not mean that the state may not support an army whose soldiers volunteer for war or advance directives permitting people to forgo life-sustaining treatment. The state may support such agreements by which people risk death, because the purpose of these agreements is something else—national defense or freedom from unwanted treatment. Moreover, death may be far from certain in those cases. Yet in the case of assisted suicide, death is the goal and certain.

67. 505 U.S. at 857.

68. 497 U.S. at 278.

69. Even Justice Stevens's statement in dissent that "[c]hoices about death touch the core of liberty" is offered in the context of saying that "the right to be free from unwanted life-sustaining medical treatment . . . presupposes no abandonment of the desire for life." 497 U.S. at 343 (Stevens, J., dissenting). Thus it appears that "[c]hoices about death" refers to choices to refuse treatment, not more broadly to choices to commit suicide and seek assistance. The intentional ending of one's life would seem to signal the end of a "desire for life." For this reason and those cited in my text, the Ninth Circuit is clearly wrong in treating *Cruzan* as a case about a "right to die." See *Compassion in Dying,* 79 F.3d at 802.

70. The Chief Justice starts with case law on "bodily integrity" and informed consent, explaining how these notions bore fruit in the termination of treatment cases. See Cruzan, 497 U.S. at 269–77. Cf. Leon R. Kass, "Is There a Right to Die?" *Hastings Center Report* 23 (January–February 1993): 34–43 (arguing no).

71. Only Justice Scalia conflates the two, but by way of saying the states can oppose both. "American law has always accorded the State the power to prevent . . . suicide—including suicide by refusing to take appropriate measures necessary to preserve one's life." 497 U.S. at 293 (Scalia, J., concurring).

72. 497 U.S. at 280 (footnote with citation omitted).

73. Miles and August, "Courts, Gender and 'the Right to Die,'" pp. 87–89.

74. See Bureau of Justice Statistics, *Selected Findings* (Washington, D.C.: U.S. Department of Justice, Office of Justice Programs, November 1994), p. 3 (by 1992, 70 percent of victims of "intimate murder" were female). See generally ibid., p. 2 ("Annually, compared to males, females experienced over 10 times as many incidents of violence by an intimate."); Council on Ethical and Judicial Affairs, American Medical Association, "Physicians and Domestic Violence: Ethical Considerations," *Journal of the American Medical Association* 267 (1992): 3190–93, 3190 ("Most evidence indicates that domestic violence is predominantly perpetrated by men against women." [footnotes with citations omitted]).

75. See, e.g., Howard I. Kushner, "Women and Suicide in Historical Perspective," in Joyce McCarl Nielsen, ed., *Feminist Research Methods: Exemplary Readings in the Social Sciences* (Boulder, Colo.: Westview Press, 1990), pp. 193–206, 198–200.

76. One might argue that if a woman's refusal of bodily invasion tends to be ignored, her request for assisted suicide will be as well. I analyze this prediction but offer substantial reasons for predicting the opposite in Wolf, "Gender, Feminism, and Death," pp. 284, 293, 308. There I maintain that one must consider the substance of what the woman is asking in each case and whether it follows or defies prevailing social patterns. When a woman refuses treatment, she is defying social patterns that encourage bodily invasion despite her no. But when she requests assisted suicide, "the history of women's subordination cuts the other way. Women have historically been seen as fit objects for bodily invasion, self-sacrifice, and death at the hands of others." P. 308.

77. 505 U.S. at 856 (citation omitted).

78. See citations in n. 5.

79. See, e.g., Susan Sherwin, *No Longer Patient: Feminist Ethics and Health*

Care (Philadelphia: Temple University Press), pp. 223–25, 227; Barbara Ehrenreich and Diedre English, *For Her Own Good: 150 Years of the Experts' Advice to Women* (New York: Doubleday, 1978).

80. Council on Ethical and Judicial Affairs, American Medical Association, "Gender Disparities in Clinical Decision Making," *Journal of the American Medical Association* 266 (1991): 559–62, esp. 561–62.

81. See Miles and August, "Courts, Gender and 'The Right to Die.'"

82. See Wolf, "Gender, Feminism, and Death," p. 289.

83. See Nicole Loraux, *Tragic Ways of Killing a Woman,* trans. Anthony Forster (Cambridge, Mass.: Harvard University Press, 1987), p. 8.

84. Kushner, "Women and Suicide in Historical Perspective," p. 195, citing Barbara Welter, "The Cult of True Womanhood: 1820–1860," *American Quarterly* 18 (1966): 151–55.

85. Carol Gilligan, *In a Different Voice: Psychological Theory and Women's Development* (Cambridge, Mass.: Harvard University Press, 1982), p. 132.

86. See Nancy S. Jecker, "Physician-Assisted Death in the Netherlands and the United States: Ethical and Cultural Aspects of Health Policy Development," *Journal of the American Geriatrics Society* 42 (1994): 672–78, 676.

87. See Wolf, "Gender, Feminism, and Death."

88. See, e.g., ibid., p. 283, *citing* Kushner, "Women and Suicide in Historical Perspective," pp. 198–200.

89. See Wolf, "Gender, Feminism, and Death," p. 291, citing Kushner, "Women and Suicidal Behavior," and a study reported in Colen, "Gender Question in Assisted Suicides."

90. See Wolf, "Gender, Feminism, and Death," pp. 289–90.

91. See Charles S. Cleeland et al., "Pain and Its Treatment in Outpatients with Metastatic Cancer," *New England Journal of Medicine* 330 (1994): 592–96.

92. See William Coryell, Jean Endicott, and Martin B. Keller, "Major Depression in a Non-Clinical Sample: Demographic and Clinical Risk Factors for First Onset," *Archives of General Psychiatry* 49 (1992): 117–25.

93. See Susan D. Block and J. Andrew Billings, "Patient Requests to Hasten Death: Evaluation and Management in Terminal Care," *Archives of Internal Medicine* 154 (1994): 2039–47; Kathleen M. Foley, "The Relationship of Pain and Symptom Management to Patient Requests for Physician-Assisted Suicide," *Journal of Pain and Symptom Management* 6 (1991): 289–97.

94. See U.S. Bureau of the Census, *Statistical Abstract of the United States: 1995,* 115th ed. (Washington, D.C., 1995), p. 118; Nancy S. Jecker, "Can an Employment-Based Health Insurance System Be Just?" *Journal of Health Politics, Policy and Law* 18 (1993): 657–73; Employee Benefit Research Institute (EBRI), *Sources of Health Insurance and Characteristics of the Uninsured: Analysis of March 1992 Current Population Survey,* EBRI Issue Brief No. 133 (Jan. 1993).

95. For income statistics, see U.S. Bureau of the Census, *Statistical Abstract,* p. 158.

96. Indeed, the court says that state regulation is "both necessary and desirable to ensure against errors and abuse, and to protect legitimate state interests." 79 F.3d at 832–33.

97. See generally Sylvia A. Law, "Physician-Assisted Death: An Essay on Constitutional Rights and Remedies," *Maryland Law Review* 55 (1996): 292–342, esp. 324–41.

98. See Eric Rakowski, "The Sanctity of Human Life," *Yale Law Journal* 103 (1994): 2049–2118, 2097 (book review); Sedler, "Constitutional Challenges to Bans on 'Assisted Suicide,'" pp. 792–93; Goebel, Note, "Who Decides If There Is 'Triumph in the Ultimate Agony?'" pp. 877–78; Note, "Physician-Assisted Suicide and the Right to Die with Assistance," *Harvard Law Review* 105 (1992): 2021–40, 2033.

99. As Kreimer puts it, "In *Roe* and *Casey,* the first issue in contest is the definition of the nature and value of the entity that is being harmed: the fetus. In contrast, the definition of the entity being harmed in suicide is clear: a fully developed human life is at stake." Kreimer, "Does Pro-Choice Mean Pro-Kevorkian?" p. 813 (footnotes with citations omitted).

100. Cf. *Cruzan,* 497 U.S. at 280 ("Missouri relies on its interest in the protection and preservation of human life, and there can be no gainsaying this interest.").

101. 79 F.3d at 820 (footnote omitted).

102. *Cruzan,* 497 U.S. at 280.

103. Ibid.

104. 79 F.3d at 820.

105. Ibid. at 825.

106. See 49 F.3d at 592–93.

107. See 79 F.3d at 825.

108. See ibid. at 825, 827, 837.

109. See, e.g., Council on Ethical and Judicial Affairs, American Medical Association, "Gender Disparities in Clinical Decision Making."

110. 79 F.3d at 825.

111. For a comparable concern, see Daniel Callahan, "Vital Distinctions, Mortal Questions: Debating Euthanasia and Health Care Costs," *Commonweal* 115 (1988): 397–404.

112. On incompetents see, e.g., Loes Pijnenborg et al., "Life-Terminating Acts without Explicit Request of Patient," *Lancet* 341 (1993): 1196–99.

On assisting suicide when the patient has no physical disease, see Tony Sheldon, "Reprimand for Dutch Doctor Who Assisted Suicide," *British Medical Journal* 310 (1995): 894–95; Alan D. Ogilvie and S. G. Potts, "Assisted Suicide for Depression: The Slippery Slope in Action?" *British Medical Journal* 309 (1994): 492–93.

On children, see Wolf, "Pediatric Euthanasia and Assisted Suicide"; James P. Orlowski et al., "Pediatric Euthanasia," *American Journal of Diseases of Children* 146 (1992): 1440–46; Henk K. A. Visser et al., "Medical Decisions concerning the End of Life in Children in the Netherlands," *American Journal of Diseases of Children* 146 (1992): 1429–31; Committee of the Section on Perinatology, Dutch Pediatric Association, "To Do or Not to Do? Boundaries of Medical Action in Neonatology" (English summary), in *Doen of laten? Grenzen van het medisch handelen in de neonatologie* (Utrecht: Nederlandse Vereniging voor Kindergeneeskunde, 1992), pp. 11–15.

113. Kreimer argues that the state prohibiting assisted suicide is generally asserting an interest in protecting the many by depriving the patient before the court of access to assistance. "In prohibiting assisted suicide and euthanasia, the State is choosing to protect the welfare of others at the cost of the plaintiff's control over her own body." Kreimer, "Does Pro-Choice Mean Pro-Kevorkian?" p. 842. His analysis is that within limits the state may constitutionally do that. The state may not reallocate rights from one person to another, as in the cases attempting to compel organ donation. But it may "sacrifice . . . the suffering of one for the aggregate good of the whole." P. 848. This relates to the applicable standard for evaluating a ban, which I discuss above in text.

114. See, e.g., *Cruzan*, 497 U.S. at 271.

115. Even using RU–486 or Methotrexate requires a prescription, medical supervision, and visits to the doctor. See, e.g., Julie Chao, "Doctors Trained in S.F. on Drug to Abort; Workshops Present Research on New Nonsurgical Process Available Soon," *San Francisco Examiner,* April 1, 1996, p. A-4; Marion Asnes, "RU–486: What You Don't Know; Medical Complications," *Working Woman* 19 (November 1994): 73. However, there are growing efforts to allow nonphysicians to perform at least some abortions. See, e.g., Chao, "Doctors Trained in S.F."; Rebecca Dresser, "What Bioethics Can Learn from the Women's Health Movement," in Wolf, ed., *Feminism and Bioethics,* p. 156; Diane Curtis, "Doctored Rights: Menstrual Extraction, Self-Help Gynecological Care, and the Law," *New York University Review of Law and Social Change* 20 (1993–94): 427–69; Janet Benshoof, "*Planned Parenthood v. Casey*: The Impact of the New Undue Burden Standard on Reproductive Health Care," *Journal of the American Medical Association* 269 (1993): 2249.

116. See Wolf, "Gender, Feminism, and Death," pp. 301, 307; Edmund D. Pellegrino, "The Place of Intention in the Moral Assessment of Assisted Suicide and Active Euthanasia," in Tom L. Beauchamp, ed., *Intending Death: The Ethics of Assisted Suicide and Euthanasia* (Upper Saddle River, N.J.: Prentice Hall, 1996), pp. 163–83; Daniel Callahan and Margot White, "The Legalization of Physician-Assisted Suicide: Creating a Regulatory Potemkin Village," *University of Richmond Law Review* 30 (1996): 1–83, 66–67; Leon R. Kass, "Neither for Love nor Money: Why Doctors Must Not Kill," *Public Interest* 94 (Winter 1989): 25–46; Wolf, "Holding the Line on Euthanasia"; Willard Gaylin et al., "'Doctors Must Not Kill,'" *Journal of the American Medical Association* 259 (1988): 2139–40.

117. See 79 F.3d at 827–28.

118. See Council on Ethical and Judicial Affairs, American Medical Association, "Gender Disparities in Clinical Decision Making."

119. Kreimer shares this expectation but then uses it to suggest that prohibiting assisted suicide burdens women more than men. Kreimer, "Does Pro-Choice Mean Pro-Kevorkian?" p. 850 n.170. But the question for my purposes is whether the state has a greater interest in making sure that persisting sexism and gender

inequities are not enacted in the differential deaths of women through assisted suicide, or in ensuring that women have equal access to the means of suicide. In addition to arguing that the former is the weightier interest, I know of no support for the proposition that ensuring anyone's access to suicide or even equal access is a recognized state interest at all.

120. See also Wolf, "Gender, Feminism, and Death."

121. I am grateful to Robert Burt for provoking this insight.

122. See generally Dorothy E. Roberts, "Reconstructing the Patient: Starting with Women of Color," in Wolf, ed., *Feminism and Bioethics,* pp. 116–43.

123. See Peter Steinfels, "Help for the Helping Hands in Death," *New York Times,* February 14, 1993, sec. 4, pp. 1, 6.

124. See, e.g., Catharine A. MacKinnon, *Feminism Unmodified: Discourses on Life and Law* (Cambridge, Mass.: Harvard University Press, 1987), p. 42.

125. See, e.g., Judith Lorber, *Paradoxes of Gender* (New Haven, Conn.: Yale University Press, 1994); Judith Butler, *Bodies That Matter: On the Discursive Limits of "Sex"* (New York: Routledge, 1993); Judith Butler, *Gender Trouble: Feminism and the Subversion of Identity* (New York: Routledge, 1990).

126. For discussion of the gendering or feminization of people as part of an effort to subordinate them, see, e.g., Nikolaus Benke, "Women in the Courts: An Old Thorn in Men's Sides," *Michigan Journal of Gender and Law* 3 (1995): 195–256, 244–50 (discussing the oppression of men by "feminizing" them, a "process . . . [in] which men are subjected to gender rules originally developed for and connected with women"; "discrimination against male homosexuals . . . reveals that gender, although based on sex and manifoldly related to sex, is not restricted to a specific sex" [footnotes omitted]); Mary Anne C. Case, "Disaggregating Gender from Sex and Sexual Orientation: The Effeminate Man in the Law and Feminist Jurisprudence," *Yale Law Journal* 105 (1995): 1–105, 34 (discussing "discrimination against all persons, male or female, who display feminine characteristics or who lack masculine ones"); Francisco Valdes, "Queers, Sissies, Dykes, and Tomboys: Deconstructing the Conflation of 'Sex,' 'Gender,' and 'Sexual Orientation' in Euro-American Law and Society," *California Law Review* 83 (1995): 1–377, 266–70 (feminization of gay men as a means of preserving male heterosexual privilege; persons associated with qualities seen as "female" or "feminine" devalued); Brande Stellings, Note, "The Public Harm of Private Violence: Rape, Sex Discrimination and Citizenship," *Harvard Civil Rights–Civil Liberties Law Review* 28 (1993): 185–216, 188–89, 196 (rape is a system of subordination; in prison rape, men often "feminize" their male victims, redefining the victim as a woman); Marc A. Fajer, "Can Two Real Men Eat Quiche Together? Storytelling, Gender-Role Stereotypes, and Legal Protection for Lesbians and Gay Men," *University of Miami Law Review* 46 (1992): 511–651, 621–23 (male homosexuals perceived as having lost their masculinity and "discriminat[ed] against . . . in a way that mirrors discrimination against women"); MacKinnon, *Feminism Unmodified,* p. 56 (rape of men by men as an act of male dominance through which the victim is feminized).

127. The Fifteenth Amendment did not secure the right to vote for all male citizens regardless of "race, color, or previous condition of servitude" until 1870,

thus postdating the original Constitution by the better part of a century. The Nineteenth Amendment did not secure the franchise for women until fifty years later, in 1920. See generally Catharine A. MacKinnon, "Reflections on Sex Equality under Law," *Yale Law Journal* 100 (1991): 1281–1328, 1281–83 & nn.2, 9. For a glimpse of the long discussion of the Constitution as a proslavery document, see, e.g., Robert M. Cover, *Justice Accused: Antislavery and the Judicial Process* (New Haven, Conn.: Yale University Press, 1975), pp. 151–52, 209.

128. See Uwe E. Reinhardt, "Reforming the Health Care System: The Universal Dilemma," *American Journal of Law and Medicine* 19 (1993): 21–36, 30.

Part V

Public Policy Options
and Recommendations

9

CONSIDERATIONS OF SAFEGUARDS PROPOSED IN LAWS AND GUIDE-LINES TO LEGALIZE ASSISTED SUICIDE

Steven Miles, M.D., Demetra M. Pappas. J.D., M.Sc., and Robert Koepp, M.A.

European and North American nations have been considering changing the law and public policy with regard to voluntary active euthanasia, physician- (or medically) assisted suicide, and euthanasia by advance directive with increasing frequency and creativity. Bills, acts, and referenda have been proposed, passed, challenged, enjoined. Doctors and lay interest groups have filed suits in civil court and invited criminal prosecution for assisting in the deaths of consenting and requesting patients. Members of the legislature and the judiciary are now in the midst of political and judicial activism precipitated by medical practitioners and by patients and groups acting for or reacting against medically assisted death.

A week in the debate of the right to assisted death yields the following. On March 6, 1996, the United States Court for the Ninth Circuit, *en banc*, held, in the strongest possible terms, that persons have a constitutionally protected liberty interest with regard to choosing the time and manner of their death. They also held that the provision of the Washington statute banning assisted suicide, as applied to competent, terminally ill adults who wish to hasten their deaths by obtaining medication prescribed by their doctors, violates the due process clause of the United States Constitution.[1] In a footnote to this part of the holding, the court proclaimed, "[w]e would add that those whose services are essential to help the terminally ill patient obtain and take that medication and who act under the supervision or direction of a physician *are necessarily covered by our ruling.*"[2]

The following day, lawyers for Dr. Jack Kevorkian, on trial in Michigan for two charges of assisting in the suicide of "patients," argued for a trial order to dismiss charges based upon the Ninth Circuit ruling. The trial court denied the motion for lack of jurisdiction. The jury then acquitted Dr. Kevorkian in eight and one-half hours. The defense upon which the acquittal was based was an exceptional clause in the temporary statute that had made it a felony to assist in a suicide; it said that "a person is not guilty of criminal assistance of suicide if that person was administering medications or procedures with the intent to relieve pain and discomfort and not to cause death," regardless of whether the treatment "may hasten or increase the risk of death."[3] This "double effect" exception enabled Dr. Kevorkian to successfully propose that his administration of carbon monoxide, a substance without painkilling or palliative properties other than by causing death, relieved pain and thus relieved the patient's suffering. Dr. Kevorkian was still to be tried in Michigan for two assisted suicides under a theory of common law felony.[4]

Moving farther east, the United States Court of Appeals for the Second Circuit, a federal court with equal power and prestige to the Ninth Circuit, issued a decision in *Quill v. Vacco,* No. 95-7028 (2d Cir.), on April 2, 1996, less than a month after the Ninth Circuit *en banc* decision. This case was brought by (among others) Dr. Timothy Quill, a respected hospice physician, who invited prosecution by publishing an account of how he assisted the suicide of one of his patients with cancer. He is a co-author of one of the proposals for regulating assisted suicide that we will be examining. The Second Circuit majority held that New York statutes criminalizing assisted suicide violate the Equal Protection Clause of the Constitution "[b]ecause to the extent that they prohibit a physician from prescribing medications to be self-administered by a mentally competent, terminally ill person in the final stages of his terminal illness, they are not rationally related to any legitimate state interests." The Second Circuit Court thereby reversed the federal district court that had expressly held that terminally ill competent adult patients do *not* have any fundamental substantive due process right to physician-assisted suicide (PAS) and that New York statutes prohibiting assisted suicide (though permitting terminally ill patients to reject life-sustaining treatment) do not violate the Equal Protection Clause of the Constitution.[5]

The various judges speaking for the majority and dissents in the Second and Ninth Circuit Courts and lower court proceedings merit more analysis than is possible in this chapter. There are differences in whether there is a right to assisted suicide, the grounding of that right, the state's interest in preventing assisted suicide, and the state's due process interests that might support broad access to suicide or be a foundation for encumbering the exercise of the right in order to ensure that the interests of others, such as vulnerable adults who might be endangered by the legalization of assisted suicide, are protected.

With regard to due process issues, for example, the Second Circuit Court majority declined to find any "cognizable basis in the Constitution's language or design" which would permit *any* due process right to be asserted on behalf of competent persons in the final stages of terminal illness who seek to hasten death. This view, that the issue is purely and simply a matter of whether there is a "right" to assisted suicide, ironically coincides with Judge Beezer's dissent in the Ninth Circuit in which he stated simply and directly that no fundamental right to commit assisted suicide existed. Second Circuit Judge Calabresi, who concurred with the majority opinion, observed that the "Ninth Circuit recognized that equal protection arguments for invalidity were 'not insubstantial'" but that they were not argued in terms of the court's view of due process. He went on to cite a "long tradition of constitutional holding that inertia will not do," to conclude that "New York's prohibitions on assisted suicide violate both the Equal Protection and the Due Process clauses of the Fourteenth amendment . . . to the extent that these laws are interpreted to prohibit a physician from prescribing lethal drugs to be self administered by a mentally competent, terminally ill person in the final stage of that illness."

In short, while the Second and Ninth Circuit Courts agree on the result of striking down statutes on assisted suicide, they do not agree on the rationale for this result. The added diversity of the lower court rulings and the heterogeneity of state legal positions (exemplified by Michigan's prosecution of Dr. Kevorkian) is an additional invitation to the Supreme Court to attempt to resolve the variously defined rights, define crimes in parallel to those rights, and erect a framework for statutes and policy that will evolve from these events.

A variety of models have been proposed for new laws or guidelines, primarily for PAS but also for voluntary active euthanasia (VAE). Given law and current policy against assisted suicide, the primary, innovative objective of PAS model guidelines or laws is to secure legal sanction for a health care provider who complies with a patient's request for assistance with suicide. Secondarily, these models propose safeguards that are intended to prevent misuse of PAS or VAE. This chapter focuses on safeguards that are proposed in some of the current models rather than on the arguments for and against legalization of PAS or VAE. Our critique focuses on (1) the Oregon Death with

Dignity Act (Measure 16),[6] (2) the Rights of the Terminally Ill Bill in the Northern Territory of Australia, and (3) the model proposed by Miller, Quill, Brody, Fletcher, Gostin, and Meier.[7]

We will consider whether the safeguards on PAS/VAE contained in these models justify a more inquiring discussion about the grounding and implications of this kind of legislation. We are concerned that these proposals to decriminalize, legalize, or regulate PAS contain novel features—intended to safeguard and enhance respect for patient autonomy—that may ironically undermine rather than underwrite that goal. While expressing a goal of safeguarding the practice of PAS to prevent the abuse or coercion of vulnerable, discouraged, or decisionally incapacitated persons, the safeguards may lay the foundation for far-reaching restrictions on personal autonomy vis-à-vis professional authority (i.e., enhance medical paternalism). We also fear that they could result in a societal scrutiny of personal motivations with regard to controversial medical decisions. They might well support new social controls rather than the exercise of rights by or on behalf of disabled persons.

A Brief Review of Public Policy on Suicide

We use these definitions of VAE, PAS, and advance directives:

• *Voluntary active euthanasia* refers to cases where there is a direct and positive act by a physician that is intended to cause the death of a patient who has said that s/he wants to die. A compelling example of this scenario would be a terminally ill cancer patient who requests and receives a lethal injection administered by the physician with the intent to kill rather than to have a palliative effect without causing death. Such an act, performed actively by the physician, would be a clear case of euthanasia.

• *Physician-assisted suicide* is a different scenario. First, as a legal matter, the patient is the principal, whereas the doctor is the "accessory." In cases of assisted suicide, the principal is the decedent (patient), i.e., the person who commits the ultimate act leading to death, while the doctor is an assistant or facilitator—most frequently by providing the means and opportunity. In the trial of *People v. Kevorkian* (the Frederick and Khalili assisted suicides), the definition issued by the court, consistent with the Michigan law prohibiting assisted suicide, was that Dr. Kevorkian would be guilty under the law if he had knowledge that the person intended to commit suicide and either provided the means or by virtue of a physical act assisted in their suicides, unless the purpose of the dispensed drugs was to relieve pain or discomfort without intent to cause death, even if death were to be hastened (by the carbon monoxide provided).[8] Assisted suicide cases, unlike those of euthanasia, thus entail the prescribing, dispensing, and instructing in the use of a lethal agent, rather than (for example) injection by the physician as is the case with euthanasia. A doctor who prescribes a lethal amount of barbiturates to a terminally or chronically ill patient who then self-administers serves as the paradigmatic example here.

•An *advanced directive* for voluntary active euthanasia would en- compass the situation in which an individual who is neither decisionally incapacitated nor wanting assisted suicide or euthanasia at the time when the advance directive is executed, but who directs that s/he be euthanized under specified circumstances of suffering if s/he were to become decisionally incapacitated. This might include, for example, a person who knows that s/he has genetic or preclinical markers for Huntington's disease and thus who expects with certainty (barring a premature death by accident, for example) to become psychotic, spastic, demented, and suffer a complete and irrevocable loss of mental and physical capacities before dying of infections. Such a patient could reasonably anticipate that s/he would become incompetent and disabled after onset and thus be excluded from the current statutory models for either PAS or VAE.

Although euthanasia and suicide have long been the topic of moral debate, the questions of decriminalization, legalization, and regulation of medically assisted death is a more recent debate. The specific debate about PAS has been a phenomenon of the latter part of this century and rampant since 1990, when Dr. Kevorkian and Dr. Quill publicly invited prosecution.

The early debate focused on the principle of the sanctity of life, a concept, as articulated by John Locke, whereby a human life is the property not of the person living that life, who is simply a tenant, but of God. To commit suicide is therefore a theft from society and an insult to God. From this is derived the fundamental tenet of every Western society and system of law that it is supremely wrong to intentionally (or recklessly or negligently) kill another human being. Thus, just as tort law and criminal law refuse to recognize a "right" to allow one to consent to enslavement or mutilation, neither does the law allow a consent to one's murder.[9] It is this axiom that advocates of personal autonomy battle most vigorously, even while allowing that, ordinarily, one cannot consent to one's own murder. Judeo-Christian thought has always allowed certain exceptions to this. Norman St. John-Stevas, writing against voluntary active euthanasia and suicide, commented in

Life, Death and the Law: A Study of the Relationship between Law and Christian Morals in the English and American Legal Systems[10] that these include divine inspiration, execution of a just death penalty, and altruistic suicide. Conclusions favoring and condemning suicidal and self-martyring acts have long rested upon diverse and complex theological, familial, and national senses of duty and virtue.

Over the past century, law decriminalized both suicide and its attempt. Prior to this shift, the crime of suicide (i.e., self-murder), like the crime of murder, was punishable by forfeiture of the assailant's (in suicide, decedent's) property to the Crown or state. In addition, those who died by suicide were not permitted to be buried on consecrated ground. These forfeitures came to be viewed as an inappropriate and unduly harsh punishment of the family of the person who had committed suicide. Finally, suicide attempts came to be viewed as incompetent, and therefore not culpable, decisions. In this perspective, it was cruel to punish acts motivated by suffering, and an abuse of civic authority to punish this self-harming conduct, however theologically damnable.

This decriminalization of suicide, commencing at the turn of the nineteenth century, was not the same as legalization. Anglo-American law (applicable in most states and in the United Kingdom) continued to hold those who assisted in a suicide subject to criminal liability, while those who attempted suicide were only subject to civil psychiatric commitment. As Judge Beezer correctly observes in his dissenting opinion in the *en banc* Ninth Circuit case, "[t]he modern consensus consists of an overall disapproval of suicide which is manifested through (1) not criminally punishing the suicide itself, but instead treating it as a medical or psychological problem, (2) allowing the state to intervene to prevent someone from committing suicide and (3) enacting criminal statutes prohibiting the aiding or assisting of suicide."[11]

The most recent stage of the debate regarding whether to decriminalize or to legalize providing lethal assistance to persons who want to receive euthanasia or assistance in committing suicide, has also come into prominence during the late nineteenth and twentieth century. It is too soon, being now in the midst of this debate, to write the full history of the dramatic rise and final outcome of the PAS/VAE debate. In part, the immense increase in longevity, the lack of adequate means of financing health care, and the problem of maintaining four- or five-generation family structures play a role. The increased prevalence of degenerative diseases also plays a role.[12] Widespread distrust in medical paternalism, a correct public perception of the inadequacy of palliative medicine at the end of life, and a largely erroneous belief that end-of-life care consists in the relentless overuse of medical technology also play a role. Finally, the articulation and successful implementation of an autonomy and privacy-based "right to die" with regard to the right to refuse life-sustaining medical treatment, and the demand that health professionals stop or disconnect such treatments, also forms part of the conceptual foundation for a right to medical assistance with an already decriminalized suicide.[13]

Those who support legalizing assisted suicide given the foregoing decriminalization of suicide claim that prohibiting assistance is an arbitrary barrier on the exercise of personal choice given social support for autonomous decisions to forgo life-sustaining treatment.[14] They further argue that physicians are forced into a position where their patients are in intractable pain and discomfort, and the physicians who treat them are disempowered and legally rendered passive.[15] Finally they claim that the failure to legalize assistance to suicide, given that suicide itself is not illegal, creates inequitable barriers to properly supported, effective, painless suicide.

The resolution in favor of decriminalizing the act of committing suicide is therefore historically, legally, and conceptually distinct from the recent proposal to legalize assisting suicide. On the one hand, it does not necessarily follow that decriminalizing the act of suicide means that assistance should therefore be legalized and/or regulated. Nor does a conclusion favoring decriminalizing assistance of itself say anything about the feasibility, design, or salutary implications of such legislation for the practice of assisted suicide or for other areas of health law. On the other hand, it is ordinarily not possible to be criminally liable for aiding and abetting in a non-crime, particularly given the legislative and moral historical reasons for decriminalizing suicide.

In this regard, we acknowledge the contrast between the "Dutch compromise" and the "Michigan paladin." In the Netherlands, euthanasia and assisted suicide are still technically crimes; the policy prohibits the general act but requires reporting—without punishment—specific instances, with cases serving as educational rather than exemplary vehicles. Thus, while compassion, understanding, and even respect for cases of "exceptional circumstances" are now typified, we do not find that the Netherlands generally condones or approves of classes of suicide by the provision of formal channels (legal or medical mechanisms) for assistance. A reverse situation is seen in Michigan. The Kevorkian cases are about de facto decriminalization in the setting of de jure criminalization. Dr. Kevorkian is widely perceived as being not convictable (even by the authorities prosecuting him for assisted suicide or related homicide charges), though he has been stripped of his medical licenses. Thus, opposite to the Dutch compromise, attempts to punish the specific instances in Michigan have failed even where there is widespread support to cease to prohibit the general.[16]

The failure to imagine a workable regulatory framework for a Dr. Kevorkian justifies concern about the safeguards for legalized PAS/VAE. This fear of an insufficiently safeguarded practice of PAS or VAE most pointedly applies to concerns that legalizing these practices would especially endanger stigmatized, vulnerable, or costly-to-care-for persons. Judge Noonan, in the first Ninth Circuit decision, expressly noted in his writing in *Compassion in Dying v. Washington*[17] that a state's interests in protecting the elderly, the infirm, the poor, the handicapped, and minorities from a premature and avoidable death, from exploitation, and from the structural pressure to prematurely end their lives which would arise from allowing PAS are profound and weighty. This was wholeheartedly embraced by Judge Beezer in a section of his dissent from the *en banc* majority, which he entitled "The Protection of the Interests of Innocent Third Parties."

PAS/VAE Safeguards That Limit Autonomy

None of the current guidelines or laws to legalize PAS or VAE support a universal, unqualified, autonomy-based right to secure assistance in the choice to die. Instead, they propose three kinds of qualifications that limit personal autonomy. First, the choice must be *authentic,* meaning that the would-be decedent's decision for PAS or VAE must be carefully considered, informed, rational, and mature. Second, the authenticity of the choice must be confirmed by the *ability* of a would-be decedent to directly and contemporaneously participate in the self-administration of the lethal substance(s). Third, the would-be decedent must have a *qualifying rationale.* The way by which the proposed models design or employ these qualifications to restrict access to PAS or VAE is to varying degrees unique and novel public policy. For this reason, the foundation of, the rationale for, and the potential implications arising from those restrictions merits scrutiny.

Authentic Decisions

The right to receive assistance after making a decision to commit suicide belongs to persons who can make an authentic choice. The various proposals require these individuals to be adults who are psychiatrically and cognitively able to make informed and uncoerced decisions. The right is not extended to minors, who are deemed incompetent on the basis of their status as presumed immature individuals.

Individuals with psychiatric or cognitive disorders that impair decisional capacity are not allowed to exercise the right to choose PAS. Those who are found to be un- or insufficiently informed or who are implicitly or explicitly coerced are also to be excluded.

In the models we review, each of the restrictions on responses to a request for PAS or VAE purports to promote respect for autonomous choices while safeguarding those who are incapable of making autonomous choices in such a grave matter. We believe that in both regards, they could undermine the rights of persons whose autonomy should be promoted and are inadequate to protect those whose capacity for an authentic choice is impaired. For this reason, this aspect of these policies should be further considered and defined in terms that are clinically usable and with anticipated exceptions delineated and justified.

First, though there is no clear agreement regarding the border between a psychiatrically or cognitively qualified request for assisted suicide from a nonqualifying or disabled one, current proposals regarding safeguards in PAS laws assert or presume that such a border is either generally known or axiomatically accepted. No significant professional organization has expressly defined the boundary between such psychocognitively capable and incapable suicides, and some have vigorously argued that this distinction should either be rejected or used cautiously in view of problems regarding the feasibility of making it precise.[18] It should be noted, however, that the capacities generally recognized as relevant to determining competence (although the terms are frequently used interchangeably) are (1) possession of a set of values and goals, (2) the ability to communicate and understand information, and (3) the ability to reason and to deliberate about one's choices.[19]

> Oregon's Measure 16 Section 1.01(6) not only presumes that such a distinction can be made but asserts that it can be dichotomously made, i.e., patients are either defined as incapable or capable. "Incapable" under the Oregon Death with Dignity Act "means that in the opinion of a court *or* in the opinion of the patient's attending physician *or* consulting physician, a patient lacks the ability to make *and* communicate health care decisions to health care providers, including communications through persons familiar with the patient's manner of communicating if those persons are available. "Capable" according to Measure 16 Section 1.01(6), simply "means not incapable."
>
> Similarly, the model guidelines put forth by Miller and his co-authors, while stating that "an acceptable policy of legalized physician-assisted death . . . is used as a treatment of last resort in response to the voluntary

requests of competent patients who are suffering from terminal or incurable illnesses,"[20] proclaims that "[i]n order to ensure that physician-assisted death is voluntary, which is the inviolable cornerstone of this policy, only adults with decision-making capacity should be eligible for physician-assisted death."[21] However, while enumerating requirements regarding written or oral witnessed consent, reporting procedures, and sanctions, capacity itself is left undefined for these purposes.

Similarly, the Rights of the Terminally Ill Bill in northern Australia issues a broad safeguard in Part II, 7 (h), stating that the medical practitioner must be "satisfied, on reasonable grounds, that the patient is of sound mind and that the patient's decision to end his or her life has been made freely, voluntarily and after due consideration."

The fact that there is no empirical foundation for the assertion in its most extreme form (as in the Oregon statute) has three significant implications with regard to the regulation of PAS. First, it significantly weakens the law's ability to define the difference between PAS and a coerced homicide. Second, the misleading presence of a safeguard for which there is no empirical foundation conceals the lack of an appropriate safeguard for the very class of abuses that this provision is intended to protect against. As Chochinov et al. put it, "[o]f all the issues that must be factored into the euthanasia [and assisted suicide] debate, psychiatric considerations are likely to be among the most controversial."[22] Third, the outright restriction of PAS/VAE to adults (Oregon's Measure 16; Section 1.01(1) and Section 2.01) is an exception to other relevant health laws and right-to-die statutes and precedents permitting life or death medical decisions to be exercised on an immature minor's behalf by parents or by mature minors themselves. Neither are there criteria or legal procedures proposed to review requests for PAS that are made by mature minors. Australia's legislation is also silent on this point.

None of the existing laws or proposals for PAS offers a cogent rationale for restricting this legislatively (or, in the Second and Ninth Circuits, judicially) created right to persons over eighteen years of age. This ungrounded and therefore fictive safeguard is obviously politically desirable with regard to the law's proponents' goal of legalizing PAS, but it has several adverse consequences. First, it fails to anticipate clinical situations which may arise with those minors who have terminal illness and intractable pain and who are incapable of having any redeeming experience with their pain that would make them want to continue to live. Second, there are minors with sophisticated understandings of their own mortality and impending death that would surely make them capable of discussing and perhaps choosing PAS or

VAE. Third, given the established right of children to be as eligible for withdrawal of life support as adults and the developing foundational analogies between the right to forgo life-sustaining treatment and the right to determine the time and manner of one's death, the absence of policy provisions addressing children opens the door to successful litigation on behalf of minors even as it conceals the lack of a thoughtfully conceived set of safeguards for this practice of PAS/VAE on children.

Autonomy and the Hurdle of Physical Ability

The right to be free from unwanted life-sustaining treatment, as articulated in *Cruzan v. Director, Missouri Department of Health*[23] and Anglo-American right-to-die law, which largely developed in cases about the care of incompetent persons, has strongly affirmed that the rights of all persons, competent and incompetent, physically disabled and nondisabled, are the same. Yet the U.S. preference for PAS embodies a striking exception to this tradition of equitable respect for autonomy because policy models that permit PAS, but not VAE, create barriers to the exercise of a right by physically disabled persons.

> The Oregon Death with Dignity Act restricts PAS to persons who are capable of executing a "written request for medication for the purpose of ending [the patient's] life in a humane and dignified manner. Presumably Oregon's decision to legalize PAS, as opposed to VAE, is that PAS imposes the safeguard of having the patient finally ratify his or her intent to take the lethal drug by self-administering it, rather than have it administered to them by a possibly coercive other. As of this date, the Ninth Circuit's *en banc* decision in *Compassion in Dying v. State of Washington* appears to allow for permissiveness not only in actors, but also in *actions*.
>
> The Australian act allows for both PAS and VAE and thus, by permitting VAE, allows for medical assistance with suicide for persons who are too physically disabled to perform the patients' roles of self-administration of a lethal substance as would be required in PAS.

No policy models allow for advance directives, substituted judgment, or best interests standards for decision making on behalf of decisionally incapable persons that could apply to medical aid to end life. Such advance directives would be helpful for persons with strong views who do not wish to avail themselves of PAS at a point in time when they are capable of making a decision about PAS and communicating that decision by creating an advance directive but who do want assistance in ending their life at some future time and circumstance when their decisional abilities are lost. By not permitting advance directives, and by further restricting the legalization of medically administered death to PAS or even VAE, the policy models presume an inequality of rights on the part of decisionally capable and incapable persons.

Considered together, the twin safeguards currently being proposed in U.S. law (legalizing PAS but not VAE, and the ban on advance directives) are designed to assure that assistance with suicide is only given to persons who contemporaneously affirm and physically confirm their decision to use assistance to die. Either may improve the ability to assess the authenticity of a physically capable and competent person's decision to die. But both do so in a manner that discriminatorily restrict who may exercise the recognized personal liberty that is the premise of this legislation. The physically disabled are thus discriminated against per se. The ban on noncontemporaneously expressed preferences postulates that decisionally capable persons have greater rights than incapable persons. This latter proposal contradicts two decades of bioethics writings, court rulings, and statutes regarding medical decision making, advance directives, and the closely related and equally consequential right to forgo life-sustaining treatment.

Neither safeguard comports with the conventionally understood "burdens of proof" that may be required as evidence of what a person's decision is with regard to the exercise of a fundamental personal right. The measures of "burden of proof" in these proposals are entirely unlike the usage of "preponderance of the evidence," "clear and convincing," or "beyond a reasonable doubt" by various jurisdictions to weigh evidence of a patient's intent to exercise a right to significant health care decisions in end-of-life medical care. What appears to be left is a standard of "physical ability to express." Such a testing of physical ability with regard to the expression of a fundamental right (at least according the Ninth Circuit *en banc*) is unlikely to pass constitutional muster in terms of due process or equal protection and fails to comport with either common law precedent or the Americans with Disabilities Act. In terms of ethics, these safeguards against coercion break with the notion of respect for autonomy as defined over the last twenty years. We predict that a law founded upon such safeguards will be rejected in view of the combined effect of the right to refuse unwanted medical treatment set forth in *Cruzan* and the "undue burden on the exercise of a constitutionally protected liberty interest," the standard espoused in *Planned Parenthood of Southeastern Pennsylvania v. Casey*.[24] In this way, the weakly grounded statutory distinction between PAS and VAE may invite the rapid judicial extension from PAS to VAE and thus destroy a safeguard that was presumably deemed necessary as assisted suicide was legalized.

Resurgent Medical Paternalism

A third set of novel features of PAS proposals is that they give physicians a new extrajudicial authority to deny assistance to suicide to legally competent persons by declaring them decisionally incapable without any recourse or appeal.

> Section 3.01(1) of Measure 16 says that the attending physician shall make the initial determination of whether a patient has a terminal disease, is capable and "has made the request voluntarily." If the attending physician or a consulting physician concludes, in accordance with Section 3.03, that a patient "*may* be suffering from a psychiatric or psychological disorder, or depression causing impaired judgment, either physician *shall* refer the patient for counseling. No medication to end a patient's life in a humane and dignified manner *shall* be prescribed until *the person performing the counseling* determines that the person is not suffering from a psychiatric or psychological disorder, or depression causing impaired judgment" (emphasis added).
>
> This concept is also embraced (more briefly) by the northern Australia legislation, in Part II:7(1)(h) as discussed earlier. However, a recent article by two Australian doctors stated that the Oregon provision did not go far enough (notwithstanding mandatory language), and that "requiring a psychiatric consultation is an essential safeguard."[25]

The trend in bioethics and mental health law has been against giving physicians extrajudicial power to overrule fundamentally personal choices by declaring patients to be incompetent to make them. The provisions in PAS laws that physicians assume such powers are a striking reversal of existing public policy which presumes patients to be competent to make decisions, including potentially self-harming medical and life-style choices, unless and until a patient is declared incompetent pursuant to a legal procedure. Emergency commitment procedures give physicians at most seventy-two hours to unilaterally suspend a competent person's rights to make decisions about their medical care, in stark contrast to the Oregon and Australia provisions, each of which allows physicians to declare patients incompetent in these decisions for an indefinite period. The ill-defined scope of this medical prerogative, the lack of an empirical foundation to distinguish rational suicide from psychiatrically impaired requests (see above), the lack of defined rights or due processes for appeals, and the lack of sanctions for abuse in the exercise of this powerful clinical prerogative are all extremely unusual, and cause for concern, and have disturbing implications for health law should they spread to other controversial medical decisions.

Assistance Restricted to Properly Motivated Requests for Suicide

A fourth set of novel restrictions on patient autonomy is the use of condition-specific restrictions on the right of a person to exercise a fundamental personal right.

Oregon Measure 16 in Section 1.01(12), defines terminally ill (and therefore within the ambit of a proper request for assisted suicide) as "an incurable and irreversible disease that has been medically confirmed and will, within reasonable medical judgment, produce death within six (6) months." In contrast to the physical ability to participate in PAS that is used to confirm the authenticity of the request, as discussed below, this restriction explicitly limits those who "*may* initiate a written request for medication" to aid in dying under Section 2.01. and thereby excludes persons who are not terminally ill.

The Australian Rights of the Terminally Ill Act is similar in restricting the right to VAE even if it is both more and less stringent as to whose rights are restricted. Under Section 3, "illness" "includes injury *or* degeneration of mental *or* physical faculties," and goes on to provide that "terminal illness" refers to "an illness which, in reasonable medical judgment will, in the normal course, without the application of extraordinary measures or of treatment unacceptable to the patient, result in the death of the patient." However, Part 2, Section 4, requires the "request for assistance to voluntary [*sic*] terminate life," to be made by "a patient who, in the course of a terminal illness, is experiencing pain, suffering, and/or distress to an extent unacceptable to the patient [who then] may request the patient's medical practitioner to assist the patient to terminate the patient's life." The Australia act also provides in Section 8 that a medical practitioner "shall not" assist the patient if, "in his or her opinion, and after considering the advice of the medical practitioner referred to in section 7(1)(c), there are palliative care options reasonably available to the patient to alleviate the patient's pain and suffering to levels acceptable to the patient." Thus the time frames are more expansive but the threshold of the degree of illness more seemingly restrictive, in that it appears to limit the right to medical aid in dying to a terminal illness "plus" standard.

The Miller and Quill proposal accepts terminal and nonimminently terminal but incurable illnesses (they cite ALS as one example) as "eligible" for PAS. They also propose that "an acceptable policy of legalized physician-assisted death must include independent monitoring to ensure that it is used *only as a treatment of last resort* in response to the voluntary requests of competent patients who are suffering from terminal or incurable illnesses."[26] They state that their "liberalized, inclusive policy with respect to these issues [is meant to reflect that] the method chosen is less important than the careful assessment that precedes assisted death."[27]

As a matter of public policy, these restrictions are novel in that the right to refuse life-sustaining treatment, or indeed to consent to (or refuse) any other medical treatment, is nowhere else contingent on terminal illness, proximity to death, or reversibility. The fundamental basis for (or support of) these restrictions on the exercise of a personal right is thus unclear given the existing framework of autonomy-based respect for patient's views on medical futility, indications for unproven and emerging therapies, and the right to refuse treatment. They would restrict the personal rights of persons with early Alzheimer disease, HIV infection, or paraplegia. One might well argue that the state is here attempting to define the "acceptable indications" for the provisions of medical treatment and that this substantively differs from an unqualified right to be free of intrusive life-sustaining treatment. However, a strong counterargument is needed as to why the state can and should be involved in defining the indications for, or legitimate access to, such treatment, given its reluctance to assert the indications for other medical treatments such as respirators or bone marrow transplants.

Physician Credentials

With the exception of the northern Australia law, the proposals for PAS do not describe the clinical skills that should be expected or required for physicians who review the capacities or decisions of patients, who counsel patients about alternatives to PAS/VAE,[28] or who engage in the clinical practice of prescribing or administering medications for assisting suicide or practicing VAE.[29-30] Without such safeguards, the proposals seem to implicitly hold that the skills for this novel clinical encounter either are indistinguishable from those held by the average practitioner, or that the physician's skills are primarily those of a morally neutral and psychiatrically untrained "technician."[31] Pathologist Dr. Kevorkian, who never practiced clinical medicine after his residency, is the paradigmatic technician of death who would be qualified to practice under these laws.

Oregon's Measure 16 does not define the expertise, training, or supervision of physicians with regard to the practice of PAS. The juxtaposition of Sections 4.01(3) (immunities regarding an "attending physician" who prescribes medication in "good faith") and 4.02(3) ("nothing in this Act limits further liability for civil damages resulting from other negligent conduct or intentional misconduct by any persons") and 4.02(4) ("the penalties in this Act do not preclude criminal penalties applicable under other laws for conduct which is inconsistent with the provisions of this Act"), appears to protect from unprofessional practice but does not say what *is* required of doctors for this new kind of clinical act.

Miller et al., in their proposal, suggest that "[i]n order to institute effective consultation, new programs for the training and certification of palliative-care consultants would need to be developed and implemented [but w]e do not envision the creation of a new medical specialty . . . [in] the creation and enforcement of this vital safeguard in the proposed policy of legalized physician-assisted death."[32]

Northern Australia's Rights of the Terminally Ill Bill attempts to describe the qualifications of physicians in Part 2—Request for and Giving of Assistance. The pertinent part, Section 7 regarding "Conditions under which medical practitioner may assist," provides (3) "Where a patient's medical practitioner has no special qualifications in the field of palliative care the information to be provided to the patient on the availability of palliative care shall be given by a medical practitioner (who may be the practitioner referred to in subsection (1) (c)[second medical opinion] or any other medical practitioner) who has such special qualifications in the field of palliative care as are prescribed." The act also states, in Section 2 (2), "[i]n assisting a patient under this Act, a medical practitioner shall be guided by appropriate medical standards and such guidelines, if any, as are prescribed, and shall consider the appropriate pharmaceutical information about any substance reasonably available for use in the circumstances."

Conclusion

Doctors who engage in medical aid in dying, whether voluntary active euthanasia or assisted suicide, walk in the shadow of the law for the most part. There has long been a silent, secret practice without any governmentally or publicly approved criteria, safeguards, or mechanisms for accountability. The United States seems to be on the verge of explicitly legalizing the practice of medically assisted death. Our concern with the safeguards in the existing proposals for PAS is not meant as an endorsement of unregulated practice. Rather, it is our concern that once the medical profession is empowered to engage in a "treatment" whose central purpose is to cause death, we depart from the standards of the profession.

There is a great deal at stake in the regulatory framework for PAS or VAE. First, there is the social permission for the newly declared right. Second, there are the regulatory procedures to ensure that the new clinical practice is accountable and contained to the instances where an autonomous choice is made. Third, there is the potentially far-reaching impact from PAS law back to other parts of health law, should novel regulatory visions be passed. Here the ideas, embodied in PAS proposals, that physicians can unilaterally and indefinitely suspend competent patients' rights, that disabled persons have fewer rights than nondisabled persons, or that certain fundamental rights pertain only to people with some medical conditions strike us as of potentially far-reaching concern. In such ways, our society's policy framework for PAS may not only force a reweaving of the right to refuse treatment decisions but stretch all the way to other controversial health care decisions (as in reproductive health care) where issues of medical paternalism or disease-specific rights have been proposed.

NOTES

1. *Compassion in Dying et al. v. State of Washington and Gregoire*, No. 94-35535, 96 C.D.O.S. 1507, slip op. at p. 40 (9th Cir., *en banc*, March 6, 1996), *rev'g*, 49 F.3d 586 (9th. Cir. 1995).

2. Ibid., footnote 140. This expressly embraced pharmacists, health care workers, family members, "or the persons who help the patient to his death bed and provide the love and comfort so essential to a peaceful death."

3. Public Act 3 of Michigan (1993).

4. "Kevorkian Faces Suicide Prosecutions without a Law Being Cited," *New York Times*, April 17, 1996, p. A20.

5. *Quill v. Koppell*, 870 F. Supp. 78 (S.D.N.Y. 1994).

6. It should be noted that under the Ninth Circuit decision rendered *en banc* in the case of *Compassion in Dying v. Washington*, the Oregon United States District Court decision in *Lee et al. v. Oregon et al.*, 891 F. Supp. 1429 (D.Or. 1995) holding invalid the voter initiative permitting doctors to prescribe medications for terminally ill patients to use in ending their lives, under, *inter alia*, equal protection grounds, is claimed to "conflict squarely with the reasoning of this (i.e., the Ninth Circuit *en banc*) opinion and with the legal conclusion we have reached. Slip. op. p. 39. However, while reversing in dicta, the court expressly declines to address the question raised in Lee whether the entire (Washington) statute or the "or aids" provision is unconstitutional, "[b]ecause *Lee* was erroneously decided [and] we need not undertake that task. *Compassion in Dying v. Washington*, footnote 138.

7. "Regulating Physician-Assisted Death," *New England Journal of Medicine* 331 (July 14, 1994): 119–24.

8. Demetra M. Pappas, Transcription of Jury Instructions issued by Hon. Jessica Cooper on March 7, 1996. These instructions were consistent with Public Act 3 (1993), codified in MCL 752.1027 (Sec. 7) and approved by the Michigan Court of Appeal prior to their issue.

9. This is perhaps the sole proposition of Circuit Judge Noonan's opinion in the

original Ninth Circuit case, *Compassion in Dying v. Washington*, 49 F.3d 586,594 (9th Cir. 1995). Further, the majority of the *en banc* panel, by repeatedly characterizing the issue as "whether there is a fundamental right to determine the time and manner of one's death" (passim) when one is terminally ill and competent, leaves the underlying tenet of theoretical criminal and tort law undisturbed.

10. Norman St. John-Stevas, *Life, Death and the Law* (London: Eyre & Spottiswoode, 1961), pp. 250–51.

11. *Compassion in Dying v. Washington* (Beezer, J. dissenting), slip op. at 49 (footnotes omitted).

12. Demetra M. Pappas, "Recent Historical Perspectives Regarding Medical Euthanasia and Physician Assisted Suicide," *British Medical Bulletin* 52 (1996): 14.1–8.

13. See, e.g., J. G. Bachman, K. H. Alcser, D. J. Doukas, et al., "Attitudes of Michigan Physicians and the Public toward Legalizing Physician-Assisted Suicide and Voluntary Euthanasia," *New England Journal of Medicine* 334 (1996): 303–309; D. J. Doukas, D. Waterhouse, D. W Gorenflo, and J. Seid, "Attitudes and Behaviors on Physician-Assisted Death: A Study of Michigan Oncologists," *Journal of Clinical Oncology* 13 (1995): 1055–61; C. A. Steverns and R. Hassan, "Management of Death, Dying and Euthanasia: Attitudes and Practices of Medical Practitioners in South Australia," *Journal of Medical Ethics* 20 (1994): 41–46; B. J. Ward and P. A. Tate, "Attitudes among NHS Doctors to Requests for Euthanasia," *British Medical Journal* 308 (1994): 1332–34.

14. Dan W. Brock, "Voluntary Active Euthanasia," *Hastings Center Report* 22 (March–April 1992): 10–22.

15. Howard Brody, "Assisted Death—A Compassionate Response to Medical Failure," *New England Journal of Medicine* 327 (1992): 1384–88.

16. For a lengthy exposition, see Bachman et al., "Attitudes of Michigan Physicians."

17. 49 F.3d 586 (9th Cir. 1995).

18. See, for example, Y. Conwell and E. D. Caine, "Rational Suicide and the Right to Die: Reality and Myth," *New England Journal of Medicine* 325 (1991): 1101–02; D. C. Marson, F. A. Schmitt, K. K. Ingram, and L. E. Harrell, "Determining the Competency of Alzheimer Patients to Consent to Treatment and Research," *Alzheimer Disease and Associated Disorders* 8 Suppl. 4 (1994): 5–18; D. Rutman and M. Silberfeld, "A Preliminary Report on the Discrepancy between Clinical and Test Evaluations of Competence," *Canadian Journal of Psychiatry* 37 (1992): 634–39; and S. H. Dinwiddie, "Physician-Assisted Suicide: Epistemological Problems," *Medicine and the Law* 11 (1992): 345–52.

19. President's Commission on the Study of Ethical Problems in Medicine and Biomedical and Behavioral Research, "Making Health Care Decisions" (1983) in I. Kennedy and A. Grubb, *Medical Text with Materials,* 2d ed. (1994), p. 130. See also "Ethical Debate: Doctors' Legal Position in Treating Temporarily Incompetent Patients," *British Medical Journal* 311 (1995): 116. Nonetheless, one can be suffering from mental incapacity and still be held competent to consent to or refuse treatment, as the 1993 *Chabot* case in the Netherlands demonstrates. In that case,

a deeply depressed woman was assisted in committing suicide, after which the doctor was effectively exonerated.

20. *NEJM* 331, no.2, p. 120.

21. Ibid., p. 121.

22. "Desire for Death in the Terminally Ill," *American Journal of Psychiatry* 152 (August 1995). See also Conwell and Caine.

23. 497 U.S. 261 (1990).

24. 112 S.Ct. 2791 (1992).

25. C. J. Ryan and M. Kaye, "Euthanasia in Australia—The Northern Territory Rights of the Terminally Ill Act," *New England Journal of Medicine* 334 (February 1, 1996): 326, 327.

26. Miller et al., "Sounding Board, Regulating Physician-Assisted Death," p. 120.

27. Ibid.

28. Steven H. Miles, "Commentary: Physicians and Their Patients' Suicides," *JAMA* 271 (June 8, 1995): 1786–88.

29. A. Alpers and Bernard Lo, "Physician-Assisted Suicide in Oregon: A Bold Experiment," *JAMA* 274 (August 9, 1995): 483, 485.

30. M. A. Lee et al., "Legalizing Assisted Suicide in Oregon," *New England Journal of Medicine* 334 (February 1, 1996): 313.

31. J. Persels, "Forcing the Issue of Physician-Assisted Suicide: The Impact of the Kevorkian Case on the Euthanasia Debate," *Journal of Legal Medicine* 14 (1993): 115.

32. Miller et al., p. 120.

10

PHYSICIAN-ASSISTED SUICIDE
EVOLVING PUBLIC POLICIES

William J. Winslade, Ph.D., J.D.

We do not choose to be born. Nor do we have a choice about whether we will die. Many of us will have no choice about when, where, or how we will die. We may die suddenly from an injury or unexpectedly from an illness. But some of us will die from a terminal illness—such as cancer or AIDS—that is diagnosed long before death ensues. Others will suffer, before they die, from debilitating conditions such as Parkinson's disease, amyotrophic lateral sclerosis, or emphysema. In such cases we will have choices to make along the way: about alternative forms of treatment, whether to sign an advance directive, whether to accept or refuse certain procedures, palliative care, or hospice care. Should physician-assisted suicide (PAS) also be among our options?

This question has provoked continuing controversy in the United States, especially since Dr. Jack Kevorkian assisted Janet Adkins's suicide in 1990. Since that time numerous cases, public opinion surveys, media stories, proposed legislation, court decisions, professional debates, and publications have explored the legal, ethical, religious, medical, psychological, and other aspects of PAS. I argue that public policy in the United States should respect the preferences of competent persons afflicted with a terminal illness or experiencing intolerable pain or suffering who request PAS. Subject to appropriate safeguards and government oversight, willing physicians should be permitted to offer assisted suicide in carefully circumscribed situations.

Public policy concerning PAS will not and should not be revised rapidly or radically because fundamental values are at stake. But the current policies in the United States that legally proscribe PAS in all cases are too restrictive. Personal liberty about a private matter such as control over one's own death should be accorded great, though not unlimited, respect. Although the general rule that assisted suicide may be proscribed should be maintained, specific exceptions should be allowed for PAS that can be justified in particular cases. Because PAS is an extreme measure involving vulnerable patients and physicians licensed by the state, public scrutiny and governmental oversight are warranted to prevent exploitation or error.

Even limited toleration of PAS, however, will provoke irreconcilable value conflicts about the permissibility of such a practice.[1] Those who believe some instances of PAS are morally permissible and should not be illegal will be unable to persuade those who believe that PAS should always be prohibited. Public policy, however, rarely rests upon unanimity. Rather it typically reflects compromise, accommodation of conflicting values, and a range of options. I argue that the option of PAS, though never a good thing in itself, is sometimes the least undesirable choice for a particular person. Public policy, and especially the law, should respect individuals who, after careful consideration and sufficient consultation, make PAS their next-to-last choice. Their last decision is to take their own life.

Before turning to the details of my policy proposals, let me add a personal note. My attitude toward PAS is ambivalent. As a psychoanalyst I know from clinical experience that many persons who seriously entertain the idea of suicide later change their minds. I also know that persons who say they want PAS may be asking for something else—reassurance that they will not be abandoned, relief from pain, permission to die, and so forth. But some competent persons sincerely believe in and have good reasons to prefer PAS to a quality of life that they experience as unacceptable and may need a physician's help to end their lives. Such persons should not be forced to ask their physician to commit a crime on their behalf. As a lawyer I believe that morally permissible acts of PAS should not be illegal. As a philosopher I believe that some cases of PAS can be morally justified. Thus, despite my ambivalence and my appreciation of the arguments against PAS, I believe that our public policy should be flexible enough to accommodate those for whom PAS provides control over their death when they no longer possess control over their life.

Public policy that permits PAS must take into consideration the interests of patients, physicians, and the larger community. A brief discussion of public opinion brings out that attitudes toward PAS vary widely. Next the interests of patients are linked with the responses of physicians. Analysis of current law and proposed revisions of the law are followed by recommendations for governmental oversight. This chapter explores the factors relevant to the construction of a social policy but does not provide a detailed blueprint. If my general arguments are sound, the next step should be the formulation of specific policies.

Public Attitudes and Opinions

Public opinion about PAS ranges across a wide spectrum. Some ardently and others ambivalently favor PAS. Some fervently and others reluctantly oppose PAS. Still others remain undecided. Much public debate about PAS is polarized and politicized, not least because the controversial conduct of Dr. Jack Kevorkian sometimes provokes reactive rather than reflective and rational discussion. (Similarly, the practice of and the response to euthanasia in the Netherlands generates widely divergent attitudes. Some believe that euthanasia is a humane and compassionate response to suffering; others view it as evil or callous indifference to human life.) Although consensus is clearly lacking, two recent surveys suggest increasing support for legalizing PAS among physicians in Oregon and Michigan and the general public in Michigan.[2] These recent surveys, like earlier ones, reflect increasing public and professional support for the idea of legalizing PAS in some circumstances. Public opinion is relevant to policy formulation precisely because it expresses communal as well as personal values. But it is far from decisive. It does not mean that those who favor changing the law would choose PAS for themselves. Nor does it necessarily mean that those who oppose legalizing PAS would never consider or choose PAS on moral grounds or for personal reasons. Many persons who believe that PAS is sometimes permissible can imagine, have experienced, or have read about cases that enable them to understand why a person might (or might not) choose PAS. In addition to general attitudes about control over personal death or the power of particularly compelling cases, other reasons support a policy that tolerates PAS.

Patients' Interests and Physicians' Responses

Persons who possess the means and the motives sometimes take their own life. Although some religious doctrines classify suicide as a sin, others do not. Some secular thinkers believe suicide is irrational, while others hold that it may be rational in some instances. Mental health professionals tend to assume that suicide is usually a product of mental illness, but many disagree. Suicide and attempted suicide are not illegal in the United States. Americans who cherish individual liberty tolerate suicide, even if they do not endorse or encourage it.

The case for tolerating suicide as a personal choice is strongest when the person is competent, rational, and has good reasons for such a decision. Terminal illness, chronic and intractable pain and suffering, or an unacceptable quality of life are some of the reasons why a person might commit suicide. Of course it is well known that suicidal ideas are sometimes transient or a product of treatable depression. We provide voluntary and may impose involuntary treatment on suicidal persons suffering from a mental disorder. But even those who oppose suicide in principle can appreciate that some persons view suicide as a lesser evil than the alternatives open to them.

The most powerful argument in favor of PAS derives from the value ascribed in the United States to personal privacy, liberty, and self-determination. In the context of terminal illness or severe pain and suffering, the key idea is control over the time, place, and manner of one's own death. Persons who know that they are dying may prefer to extend their lives as long as possible or to refuse procedures that prolong the dying process. Such measures may delay or hasten the dying process but do not necessarily provide as much control as PAS. The option of PAS offers patients specific control of how, when, and where they will die.

Several objections can be raised against the preceding proposals. First, one might challenge the alleged value of control. Perhaps the idea that we can control our own death is a grandiose delusion. Maybe we should accept our limitations and realize that just as we cannot ultimately prevent death, we cannot effectively orchestrate it either. But PAS in fact increases patients' limited choices. Janet Adkins, Diane, and other cases of PAS illustrate that patients' need for control varies widely. It is hard to deny that PAS in fact enhances personal control over dying and death. For persons whose future outlook is bleak, control in the present becomes more significant.[3]

Another objection is that the degree of pain and suffering of terminally ill or chronically disabled patients is exaggerated. With proper palliative care and pain control, fewer patients will desire or seek PAS.[4] This argument is surely apt in some cases; but some patients may prefer to reject palliative care because of a desire not to prolong suffering. Although some commentators argue that some dying patients may find meaning in suffering,[5] the desire to end one's suffering is rational and may give greater meaning to death itself. Quite apart from pain and suffering, however, some patients may simply prefer not to live any longer. Do such persons have a duty to live a quality of life they do not want? This in the end should be a personal matter and a private decision.

Patients with a terminal illness, chronic and intractable pain or suffering, or a quality of life that they are unwilling to endure may prefer to end their life. Some persons act solely on their own; others seek help to carry out their decision. Is it reasonable and appropriate for such patients to ask their physicians to provide PAS? It is not uncommon for patients to turn to physicians, not only because they have the means and the knowledge but also because physicians occupy a privileged position in regulating life and death. Physicians strive to preserve the length and quality of life as primary goals of medicine. They seek to prevent death and can sometimes postpone it, but they can also help bring it about painlessly and effectively. Physicians are special gatekeepers at the borders of life and death. Their knowledge and their power impose upon them extraordinary duties of discretion and restraint. Because of their power, authority, and knowledge, physicians are regulated not only by their profession but also by the government that gives physicians a license to practice.

Physicians have an obligation to respond with empathy to their patients who request PAS.[6] Physicians also have a duty to make reliable diagnoses and prognoses, to evaluate patients' psychological needs properly, and to offer pain control, palliative care, counseling, and emotional support. Assisting patient suicide is not a requirement of standard medical care. Physicians may for personal or professional reasons refuse a request for PAS; it nevertheless may arise out of the physician-patient relationship as an understandable patient request. When a competent patient with a terminal illness or intolerable pain or suffering voluntarily asks a physician for PAS, it is obligatory for a physician to take the request seriously. It is morally permissible, but not a duty, to honor the request in some circumstances.

If a patient seeks PAS, physicians who are willing to help should not rely solely on their own discretion. They should consult with colleagues to confirm medical facts, to explore psychological issues, and to review ethical considerations, legal matters, and other contextual features, such as family relationships and economic factors, that might be unduly influencing a patient's request for PAS. A physician should thoroughly explore all the patient's options to be sure that a request for PAS is authentic and a last resort under the circumstances.[7]

Some commentators believe that few physicians know their patients well enough as persons or as friends to be sure that PAS is an authentic decision in a particular case.[8] I agree that no physician should provide PAS based on superficial interactions such as those that seem typical of Dr. Jack Kevorkian.[9] But Dr. Timothy Quill presents a different example, a physician who has intimate personal knowledge of his patients and a deep understanding of their needs and desires.[10] A physician who is willing to offer PAS shoulders a heavy burden of responsibility to understand fully patients' explicit requests as well as the tacit dimensions of their lives. Less than such a deep understanding is insufficient to justify the extraordinary offer of PAS.

Physicians who are willing, even if reluctant, to assist their patient's suicide must also examine their own motives and feelings. As Steven Miles points out,[11] the emotional dimensions of caring for dying patients deeply affect physicians' psyches. Physicians who are willing to provide PAS must not do so to meet their own conscious or unconscious needs, frustrations, or despair. It must be a compassionate response to the patient's voluntary, informed, carefully considered request. Physicians who render such assistance do so not as a moral duty to their patients but because it is a morally permissible response to their patients' personal preferences, needs, and desires for control over their death. Physicians who decline to provide PAS should not abandon their patients in other respects but should help them cope with their situation and refer them to a physician who might be willing to consider PAS.

It is important to point out, however, that even when a physician provides the means for a patient's suicide, it does not necessarily follow that the patient will carry it out. The knowledge that PAS is an option may serve as the support that a patient needs to cope with suffering.[12] Physicians should continue to work with their patients, to provide counseling, pain control, and palliative care. Some patients may be satisfied to have available but not exercise their option for suicide. The duties of physicians are to preserve the integrity of their relationship and to respect their patients' autonomous decisions.

Some critics argue that PAS is a violation of the professional aspirations, duties, and standards of physicians.[13] Others reply that PAS is compatible with professional integrity, and I agree.[14] It is my position that PAS is neither a violation of nor an essential part of physicians' duties to patients or their profession. Nor is PAS simply a supererogatory act. Rather it may be an act of respect for patients' values and preferences that arises out of but then goes beyond the duties encompassed in the physician-patient relationship. It is to some degree a response of personal compassion and to some degree a response of professional discretion. Given the nature of the situation, it is not surprising that it is difficult to characterize PAS simply as an act of duty or of compassion. Because it lies at or partly beyond the boundary of the physician-patient relationship, our attempts to characterize PAS are inherently difficult and uncertain.

PAS is not a wholly private matter between physicians and patients that should be left solely to their mutual discretion. Individual liberty supports patients' rights to ask for but not demand PAS. Physicians who provide it engage in conduct which must be shown to be justified in a particular case. Physicians, licensed by the state, have an obligation to subject their proposed conduct to external review. The public has an interest in preventing exploitation of vulnerable patients, mistaken reactions to impulsive or unreasonable patients' requests, or precipitous responses by physicians.

PAS and the Law

Just as public opinion surveys and other studies[15] reveal divided opinions about PAS, so also the law reflects our societal ambivalence. Many states' criminal statutes make assisted suicide a felony; other states treat it as a common law crime. Even when PAS is illegal and known to occur, prosecutions are rare and no convictions of physicians for PAS have been reported.[16] Dr. Kevorkian, who repeatedly defies authorities' attempts to restrict his efforts and is frequently subjected to prosecution, has not as of early 1997 been convicted of a crime. A published report of PAS by Dr. Quill resulted in a criminal proceeding that was dropped after a grand jury failed to indict him.[17] Furthermore, the practice of PAS is an open secret in the medical community, although the precise frequency of the practice is unknown.

Two recent ground-breaking federal appellate court decisions have invalidated state statutes in Washington and New York that impose a total ban on assisted suicide so far as the statutes applied to physicians.[18] Both decisions reach the same legal conclusion: that mentally competent, terminally ill patients have a right to ask their physician to prescribe medication to enable such patients to control the time and manner of their death. These courts also agree that state laws may, and indeed should, carefully regulate physician conduct to prevent mistakes or abuse. The courts differ, however, in their legal opinions about the nature of patients' liberty interest that gives rise to the right to request PAS. The United States Court of Appeals for the Ninth Circuit ruled that the liberty interest is a constitutionally recognized "right to die" protected by the Due Process Clause of the Fourteenth Amendment. The United States Court of Appeals for the Second Circuit held that the liberty interest in question, although not a substantive constitutional right, permits terminally ill patients to ask their physicians for medication to hasten death. Those state laws (subject to the federal jurisdiction of the Ninth and Second Circuits) that make it a crime for physicians to assist their patients in this way are invalid either because they infringe upon a constitutional due process liberty interest of patients or are not sufficiently rationally related to any state interest to justify treating PAS differently than requests to withhold or withdraw life-sustaining treatment.

Both courts consider and carefully weigh patients' liberty interest and the states' interest in preserving life, preventing suicide, maintaining the integrity of the medical profession, and avoiding mistakes or abuse of vulnerable patients. Both courts believe that states may preserve these state interests by carefully regulating physicians, rather than totally prohibiting them from prescribing medication that enables patients to hasten their impending death. Thus state laws that criminalize assisted suicide are invalid to the extent that they permit no exceptions in such circumstances.

The holdings in both cases are strictly limited to the liberty interests of competent terminally ill adults who seek lethal medication from their physicians, the only issue presented in the pleadings. The Ninth Circuit opinion acknowledges but does not specifically address the liberty interests of nonterminally ill persons confronted with intractable pain or suffering or irreversible unconsciousness. The Ninth Circuit opinion also recognizes that physician-administered medication, especially for conscious but physically incapacitated patients, may be as justifiable as physician-prescribed medication for persons who are able to help themselves. But that issue was not before the court. The Second Circuit opinion clearly rules out physician-administered medication as impermissible euthanasia; it allows prescriptions only for patients who can self-administer lethal medications.

The legal finality of these narrowly formulated but highly controversial opinions is unsettled. The United States Supreme Court has agreed to hear the appeals of the Ninth and Second Circuits' decisions on PAS.[19] Depending on the Supreme Court's decision, the legal status of PAS may be modified and the authority of states to regulate or prohibit PAS may be changed. Another kind of decision would leave the opinions of the Ninth and Second Circuits binding on the states within their jurisdiction. For example, California's assisted suicide statute, which is very similar to Washington's, would unconstitutionally infringe patients' liberty interests. The Ninth Circuit opinion also observed that the injunction issued by a federal district court blocking the implementation of Oregon's Death with Dignity Act passed by a voter referendum is inconsistent with the Ninth Circuit's holding in *Compassion in Dying* (more fully discussed in the next section). The Second Circuit ruling makes PAS legal, subject to appropriate state regulation, not only in New York but also in Vermont and Connecticut.

Until we know the Supreme Court's decision, it is uncertain how the issues will be formulated or interpreted. The Supreme Court might accept or reject the constitutional liberty interest reasoning of the Ninth Circuit, the nonconstitutional liberty interest invoked by Second Circuit, or the view that there is no liberty interest at all in PAS. Predictions about what the high court will do are perilous and often mistaken.

Legislation or Voter Initiatives Legalizing Physician-Assisted Suicide

One way that some states have sought to accommodate patients who request PAS is to pass laws that legalize it under certain conditions, such as Oregon's Death with Dignity Act (ODDA).[20] Under this statute a terminally ill person is permitted to request a physician's prescription for a lethal dose of medication for the purpose of ending the patient's life. The passage of the ODDA following the defeat of similar voter initiatives or referendums in other states arguably reflects increasing social tolerance of PAS. The ODDA has not yet taken effect because a federal district court found that the statute violates the Equal Protection Clause of the Fourteenth Amendment of the U.S. Constitution.[21]

The United States Court of Appeals for the Ninth Circuit, however, rejected the opinion of the Federal District Court.

> The Oregon District Court's reasoning conflicts squarely with the reasoning of this opinion and with the legal conclusions we have reached. Here, we determine that a statute that prohibits doctors from aiding terminally ill persons to hasten their deaths by providing them with prescription medications unconstitutionally burdens the liberty interests of the terminally ill. The benefit we conclude the terminally ill are entitled to receive in this case—the right to physician-assisted suicide—is precisely what Judge Hogan determined to be a burden and thus unlawful. In short, *Lee* treats a burden as a benefit and a benefit as a burden. In doing so, Judge Hogan clearly erred. *Lee* not only does not aid us in reaching our decision, it is directly contrary to our holding.[22]

Physician-Assisted Suicide Policies

In view of the rapidly changing but unsettled state of the law, how should policymakers respond? The first step is to wait until the United States Supreme Court announces its decision regarding the federal appellate court findings. Even then, the Court's decision may not settle whether states should permit and, if so, how they should regulate PAS. States outside the jurisdiction of the Second and Ninth Circuits currently have criminal statutes or common law rules that generally prohibit PAS. What policy changes, if any, should those states consider? Increasing public and professional sentiment favors some form of toleration of, if not recognition of a right to, PAS. In this section I offer two alternative policy approaches. The first is a policy of toleration that retains the general prohibition against assisted suicide but provides a legal excuse for PAS in certain circumstances. The second policy approach recognizes a right of patients to seek PAS but regulates the conduct of physicians to prevent error or exploitation of vulnerable patients.

Legally Excusing Physician-Assisted Suicide

A conservative way to accommodate patients who request PAS while addressing the concerns PAS raises is to slightly modify laws that criminalize assisted suicide.[23] This can be accomplished by providing physicians with a legal excuse to a charge of assisted suicide in limited circumstances. The concept of excuse is based upon the principle that a particular defendant is personally blameless for conduct otherwise considered wrongful.[24] Assisted suicide would remain a chargeable criminal offense. Such a revision to criminal law would not, however, be based upon recognizing a person's right to assisted suicide.

This approach would require physicians charged with the crime of assisted suicide to be prepared to demonstrate that their conduct was legally excused in the particular circumstances. Failure to make such a showing may subject the physician to liability. The potential for punishment would caution physicians to provide suicide assistance in only the most compelling cases, thereby minimizing the risk of mistake or abuse. Community standards would establish the criteria that must be satisfied to establish a sufficiently compelling case for a legal excuse. Prosecutors would exercise their discretion in determining whether a physician should be charged based upon the circumstances of each case. Courts would determine whether a particular physician produced sufficient evidence to warrant an excuse for an otherwise criminal act of assisted suicide.

The legal excuse approach resembles cases in which physicians were charged with but not indicted or convicted for assisting their patients with suicide.[25] Based upon considerable and growing public support for PAS, courts may be receptive to a physician's defense of excuse to a charge of assisted suicide if the physician has made a showing sufficient for the court to find the physician personally blameless for his or her conduct.

Some critics might object that this narrow legal exception will provide little comfort to physicians who are otherwise willing to provide PAS. Physicians may be discouraged from helping their patients for fear of being prosecuted, even more so than at present when the practice of PAS is illegal but clandestine and rarely investigated. Perhaps PAS should be offered only in exceptional cases by physicians who are willing to subject their conduct to full legal review and public scrutiny. In this case the law would neither encourage nor facilitate PAS, but only tolerate it. Aiding in the killing of another person, even as a last resort in dire circumstances, is still wrong but physicians can establish that they are personally blameless. The narrowness of this proposed legal exception provides a strong safeguard against PAS deteriorating into discrimination against or callous indifference toward vulnerable, suffering, or dying patients.

Regulating a Right to Physician-Assisted Suicide

If PAS is a legal right of terminally ill patients, as two federal appellate courts have ruled, what regulations are necessary to protect the interests of patients, physicians, and the public? At first glance one might think that only patients and their physicians should decide how much, if at all, to expose the physician-patient relationship to public oversight and regulation. This maximizes the privacy of their relationship, but also increases the potential for mistake or abuse. It also fails to remedy fully the current clandestine practice of PAS. Still, it would be possible for patients and their physicians to create a record of documents, witnesses, videotaped interviews, or other evidence available for postmortem review by public officials or professional organizations. In my opinion, postmortem review ordinarily is not enough. It is preferable to also utilize some form of prior review.

Because physicians are licensed by the state as well as subject to review by their professional organizations, their conduct is already subject to public scrutiny. It might be desirable, for example, to certify physicians' competence in pain management and palliative care as a prerequisite to their authority to offer PAS to their patients. It is especially appropriate to review cases of PAS because the practice is so clearly sensitive and controversial. To meet the objections of critics who fear that unmonitored PAS will open the floodgates to discrimination against poor, weak, or vulnerable patients, I believe that explicit guidelines should be established to protect the interests of patients, physicians, and the public. Such guidelines must, however, recognize and respond to the wide variety of fact patterns, psychological nuances, and existential complexities that arise in PAS cases. Practical guidelines can help to show that an instance of PAS is legally defensible and morally permissible; the guidelines should include evidence of appropriate prior review and consultation (especially with regard to patients' capacity, consent, and voluntariness), sufficient documentation for effective postmortem review, and required reporting of cases of PAS. In addition, public health research to track patterns of PAS is an important aspect of public scrutiny.

I do not believe that any single model for prior consultation and review will be suited to every case. The circumstances of the cases may involve multiple variables and values with differing, or even shifting, significance. A pluralistic approach to prior review provides the best opportunity for patients and physicians to meet their personal needs as well as the public's concerns. In some cases, for instance, a patient's terminal illness, capacity for voluntary and informed choice, a well-established physician-patient relationship, and the absence of confounding factors (family conflict, economic pressures, etc.) may make it relatively easy for an adequate record to be prepared. Still, to avoid any appearance of impropriety and to reassure the public, it is advisable, and perhaps should be mandatory, to seek outside consultation and review. Depending upon the context of the case, other health care consultants, family members or friends, ethics consultants or ethics committees, palliative care consultants or committees, clergy, or even a community "council of sages"[26] might be helpful. The evidence of adequate outside consultation will go a long way toward convincing public officials—prosecutors, grand juries, judges, and legislators—that an instance of PAS is permissible in a particular situation.

A requirement of appropriate outside consultation and review can also provide patients and their physicians with an opportunity to reflect on their reasons, examine their needs and motives, and give due consideration to other available options. PAS is an extreme measure that may be morally justified and legally permissible when sufficient precautions and adequate safeguards are in place. However, even competent patients and caring physicians may make mistakes. To prevent irreversible but avoidable errors, the patient-physician dyad in the context of PAS should, except in rare circumstances, be visible to a broader community of concerned persons. The illumination of publicity need not be a blinding glare, but can be a source of guiding light. The shadows of secrecy that currently shroud PAS create a suspicion of abuse or mistake even if the reality is that physicians' conduct is beyond reproach.

The record of outside consultation and review should be submitted along with required reporting of PAS to appropriate public officials. Physicians willing to help but anxious about liability might seek a more formal prior review. The record for a particular case could be submitted before PAS occurs for something analogous to a judicial declaratory judgment that PAS meets the criteria for immunity from liability. However, to protect patients' privacy in special cases, physicians might be willing to forgo prior review by state officials. In those cases the record could be submitted after PAS to permit authorities to conduct a full postmortem review. Obviously a prior review conducted in a timely manner protects patients from mistakes and physicians from subsequent accusations of misconduct. Establishing a suitable public forum for prior review ought to be a matter for open public discussion and creative policy development.

Some of the recent proposals that have appeared in the literature are promising but do not adequately take into consideration the diversity of personal preferences, physician practices, and community values that deserve careful consideration. For example, the ODDA discussed previously fails to provide for adequate outside review. It also establishes a bureaucratic recipe with many gaps and problems, as others have already pointed out.[27] An alternative thoughtful proposal for regulating PAS recommends the use of regional palliative care consultants with a larger community committee available for appeals.[28] This proposal may place too much discretion and power in the hands of the regional palliative care consultants and review committees. Although for some situations this alternative review process may be very helpful, for others it may be cumbersome or even intrusive. Furthermore, it eliminates the oversight of the law.

A revision of public policy about an issue so laden with symbolic value must be approached with extreme caution. The concerns expressed by those who oppose all forms of PAS because of threats to the sanctity of life and professional integrity, or potential for abuse and mistake must be taken seriously. Even though total opposition to PAS seems to me to be excessive, the concerns that give rise to it are legitimate. But we must not shirk our responsibility to make changes that are urgently needed. The wisdom of Alfred North Whitehead is an appropriate reminder:

> The art of free society consists first in the maintenance of the symbolic code; and secondly in fearlessness of revision, to secure that the code serves those purposes which satisfy an enlightened reason. Those societies which cannot combine reverence to their symbols with freedom of revision, must ultimately decay either from anarchy, or from the slow atrophy of a life stifled by useless shadows.[29]

Conclusion

Dying is often not easy, even when it is desired. For some persons the knowledge that terminal illness or intractable suffering can be ended by PAS enhances the value of their remaining life and their personal relationships. For others, suffering until natural death occurs may have greater meaning. Just as physicians can sometimes postpone an unwanted death, so also can they bring about a death that is chosen. A decision about such personal and sensitive matters belongs to individuals and, if they choose, to their physicians as helpers and friends, but subject also to the oversight of the law.[30]

NOTES

1. William J. Winslade, "Irreconcilable Conflicts in Bioethics," *Bioethics Forum* (Fall 1995): 23–27. I do not discuss in this chapter numerous related topics, such as euthanasia or terminating treatment of permanently unconscious patients, that also generate irreconcilable value conflicts. My assignment for this volume was to develop policy arguments in favor of PAS, not to discuss a wide spectrum of end-of-life controversies.

2. Jerald G. Bachman et al., "Attitudes of Michigan Physicians and the Public toward Legalizing Physician-Assisted Suicide and Voluntary Euthanasia," *New England Journal of Medicine* 334 (February 1, 1996): 303–9; Melinda A. Lee et al., "Legalizing Assisted Suicide—Views of Physicians in Oregon," *New England Journal of Medicine* 334 (February 1, 1996): 310–15.

3. Lonnie Shavelson, *A Chosen Death: The Dying Confront Assisted Suicide* (New York: Simon and Schuster, 1995); A. Solomon, "A Death of One's Own," *New Yorker,* May 22, 1995, pp. 54–69.

4. Kathleen M. Foley, "Pain, Physician-assisted Suicide and Euthanasia," *Pain Forum* 4 (1995): 163–78.

5. See generally Daniel Callahan, *The Troubled Dream of Life: In Search of a Peaceful Death* (New York: Simon and Schuster, 1993), pp. 135–40. Callahan writes: "For many religious believers, the idea of redemptive suffering is powerful. Acceptance and suffering, or understanding suffering as part of a religious interpretation of life, can provide a rationale for the suffering. It remains difficult to bear, but it is not meaningless or pointless if wisely understood" (p. 135).

6. Ellen Singer More and Maureen A. Milligan, *The Emphatic Practitioner* (New Brunswick, N.J.: Rutgers University Press, 1994).

7. Timothy E. Quill, "Doctor, I Want to Die. Will You Help Me?" *JAMA* 270 (August 18, 1993): 870–76.

8. Ronald A. Carson, "Why Physicians Should Not Assist in Suicide," *Texas Medicine,* forthcoming.

9. William J. Winslade and Kyriakos S. Markides, "Assisted Suicide and Professional Responsibilities," *Society* 29 (July–August 1995): 16–19.

10. Timothy E. Quill, *Death and Dignity: Making Choices and Taking Charge* (New York: Norton, 1994).

11. Steven H. Miles, "Physicians and Their Patients' Suicides," *JAMA* 271 (June 8, 1994): 1786–88.

12. Sherwin B. Nuland, *How We Die* (New York: Knopf, 1993), p. 257. See also Richard Posner, *Age and Old Age* (Cambridge, Mass.: Harvard University Press, 1995), p. 224.

13. Steven H. Miles, "Physician-Assisted Suicide and the Profession's Gyro-compass," *Hastings Center Report* 25 (May–June 1995): 17–19.

14. Franklin G. Miller and Howard Brody, "Professional Integrity and Physician-Assisted Death," *Hastings Center Report* 25 (May–June 1995): 8–17.

15. Society for Health and Human Values, "Physician-Assisted Suicide: Toward a Comprehensive Understanding," *Academic Medicine* 70 (July 1995): 538–90.

16. T. Howard Stone and William J. Winslade, "Physician-Assisted Suicide and Euthanasia in the United States," *Journal of Legal Medicine* 16 (1995): 481–507.

17. Timothy E. Quill, "Death and Dignity: A Case of Individual Decision Making," *New England Journal of Medicine* 324 (March 7, 1991): 691.

18. *Compassion in Dying v. State of Washington*, 1996 WL 94848 79 F. 3d 790 (9th Cir. 1996), *mot. cert. granted sub. nom.*, 1996 U.S. Lexis 4540 (U.S. Oct. 1, 1996); *Quill et al. v. Vacco et al.*, 80 F. 3d 716 (2d Cir. 1996), *cert. granted*, 1996 U. S. Lexis 4536 (U.S. October 1, 1996). These decisions warrant a careful critique of the problematic conceptual analysis and legal reasoning on which they are based. In this chapter I seek only to summarize the main conclusions reached by the courts. A more complete discussion lies beyond the scope of this chapter.

19. "Court Overturns Ban in New York on Aided Suicides," *New York Times*, April 3, 1996, p. A1. It was reported in *Newsweek*, April 15, 1996, p. 27, that "Supreme Court Justice Antonin Scalia, on whether the high court should tackle the issue of doctor-assisted suicide," quipped, "Why would you leave that to nine lawyers, for heaven's sake?" Nonetheless, the Supreme Court granted certiorari. *Vacco v. Quill*, 1996 U.S. Lexis 4536 (U.S. Oct. 1, 1996); *Washington v. Glucksberg*, 1996 U.S. Lexis 4540 (U.S. Oct. 1, 1996).

20. *Lee v. Oregon*, 81 F.Supp., p. 1431.

21. Ibid., pp. 1437–38.

22. *Compassion in Dying*, p. 838. See also Arthur A. Povelones, Jr., "When the Majority Says You May Die: Aid-in-Dying Initiatives," *Notre Dame Journal of Law, Ethics and Public Policy* 9 (1995): 537–64.

23. See, e.g., Robert F. Weir, "The Morality of Physician-Assisted Suicide," *Law, Medicine and Health Care* 20 (1992): 125. Weir suggests the development of model legislation on PAS to provide physicians with greater certainty regarding the legal status of PAS. Weir also suggests that PAS be decriminalized. Weir's proposal is an attractive one because the development of model regulations may help public officials fashion laws that may withstand the fatal judicial or public scrutiny that have undermined previous attempts at legalization and that may more effectively prevent abuse or mistake.

24. George P. Fletcher, "Excuse: Theory," pt. 1, *Encyclopedia of Crime and Justice,* vol. 2 (1983).

25. *Hobbins v. Attorney General of Michigan,* 527 N.W.2d 714, 729 (Mich. 1994), *cert. denied* 115 S.Ct. 1795, 1995 U.S. Lexis 2903 (April 24, 1995). See also Celo Cruz, "Aid-in-Dying: Should We Decriminalize Physician-Assisted Suicide and Physician-Committed Euthanasia?" *American Journal of Law and Medicine* 18 (1992): 369, 379 and n. 77.

26. Sherwin Nuland, "The Debate over Dying," *USA Weekend* February 3–5, 1995, pp. 4–6.

27. Ann Alpers and Bernard Lo, "Physician-Assisted Suicide in Oregon," *JAMA* 274 (August 9, 1995): 483–87.

28. Frank G. Miller et al., "Regulating Physician-Assisted Suicide," *New England Journal of Medicine* 331 (July 14, 1994): 119–23.

29. Alfred North Whitehead, *Symbolism: Its Meaning and Effect* (New York: Capricorn Books, 1959), p. 88.

30. I am especially indebted to Howard Stone and Kristi Schrode for their research and editorial assistance with this essay. In addition, Ron Carson, Chester Burns, Joan Lang, Ellen More, Charles Hinkley, and Peter Williams made helpful suggestions. An early version of this chapter was presented at the Second Annual Pitts Memorial Lectureship dealing with Issues in Medical Ethics, "Dying in America: Choices at the End of Life," at the Medical University of South Carolina.

Appendixes

People v. Kevorkian
Supreme Court of Michigan
447 Mich. 436, 527 N.W.2nd 714 (1994)

*[Editor's introduction: Jack Kevorkian, M.D., a retired patholo-
gist living in Michigan, assisted in the suicide of Janet Adkins in
June 1990, by means of a "suicide machine" he had developed.
In early 1991, a trial court permanently enjoined Dr. Kevorkian
from using the machine again. When he continued to assist in
suicides using different methods, the Michigan legislature intervened. In late 1992, Michigan enacted a time-limited law that (1)
established a state commission to study assisted suicide and (2)
defined a new crime of "assistance to suicide" directed against
Kevorkian's acts of PAS. During the twenty months the law was
in effect (ending in November 1994), a circuit court in Wayne
County declared the law unconstitutional, the same circuit court
dismissed criminal charges against Kevorkian, a circuit court in
Oakland County also declared the law unconstitutional and
twice dismissed criminal charges against Kevorkian, and the trial
court decisions were appealed. In May 1994, a Detroit jury
acquitted Kevorkian of violating the state statute. That same
month the Michigan Court of Appeals issued its opinion. The
majority of judges found the assisted suicide statute to be unconstitutional, but also stated that a different state law might be
consistent with the U.S. Constitution. The excerpts printed here
are from the 1994 decision by the Supreme Court of Michigan, a
decision that reverses the Court of Appeals and declares that the
former state law was not unconstitutional. Subsequent to this
decision, Kevorkian was acquitted by Detroit juries of violating
Michigan common law against suicide in two 1996 trials.]*

CAVANAGH, Chief Justice:

These cases raise three issues with regard to the state's imposition of
criminal responsibility on persons who assist others in committing
suicide. . . . (1) Whether the Michigan assisted suicide statute . . . was
enacted in violation of [the Michigan Constitution] . . . (2) Whether the
criminal provisions of [the statute] violate the United States Constitution . . . (3) Whether the circuit court erred in quashing the information
charging the defendant with murder. . . .

Having found that Michigan's assisted suicide statute does not
violate [the Michigan Constitution] . . . we now address whether the
statute runs afoul of the United States Constitution. In its opinion of
May 10, 1994, the Court of Appeals rejected this argument. So do we.

The Due Process Clause of [the U.S. Constitution] commands the states not to "deprive any person of life, liberty, or property, without due process of law. . . ." Thus, the threshold question in this case is whether the clause encompasses a fundamental right to commit suicide and, if so, whether it includes a right to assistance.

Those who assert that there is such a right rely heavily on decisions of the United States Supreme Court in abortion and so-called "right to die" cases. Focusing especially on Planned Parenthood of Southeastern Pennsylvania v. Casey . . . these advocates argue that the right to end one's own life is a fundamental liberty interest, grounded in the notion of personal autonomy and springing from common-law concepts of bodily integrity and informed consent. They further contend that an integral part of this protected interest is the right to assistance, hence the term "assisted suicide.". . .

The distinction between the withdrawal of life-sustaining medical treatment and suicide is recognized in the Guidelines for State Court Decision Making In Life-Sustaining Medical Treatment, National Center for State Courts (2d ed.), pp. 143–145 (1992). . . .

We agree that persons who opt to discontinue life-sustaining medical treatment are not, in effect, committing suicide. There is a difference between choosing a natural death summoned by an uninvited illness or calamity, and deliberately seeking to terminate one's life by resorting to death-inducing measures unrelated to the natural process of dying.
. . .

[W]e must determine whether the asserted right to commit suicide arises from a rational evolution of tradition, or whether recognition of such a right would be a radical departure from historical precepts. We conclude that the principles that guide analysis of substantive due process do not support the recognition of a right to commit suicide.
. . .

On the basis of the foregoing analysis, we would hold that the right to commit suicide is neither implicit in the concept of ordered liberty nor deeply rooted in this nation's history and tradition. It would be an impermissibly radical departure from existing tradition, and from the principles that underlie that tradition, to declare that there is such a fundamental right protected by the Due Process Clause.

We are keenly aware of the intense emotions and competing moral philosophies that characterize the present debate about suicide in general, and assisted suicide in particular. The issues do not lend themselves to simple answers. However, while the complexity of the matter does not permit us to avoid the critical constitutional questions, neither does it, under the guise of constitutional interpretation, permit us to expand the judicial powers of this Court, especially where the question clearly is a policy one that is appropriately left to the citizenry for resolution, either through its elected representatives or through a ballot initiative. . . .

We would hold that the Due Process Clause of the federal constitution does not encompass a fundamental right to commit suicide, with or without assistance, and regardless of whether the would-be assistant is a physician.

Compassion in Dying v. State of Washington
United States Court of Appeals,
Ninth Circuit
1996 WL 94848 (Wash.)

[Editor's introduction: In 1991 voters in the state of Washington, by a margin of 54 percent to 46 percent, rejected a proposed law that would have legalized PAS and voluntary euthanasia in that state. In 1994 three anonymous, terminally ill patients, five physicians, and a nonprofit organization, Compassion in Dying, challenged the state law that made assisted suicide a felony. Judge Barbara Rothstein, sitting in the U.S. District Court in Seattle, held that the state's total ban of assisted suicide "places an undue burden on the exercise of a protected Fourteenth Amendment liberty interest by terminally ill, mentally competent adults acting knowingly and voluntarily. . . ." (Compassion in Dying v. State of Washington, 850 F.Supp. 1454, 1467 [W.D. Wash. 1994]). The case was appealed, and a three-judge panel of the U.S. Court of Appeals, Ninth Circuit, reversed the decision in a 2–1 vote. Writing for the court, Circuit Judge John Noonan cited the state's important interests in not placing physicians in "the role of killers" of vulnerable patients (Compassion in Dying v. State of Washington, 49 F.3d 586, 592 [9th Cir. 1995]). The excerpts printed here are from the second hearing of this case by the full panel of eleven circuit judges in the Ninth Circuit, located in San Francisco, with an 8–3 majority agreeing with Circuit Judge Stephen Reinhardt's written opinion to set aside the court's first decision because the judges are convinced that the Washington statute violates the Due Process Clause of the Fourteenth Amendment. This decision, along with the decision by the U.S. Court of Appeals, Second Circuit, is currently before the U.S. Supreme Court.]

REINHARDT, Circuit Judge:

This case raises an extraordinarily important and difficult issue. It compels us to address questions to which there are no easy or simple answers, at law or otherwise. It requires us to confront the most basic of human concerns—the mortality of self and loved ones—and to balance the interest in preserving human life against the desire to die peacefully and with dignity. . . .

Today, we are required to decide whether a person who is terminally ill has a constitutionally-protected liberty interest in hastening what might otherwise be a protracted, undignified, and extremely painful death. If such an interest exists, we must next decide whether or not the state of Washington may constitutionally restrict its exercise by banning a form of medical assistance that is frequently requested by terminally ill people who wish to die. We first conclude that there is a constitutionally-protected liberty interest in determining the time and manner of one's own death, an interest that must be weighed against the state's legitimate and countervailing interests, especially those that relate to the preservation of human life. After balancing the competing interests, we conclude by answering the narrow question before us: We hold that insofar as the Washington statute prohibits physicians from prescribing life-ending medication for use by terminally ill, competent adults who wish to hasten their own deaths, it violates the Due Process Clause of the Fourteenth Amendment. . . .

We now affirm the District Court's decision and clarify the scope of the relief. We hold that the "or aids" provision of [the] Washington statute, as applied to the prescription of life-ending medication for use by terminally ill, competent adult patients who wish to hasten their deaths, violates the Due Process Clause of the Fourteenth Amendment. Accordingly, we need not resolve the question whether that provision, in conjunction with other Washington laws regulating the treatment of terminally ill patients, also violates the Equal Protection Clause. . . .

While some people refer to the liberty interest implicated in right-to-die cases as a liberty interest in committing suicide, we do not describe it that way. We use the broader and more accurate terms, "the right to die," "determining the time and manner of one's death," and "hastening one's death" for an important reason. The liberty interest we examine encompasses a whole range of acts that are generally not considered to constitute "suicide." Included within the liberty interest we examine, is for example, the act of refusing or terminating un-wanted medical treatment. . . .

There is one further definitional matter we should emphasize. Following our determination regarding the existence of a liberty interest in hastening one's death, we examine whether the Washington statute unconstitutionally infringes on that liberty interest. Through-out that examination, we use the term "physician-assisted suicide," a term that does not appear in the Washington statute but is frequently employed in legal and medical discussions involving the type of question before us. For purposes of this opinion, we use physician-assisted suicide as it is used by the parties and district court and as it is most frequently used: the prescribing of medication by a physician for the purpose of enabling a patient to end his life. It is only that conduct that the plaintiffs urge be held constitutionally protected in this case. . . .

The essence of the substantive component of the Due Process Clause is to limit the ability of the state to intrude into the most important matters of our lives, at least without substantial justification. In a long line of cases, the Court has carved out certain key moments and decisions in individuals' lives and placed them beyond the general prohibitory authority of the state. The Court has recognized that the Fourteenth Amendment affords constitutional protection to personal decisions relating to marriage . . . , family relationships . . . , child rearing and education. . . , and intercourse for purposes other than procreation . . . . The Court has recognized the right of individuals to be free from government interference in deciding matters as personal as whether to bear or beget a child. . . , and whether to continue an unwanted pregnancy to term. . . .

A common thread running through these cases is that they involve decisions that are highly personal and intimate, as well as of great importance to the individual. Certainly, few decisions are more personal, intimate or important than the decision to end one's life, especially when the reason for doing so is to avoid excessive and protracted pain. Accordingly, we believe the cases from Pierce through Roe provide strong general support for our conclusion that a liberty interest in controlling the time and manner of one's death is protected by the Due Process Clause of the Fourteenth Amendment.

Casey and Cruzan provide persuasive evidence that the Constitution encompasses a due process liberty interest in controlling the time and manner of one's death—that there is, in short, a constitutionally recognized "right to die." Our conclusion is strongly influenced by, but not limited to, the plight of mentally competent, terminally ill adults. We are influenced as well by the plight of others, such as those whose existence is reduced to a vegetative state or a permanent and irreversible state of unconsciousness. See note 68 supra.

Our conclusion that there is a liberty interest in determining the time and manner of one's death does not mean that there is a concomitant right to exercise that interest in all circumstances or to do so free from state regulation. To the contrary, we explicitly recognize that some prohibitory and regulatory state action is fully consistent with constitutional principles.

In short, finding a liberty interest constitutes a critical first step toward answering the question before us. The determination that must now be made is whether the state's attempt to curtail the exercise of that interest is constitutionally justified. . . .

We analyze the factors in turn, and begin by considering the first: the importance of the state's interests. We identify six related state interests involved in the controversy before us: (1) the state's general interest in preserving life; (2) the state's more specific interest in preventing suicide; (3) the state's interest in avoiding the involvement of third parties and in precluding the use of arbitrary, unfair, or undue influence; (4) the state's interest in protecting family members and loved ones; (5) the state's interest in protecting the integrity of the medical profession; and, (6) the state's interest in avoiding adverse consequences that might ensue if the statutory provision at issue is declared unconstitutional.

We acknowledge that in some respects a recognition of the legitimacy of physician-assisted suicide would constitute an additional step beyond what the courts have previously approved. We also acknowledge that judicial acceptance of physician-assisted suicide would cause many sincere persons with strong moral or religious convictions great distress. Nevertheless, we do not believe that the state's interest in preventing that additional step is significantly greater than its interest in preventing the other forms of life-ending medical conduct that doctors now engage in regularly. More specifically, we see little, if any, difference for constitutional or ethical purposes between providing medication with a double effect and providing medication with a single effect, as long as one of the known effects in each case is to hasten the end of the patient's life. Similarly, we see no ethical or constitutionally cognizable difference between a doctor's pulling the plug on a respirator and his prescribing drugs which will permit a terminally ill patient to end his own life. In fact, some might argue that pulling the plug is a more culpable and aggressive act on the doctor's part and provides more reason for criminal prosecution. To us, what matters most is that the death of the patient is the intended result as surely in one case as in the other. In sum, we find the state's interests in preventing suicide do not make its interests substantially stronger here than in cases involving other forms of death-hastening medical intervention. To the extent that a difference exists, we conclude that it is one of degree and not of kind. . . .

The state has a legitimate interest in assuring the integrity of the medical profession, an interest that includes prohibiting physicians from engaging in conduct that is at odds with their role as healers. We do not believe that the integrity of the medical profession would be threatened in any way by the vindication of the liberty interest at issue here. Rather, it is the existence of a statute that criminalizes the provision of medical assistance to patients in need that could create conflicts with the doctors' professional obligations and make covert criminals out of honorable, dedicated, and compassionate individuals.

The assertion that the legalization of physician-assisted suicide will erode the commitment of doctors to help their patients rests both on an ignorance of what numbers of doctors have been doing for a considerable time and on a misunderstanding of the proper function of a physician. As we have previously noted, doctors have been discreetly helping terminally ill patients hasten their deaths for decades and probably centuries, while acknowledging privately that there was no other medical purpose to their actions. They have done so with the tacit approval of a substantial percentage of both the public and the medical profession, and without in any way diluting their commitment to their patients.

In addition, as we also noted earlier, doctors may now openly take actions that will result in the deaths of their patients. They may terminate life-support systems, withdraw life-sustaining gastrostomy tubes, otherwise terminate or withhold all other forms of medical treatment, and may even administer lethal doses of drugs with full knowledge of their "double effect." Given the similarity between what doctors are now permitted to do and what the plaintiffs assert they should be permitted to do, we see no risk at all to the integrity of the profession. This is a conclusion that is shared by a growing number of doctors who openly support physician-assisted suicide and proclaim it to be fully compatible with the physicians' calling and with their commitment and obligation to help the sick. . . .

Whether or not a patient can be cured, the doctor has an obligation to attempt to alleviate his pain and suffering. If it is impossible to cure the patient or retard the advance of his disease, then the doctor's primary duty is to make the patient as comfortable as possible. When performing that task, the doctor is performing a proper medical function, even though he knows that his patient's death is a necessary and inevitable consequence of his actions. . . .

Washington's statute prohibiting assisted suicide has a drastic impact on the terminally ill. By prohibiting physician assistance, it bars what for many terminally ill patients is the only palatable, and only practical, way to end their lives. Physically frail, confined to wheelchairs or beds, many terminally ill patients do not have the means or ability to kill themselves in the multitude of ways that healthy individuals can. Often, for example, they cannot even secure the medication or devices they would need to carry out their wishes.

Some terminally ill patients stockpile prescription medicine, which they can use to end their lives when they decide the time is right. The successful use of the stockpile technique generally depends, however, on the assistance of a physician, whether tacit or unknowing (although it is possible to end one's life with over-the-counter medication). Even if the terminally ill patients are able to accumulate sufficient drugs, given the pain killers and other medication they are taking, most of them would lack the knowledge to determine what dose of any given drug or drugs they must take, or in what combination. Miscalculation can be tragic. It can lead to an even more painful and lingering death. Alternatively, if the medication reduces respiration enough to restrict the flow of oxygen to the brain but not enough to cause death, it can result in the patient's falling into a comatose or vegetative state. . . .

By adopting appropriate, reasonable, and properly drawn safeguards Washington could ensure that people who choose to have their doctors prescribe lethal doses of medication are truly competent and meet all of the requisite standards. Without endorsing the constitutionality of any particular procedural safeguards, we note that the state might, for example, require: witnesses to ensure voluntariness; reasonable, though short, waiting periods to prevent rash decisions; second medical opinions to confirm a patient's terminal status and also to confirm that the patient has been receiving proper treatment, including adequate comfort care; psychological examinations to ensure that the patient is not suffering from momentary or treatable depression; reporting procedures that will aid in the avoidance of abuse. Alternatively, such safeguards could be adopted by interested medical associations and constitutional violation is enough to support the judgment that we reach here.

We hold that a liberty interest exists in the choice of how and when one dies, and that the provision of the Washington statute banning assisted suicide, as applied to competent, terminally ill adults who wish to hasten their deaths by obtaining medication prescribed by their doctors, violates the Due Process Clause. We recognize that this decision is a most difficult and controversial one, and that it leaves unresolved a large number of equally troublesome issues that will require resolution in the years ahead. We also recognize that other able and dedicated jurists, construing the Constitution as they believe it must be construed, may disagree not only with the result we reach but with our method of constitutional analysis. Given the nature of the judicial process and the complexity of the task of determining the rights and interests comprehended by the Constitution, good faith disagreements within the judiciary should not surprise or disturb anyone who follows the development of the law. For these reasons, we express our hope that whatever debate may accompany the future exploration of the issues we have touched on today will be conducted in an objective, rational, and constructive manner that will increase, not diminish, respect for the Constitution.

There is one final point we must emphasize. Some argue strongly that decisions regarding matters affecting life or death should not be made by the courts. Essentially, we agree with that proposition. In this case, by permitting the individual to exercise the right to choose we are following the constitutional mandate to take such decisions out of the hands of the government, both state and federal, and to put them where they rightly belong, in the hands of the people. We are allowing individuals to make the decisions that so profoundly affect their very existence—and precluding the state from intruding excessively into that critical realm. The Constitution and the courts stand as a bulwark between individual freedom and arbitrary and intrusive governmental power. . . . Those who believe strongly that death must come without physician assistance are free to follow that creed, be they doctors or patients. They are not free, however, to force their views, their religious convictions, or their philosophies on all the other members of a democratic society, and to compel those whose values differ with theirs to die painful, protracted, and agonizing deaths.

Quill v. Vacco
United States Court of Appeals,
Second Circuit
1996 WL 148605 (N.Y.)

[Editor's introduction: In 1991 the New England Journal of Medicine published an article by Timothy Quill, M.D., in which he described his assistance in the suicide of a patient who had acute leukemia, even though he knew he was breaking a New York law that prohibited acts of assisted suicide. In 1994, Dr. Quill, joined by two other physicians and three terminally ill patients, challenged the state law in the U.S. District Court. The patients indicated that they wanted "medical assistance in the form of medications prescribed by physicians to be self-administered for the purpose of hastening death." The physicians said the "proper and human medical practice should include the ability to prescribe medication [in circumstances like these three cases] which will enable a patient to commit suicide" (Quill v. Koppell, 870 F.Supp. 78, 80 [S.D.N.Y. 1994]). All three patients, one with thyroid cancer and two with end-stage AIDS, died months before the court denied their motion and dismissed the case. The case was appealed, and a three-judge panel of the U.S. Court of Appeals, Second Circuit, reversed the district court decision. Written by Circuit Judge Roger Miner, the Second Circuit opinion ruled that the New York law violates the Equal Protection Clause of the Fourteenth Amendment. Circuit Judge Guido Calabresi agreed that the New York law is unconstitutional but indicated in a separate written opinion that New York or some other state might in the future enact a law regulating assisted suicide that could be constitutional. In October 1996, the U. S. Supreme Court agreed to review together the decisions of the Second and Ninth Circuits.]

MINER, Circuit Judge:
  Plaintiffs-appellants Timothy E. Quill, Samuel C. Klagsbrun and Howard A. Grossman appeal from a summary judgment entered in the United States District Court for the Southern District of New York. . . . The action was brought by plaintiffs-appellants, all of whom are physicians, to declare unconstitutional in part two New York statutes penalizing assistance in suicide. The physicians contend that each statute is invalid to the extent that it prohibits them from acceding to the requests of terminally-ill, mentally competent patients for help in hastening death. . . . We reverse in part, holding that physicians who

are willing to do so may prescribe drugs to be self-administered by mentally competent patients who seek to end their lives during the final stages of a terminal illness. . . .

The action giving rise to this appeal was commenced by a complaint filed on July 20, 1994. The plaintiffs named in that complaint were the three physicians who are the appellants here and three individuals then in the final stages of terminal illness: Jane Doe (who chose to conceal her actual identity), George A. Kingsley and William A. Barth. . . .

As in Bowers [Bowers v. Hardwick] the statutes plaintiffs seek to declare unconstitutional here cannot be said to infringe upon any fundamental right or liberty. As in Bowers, the right contended for here cannot be considered so implicit in our understanding of ordered liberty that neither justice nor liberty would exist if it were sacrificed. Nor can it be said that the right to assisted suicide claimed by plaintiffs is deeply rooted in the nation's traditions and history. . . .

The right to assisted suicide finds no cognizable basis in the Constitution's language or design, even in the very limited cases of those competent persons who, in the final stages of terminal illness, seek the right to hasten death. We therefore decline the plaintiffs' invitation to identify a new fundamental right, in the absence of a clear direction from the Court whose precedents we are bound to follow. . . .

According to the Fourteenth Amendment, the equal protection of the laws cannot be denied by any State to any person within its jurisdiction. . . . This constitutional guarantee simply requires the states to treat in a similar manner all individuals who are similarly situated.

Applying the foregoing principles to the New York statutes criminalizing assisted suicide, it seems clear that: 1) the statutes in question fall within the category of social welfare legislation and therefore are subject to rational basis scrutiny upon judicial review; 2) New York law does not treat equally all competent persons who are in the final stages of fatal illness and wish to hasten their deaths; 3) the distinctions made by New York law with regard to such persons do not further any legitimate state purpose; and 4) accordingly, to the extent that the statutes in question prohibit persons in the final stages of terminal illness from having assistance in ending their lives by the use of self-administered, prescribed drugs, the statutes lack any rational basis and are violative of the Equal Protection Clause. . . .

In view of the foregoing, it seems clear that New York does not treat similarly circumstanced persons alike: those in the final stages of terminal illness who are on life-support systems are allowed to hasten their deaths by directing the removal of such systems; but those who are similarly situated, except for the previous attachment of life-sustaining equipment, are not allowed to hasten death by self-admin-istering prescribed drugs. . . .

[T]he writing of a prescription to hasten death, after consultation with a patient, involves a far less active role for the physician than is required in bringing about death through asphyxiation, starvation and/or dehydration. Withdrawal of life support requires physicians or those acting at their direction physically to remove equipment and, often, to administer palliative drugs which may themselves contribute to death. The ending of life by these means is nothing more nor less than assisted suicide. It simply cannot be said that those mentally compe-tent, terminally-ill persons who seek to hasten death but whose treatment does not include life support are treated equally.

A finding of unequal treatment does not, of course, end the inquiry, unless it is determined that the inequality is not rationally related to some legitimate state interest. The burden is upon the plaintiffs to demonstrate irrationality. . . . But what interest can the state possibly have in requiring the prolongation of a life that is all but ended? Surely, the state's interest lessens as the potential for life diminishes. . . . And what business is it of the state to require the continuation of agony when the result is imminent and inevitable? What concern prompts the state to interfere with a mentally competent patient's "right to define [his] own concept of existence, of meaning, of the universe, and of the mystery of human life," Planned Parenthood v. Casey . . . , when the patient seeks to have drugs prescribed to end life during the final stages of a terminal illness? The greatly reduced interest of the state in preserving life compels the answer to these questions: "None.". . .

The New York statutes prohibiting assisted suicide, which are similar to the Washington statute, do not serve any of the state interests noted, in view of the statutory and common law schemes allowing suicide through the withdrawal of life-sustaining treatment. Physicians do not fulfill the role of "killer" by prescribing drugs to hasten death any more than they do by disconnecting life-support systems. Like-wise, "psychological pressure" can be applied just as much upon the elderly and infirm to consent to withdrawal of life-sustaining equip-ment as to take drugs to hasten death. There is no clear indication that there has been any problem in regard to the former, and there should be none as to the latter. In any event, the state of New York may establish rules and procedures to assure that all choices are free of such pressures. . . .

Finally, it seems clear that most physicians would agree on the definition of "terminally ill," at least for the purpose of the relief that plaintiffs seek. The plaintiffs seek to hasten death only where a patient is in the "final stages" of "terminal illness," and it seems even more certain that physicians would agree on when this condition occurs. Physicians are accustomed to advising patients and their families in this regard and frequently do so when decisions are to be made regarding the furnishing or withdrawal of life-support systems. Again, New York may define that stage of illness with greater particularity, require the opinion of more than one physician or impose any other obligation upon patients and physicians who collaborate in hastening death.

The New York statutes criminalizing assisted suicide violate the Equal Protection Clause because, to the extent that they prohibit a physician from prescribing medications to be self-administered by a mentally competent, terminally-ill person in the final stages of his terminal illness, they are not rationally related to any legitimate state interest.

CONTRIBUTORS

Darrel W. Amundsen, Ph.D., is Professor of Classics at Western Washington University. He is the author of *Medicine, Society, and Faith in the Ancient and Medieval Worlds*.

Dan W. Brock, Ph.D., is Professor of Philosophy and Director of the Center for Biomedical Ethics in the School of Medicine at Brown University. He is the author of *Life and Death: Philosophical Essays in Biomedical Ethics*.

Howard Brody, M.D., Ph.D., is Professor of Family Practice and Philosophy and Director of the Center for Ethics and Humanities in the Life Sciences, Michigan State University. He has been involved with the issue of physician-assisted suicide as Chair of the Committee on Bioethics of the Michigan State Medical Society and as Chair of the Commission on Death and Dying established by the Michigan legislature to study this problem in 1993–94.

Ira R. Byock, M.D., has worked in hospice care for over seventeen years and is currently Director of the Palliative Care Service in Missoula, Montana. He has chaired the Ethics Committee and serves on the Board of Directors of the Academy of Hospice Physicians.

Daniel Callahan, Ph.D., is co-founder and president of the Hastings Center. He is the author, most recently, of *The Troubled Dream of Life: In Search of a Peaceful Death*.

Christine K. Cassel, M.D., FACP, is Chairman of the Department of Geriatrics and Adult Development of Mount Sinai Medical Center and Professor of Geriatrics and Medicine. Among her publications is the edited textbook *Geriatric Medicine: Principles and Practice*.

Carol J. Gill, Ph.D., is President of the Chicago Institute of Disability Research. She is also an Adjunct Assistant Professor of Physical Medicine and Rehabilitation at Northwestern University Medical School.

Kristi L. Kirschner, M.D., holds the Coleman Foundation Chair in Rehabilitation Medicine at the Rehabilitation Institute of Chicago. She is an attending physician and director of the Disability Ethics Program at the Rehabilitation Institute.

Robert Koepp, M.A., is an Administrative Fellow at the Center for Biomedical Ethics and a graduate student in the Philosophy Department at the University of Minnesota.

Steven Miles, M.D., is an Associate Professor of Medicine in the Department of Medicine and a Faculty Associate at the Center for Biomedical Ethics at the University of Minnesota. He is also an attending physician with the Department of Geriatric Medicine at St. Paul Ramsey Medical Center in St. Paul.

Demetra M. Pappas, J.D., M.Sc., is a Research Fellow at the Center for Biomedical Ethics at the University of Minnesota and a doctoral candidate in the Departments of Sociology and Law at the London School of Economics and Political Science.

Harold Y. Vanderpool, Ph.D., Th.M., is Professor of the History and Philosophy of Medicine, Institute for the Medical Humanities, University of Texas Medical Branch in Galveston.

Robert F. Weir, Ph.D., is Professor of Pediatrics and Religious Studies and Director of the Program in Biomedical Ethics and Medical Humanities at the University of Iowa College of Medicine. He is the author of *Abating Treatment with Critically Ill Patients*.

William J. Winslade, Ph.D., J.D., is James Wade Rockwell Professor of Philosophy in Medicine at the Institute for the Medical Humanities, University of Texas Medical Branch, Galveston, where he is Professor of Preventive Medicine and Community Health and Professor of Psychiatry and Behavior Sciences. He is also Distinguished Visiting Professor of Law at the University of Houston Law and Policy Institute at the Law Center.

Susan M. Wolf, J.D., is an Associate Professor of Law and Medicine in the College of Law and a Faculty Associate at the Center for Biomedical Ethics at the University of Minnesota. She is also the editor of *Feminism and Bioethics*.

INDEX

abating life-sustaining treatment, viii–ix, 77–
  80, 155–58, 168, 170–84, 188, 231
abortion, 25, 27, 167–88
Academy of Hospice and Palliative Medi-
  cine, xiii
Adkins, Janet, 56, 87, 224, 227, 243
advanced directive, 209
"aid in dying," viii, 57
AIDS, x–xi, 224
Alcser, K., 151n, 222n
Alden, Timothy, 59n
Alpers, Ann, 223n, 239n
ALS (amyotrophic lateral sclerosis), 76, 78,
  92–93, 123, 127, 218, 224
Alvarez, Alfred, 4–8, 27, 28n, 41, 43
Alvarez, Walter, 61–62n
Alzheimer's disease, 55
Ambrose, 12, 19–20, 30–31n
American Association of Progressive Medi-
  cine, 42
American Geriatrics Society, viii, xvn
American Medical Association, viii, xvn,
  35–37, 40, 177, 198n
Americans with Disabilities Act, 216
Amundsen, Darrel, xiii, xvn, 3–30, 59n
Angell, Marcia, 60–61n, 103n
Annas, George, 66n
Aronstan, N. E., 40, 60–61n
Asnes, Marion, 199n
assisted suicide, viii, xiii
  American views, xiii
  possible legal right, 207
August, Allison, 176, 178, 190n, 196–97n
Augustine, 6–9, 11–16, 20–25, 31n
Australia: Rights of the Terminally Ill Bill in
  the Northern Territory, 208, 215–20
Ayd, Frank, 46, 63n

Bach, John, 165n
Bachman, Jerald, xvin, 151n, 222n, 237n
Back, Anthony, xvin
Bacon, Francis, 59n
Baldwin, Simeon, 62n
Barnes, Timothy, 30n
Baron, Charles, 191n

Barth, William, x, 254
Bartling v. Superior Court, 132n, 165n
Barton, Rebecca, 165n
Battin, Margaret, 7, 28–29n, 32n, 150n
Bayer, Edward, 64n
Bayles, Michael, 132n
Beauchamp, Tom, xivn, 64n, 134n, 199n
Behnke, John, 58n, 64n
Bell, Clark, 61–62n
Bender, Leslie, 189n
Benke, Nikolaus, 200n
Benrubi, G., 150n
Benshoof, Janet, 199n
Berde, C., 133n
Bergen, Ronald, 134n
Bernat, James, 103n
Billings, Andrew, 197n
Bjorck, Catherine, 66n
Blackmun, Justice Harry, 3, 5, 26–27, 28n,
  193n
Blank, Robert, 65n
Blatt, S., 133n
Blendon, Robert, xvin
Bloch, Kate, 194n
Block, Susan, 197n
Bok, Sissela, 56, 58n, 64n, 66n
Bonnicksen, Andrea, 65n
Bostrom, Barry, 165n
Bouvia, Elisabeth, 160–61, 163
Bouvia v. Glenchur, 166n
Bouvia v. Superior Court, 56, 132n
Bowers v. Hardwick, 194n
Bowlby, J., 133n
Boyko, E., 151n
Breezer, Judge Robert, 207, 210, 212
Brennan, Justice William, 171
Breo, Dennis, 61n
Brill, A. A., 39, 61n
Brock, Dan, xiii–xiv, 64n, 86–103, 103n,
  113, 133n, 192n, 222n
Brody, Baruch, xvn, 29n
Brody, Howard, xiii, xvn, 115, 117, 133–
  34n, 136–50, 150–51n, 222n, 238n
Buckman, R., 150n
Bunster-Burotto, Ximena, 194n

Burman, David, 189*n,* 192*n*
Burt, Robert, 200*n*
Butler, Judith, 200*n*
Byock, Ira, xiii, xv*n,* 107–32, 133–35*n,*
    151*n*

Caine, E., 151*n,* 222–23*n*
Calabresi, Judge Guido, 194–95*n,* 207
California: referendum on PAS, viii
Callahan, Daniel, xiii, 64*n,* 69–85, 151*n,*
    198–99*n,* 237*n*
Callanan, M., 134*n*
Campbell, Courtney, 135*n*
cancer, ix–xi, 224
Cantor, Norman, 49, 63*n*
Caplan, Richard, xiv
Capron, Alexander, 65*n,* 190*n*
Caralis, P., xvi*n*
Cardozo, Justice Benjamin, 110, 155
care of dying patients, 41, 114, 123–25
"Care of the Hopelessly Ill," 115
Carney, Tom, xvi*n*
Carr, D., 133*n*
Carrel, Alexis, 42
Carrick, Paul, xv*n*
Carson, Ronald, 237*n*
Case, Mary Anne, 200*n*
Cassel, Christine, xiv, xv*n,* 127, 133*n,* 155–
    64, 165*n,* 191*n*
Cassell, Eric, 103*n,* 134*n*
CeloCruz, Maria, 65*n*
Chao, Julie, 199*n*
Chapman, Nathaniel, 34
Chassman, J., 192*n*
Cherny, N., 134*n*
Childress, James, xiv*n,* 64*n,* 134*n*
Chrysostom, John, 18–19, 24, 31*n*
City of God, 13, 20, 22, 24
Clausen, Sara, 58*n*
Cleeland, Charles, 151*n,* 197*n*
Clement of Alexandria, 16, 24, 30*n*
Close, L., 135*n*
Code of Ethics, American Medical Associa-
    tion, 35–37, 40
Cohen, Adam, 189*n*
Cohen, J., xvi*n,* 151*n*
Cohen, Marshall, 195*n*
Colburn, Don, 165*n*
Coleman, Diane, 166*n*
Colen, B., 189*n,* 197*n*
comfort care, 45, 114

*Compassion in Dying v. State of Washing-
    ton,* xii, xvii*n,* 134*n,* 137, 169, 181–82,
    184–85, 189*n,* 191*n,* 192*n,* 194*n,* 196*n,*
    212, 215, 221–22*n,* 238*n,* 246-52
Conroy, Claire, 50
Constitution, U.S. *See* Fourteenth Amend-
    ment
Conwell, Y., 151*n,* 222–23*n*
Cook, E., 132*n*
Cooper, John, xv*n,* 29*n*
Cornell, Drucilla, 194*n*
Coryell, William, 197*n*
Costigan, Gregory, 62*n*
Cotton, Paul, 165*n*
Council on Ethical and Judicial Affairs,
    American Medical Association, 177
Courtwright, David, 58–60*n*
Cover, Robert, 201*n*
Covinsky, K., 132*n*
Cowley, L., xv*n*
Cranford, Ronald, 133*n*
Crosby, C., xvi*n*
Cross, Barbara, 59*n*
Crown, W., 135*n*
Cruz, Celo, 239*n*
*Cruzan v. Director, Missouri Department
    of Health,* 170–77, 181, 186, 192–
    96*n,* 198–99*n,* 215
Curran, William, xv*n,* 63*n*
Curtis, Diane, 199*n*
Cyprian, 22–23, 31*n*

Daniels, Norman, 113, 133*n*
Davies, Miranda, 194*n*
Davis, W., 133*n*
De patientia, 21
Deichgräber, Karl, 29*n*
Dendy, W. C., 60*n*
Dennis v. Vaaco, 189*n*
depression, viii, 83, 89–90, 118–19, 123,
    127, 142, 156, 161, 167, 179, 185,
    217, 227
DeVore, Melanie, xiv
"Diane," 56, 120, 127, 227
Dickson, Samuel, 60*n*
Diekstra, René, 118, 134*n*
Dillon, P., 103*n*
Dinwiddie, S., 222*n*
Divine Institutes, 16, 24
"Doctors Must Not Kill," 92

"Doe, Jane," ix, 254
Donnelly, John, 66*n*
Donovan, M., 103*n*
Doughtery, Margot, 164*n*
Doukas, David, xvi*n*, 151*n*, 222*n*
Downie, Jocelyn, 189*n*
Dresser, Rebecca, 199*n*
Droge, Arthur, 9, 29–31*n*
DuBose, Edwin, 58*n*, 66*n*
Durkheim, Emile, 8–11, 29*n*
Dworkin, Ronald, 189*n*, 192*n*, 195*n*
Dyck, Arthur, xv*n*, 39, 61*n*, 63*n*, 65*n*
dying at home, 33–37
dying in hospitals, 43–47

Edelstein, Ludwig, 5, 28*n*
Edwards, M., 150*n*
Ehrenreich, Barbara, 197*n*
Eissler, K., 64*n*
Emanuel, Ezekiel, 58*n*, 63*n*
Emanuel, Linda, 63*n*, 192*n*
emphysema, 224
Endicott, Jean, 197*n*
English, Diedre, 197*n*
Epistle to Diognetius, 15
Epitome, 16, 24
Erikson, Erik, 112, 133*n*
Estes, C., 135*n*
Ethical Issues in Suicide, 7
"The Ethics of Terminal Care," 113
Eusebius, 12–13, 17–18, 30–31*n*
euthanasia, ix, xi, 8, 35, 37–43, 45, 51–55,
       70–80, 114, 117, 191*n*, 218, 231
    legalization, xi
    "nonvoluntary," 81
    voluntary, viii, xiii, 86–102, 168–70, 205,
       208, 215–16, 220
Euthanasia Society of America, 40, 42, 52

Fajer, Marc, 200*n*
Federrman, D., 133*n*
Ferngren, Gary, 31*n*
Fihn, S., 151*n*
Final Exit, 57
Fletcher, George, 239*n*
Fletcher, Joseph, 52–53, 61*n*, 64–66*n*, 151*n*
Fogarty, Thomas, xvi*n*
Foley, Kathleen, 151*n*, 197*n*, 237*n*
Fourteenth Amendment (to U.S. Constitu-
       tion), 3, 169–70, 186–88, 230
Frankena, William, 29*n*

Frankl, Victor, 134*n*
Fraser, C., 65*n*
French, Roger, 29*n*
Frend, W. H. C., 30–31*n*
Frickey, Phil, 193*n*
Fried, T., xvi*n*
Furlow, Thomas, 53, 65*n*
Fye, W., xv*n*, 58*n*, 60*n*

Garrison, Elise, 29*n*
Gaylin, Willard, 65*n*, 91, 103*n*, 150*n*, 199*n*
Gerhart, Kenneth, 165*n*
Gert, Bernard, 103*n*
Geyer-Kordesch, Johanna, 29*n*
Gianelli, Diane, xvi*n*
Gill, Carol, xiv, 155–64, 166*n*
Gilligan, Carol, 197*n*
Ginsburg, Ruth, 190*n*
Glaser, Barney, 44, 62*n*
Goebel, Brian, 189*n*, 192*n*, 198*n*
Goethe, C., 134*n*
Goldman, L., 103*n*
Gomez, Carlos, 134*n*
Gonin, R., 151*n*
Goodman, Ellen, 189*n*
Gorenflo, D., 151*n*, 222*n*
Gostin, Larry, 151*n*
Gourevitch, Danielle, xv*n*, 31*n*
Graber, Glenn, 192*n*
Graber, Mark, xvii*n*
"Great Persecution," 12–21
Greene, W., 133*n*
Grier, C., 133*n*
Griffin, Miriam, 29*n*
Grossman, Howard, 254
Grubb, A., 222*n*
Guisinger, S., 133*n*

Hahn, Harlan, 166*n*
Hamel, Ron, 58*n*, 66*n*
Hamilton, P., 134*n*
Hammond, J., xvi*n*
Hanson, M. J., 132*n*
Hare, J., 135*n*
Harrell, L., 222*n*
Harris v. McRae, 191*n*
Hassan, R., 222*n*
Hastings Center, 132*n*
Hatfield, A., 151*n*
Hegland, Kenney, 63*n*
Hemlock Society, 10, 56-57

Hendin, Herbert, 134*n*
Hermreck, Arlo, 62*n*
Herr, Stanley, 165*n*
Hippocratic Oath, vii, 5, 26–27, 109, 140,
   185
Hirzel, R., 29*n*
Hitchcock, Frank, 40, 60–61*n*
Hobbins v. Attorney General of Michigan,
   239*n*
Hoffman, M., 133*n*
Holden, C., 135*n*
Homilies, 15
Hooker, Worthington, 36–37, 59–60*n*
hospice care:
   as alternative to physician-assisted sui-
      cide, xiii, 111–17, 126–32, 144–45,
      187
   benefits, xiii, 107–32, 143–45, 149, 187
Hughes, E. C., 132*n*
Hume, David, 38
Humphrey, Derek, 10, 56-57, 65–66*n*
Huntington disease, 209

ICD Survey of Disabled Americans, 165*n*
In re A.C., 193*n*
Ingram, K., 222*n*
Iowa:
   survey of patients, xii
   survey of physicians, xi
"It's Over, Debbie," 54, 91

Jackson, Charles, 58*n*
Jacoby, George, 62*n*
Jacox, A., 133*n*
Jean's Way, 56
Jecker, Nancy, 66*n*, 197*n*
Jennings, Bruce, 132*n*
Jerome, 12, 19–20, 24, 30–31*n*
Jesus, 14
Job, 21
Jonsen, Albert, 58*n*, 65*n*, 151*n*
Judas, 10, 14, 18
Justin, 14–15, 24

Kadish, Sanford, 29*n*
Kamisar, Yale, xv*n*, 190*n*
Kaplan, David, xv*n*
Karnofsky, David, 41
Karst, Kenneth, 190*n*
Kass, Leon, 101–102, 103*n*, 150*n*, 196*n*,
   199*n*
Kaufman, Judge Richard, 3–7, 26–27, 28*n*

Kaufmann, G., 135*n*
Kaye, M., 223*n*
Kearney, M., 134*n*
Keller, Martin, 197*n*
Kelley, P., 134*n*
Kempster, Walter, 62*n*
Kennedy, Justice Anthony, 171, 193*n*
Kennedy, Ian, 222*n*
Kevorkian, Jack, vii, xii, 3, 56–57, 87, 150*n*,
   189*n*, 206–12, 224, 226, 230, 243
Kingsley, George, 254
Kirschner, Kristi, xiv, 155–64
Klagsbrun, Samuel, 253
Klastersky, J., 63*n*
Klein, Catherine, 194*n*
Kline, Robert, 189*n*, 192*n*
Knox, Richard, xvi*n*
Koepp, Robert, xiv, 205–20
Kohl, Marvin, 61*n*, 65*n*
Kohn, Lawrence, 63–64*n*
Koziol-McLain, Jane, 165*n*
Kreimer, Seth, 188*n*, 192*n*, 198–99*n*
Kübler-Ross, Elisabeth, 48, 63*n*, 134*n*
Kudlien, Fridolf, 29*n*
Kurtz, Paul, 65*n*
Kushner, Howard, 196–97*n*

Lactantius, 16, 24, 30*n*
Ladd, John, 103*n*
Law, Sylvia, 189–90*n*, 198*n*
Lee, Melinda, xvi*n*, 223*n*, 237*n*
Lee v. State of Oregon, xvii*n*, 221*n*, 238*n*
legal minors, 212, 214
Lessenberry, Jack, 189*n*
Let Me Die before I Wake, 56
Lichtenstein, R., 151*n*
Lichtenthaeler, Charles, 29*n*
Life, Death, and the Law, 210
Linkins, K., 135*n*
Livingston, William, 33, 58*n*
Lo, Bernard, 223*n*, 239*n*
Locke, John, 209
Loewy, Eric, 192*n*
Longmore, Paul, 164–66*n*
Loraux, Nicole, 197*n*
Lorber, Judith, 200*n*
Loving v. Virginia, 190n
Lowenstein, Steven, 165*n*
Lynn, Joanne, 64*n*, 103*n*, 151*n*

MacBride, Jonathan, 190*n*
MacDonald, Arthur, 60–62*n*

MacKinnon, Catharine, 200–201*n*
Management of Cancer Pain Guideline Panel, 151*n*
Mann, Horace, 60*n*
Mappes, Thomas, 64*n*
Marker, Rita, 58*n*
Markides, Kyriakos, 238*n*
Marshall, Justice Thurgood, 171
Marson, D., 222*n*
Martyr, Justin, 30*n*
martyrdom, 8–9, 11–20, 25
Marx, C. F. H., 59–60*n*
Marzen, Thomas, 190*n,* 194*n*
Massachusetts: survey of physicians, xi
Materson, Richard, 166*n*
Matthews, P., 135*n*
Maximilla, 18
May, D., 28*n*
McAfee, Larry, 156–63, 165*n*
McCarrick, Pat, 65*n*
McCue, Jack, 65*n*
Mcguire, L., 103*n*
McNeil, John, 165*n*
Meier, Diane, xiv, xv*n,* 127, 133*n,* 151*n,* 165*n,* 191*n*
Meisel, Alan, 194*n*
Mero, Ralph, 65*n*
Michigan: survey of physicians, xi
Michigan State Medical Society, xiii
Migne, Jacques, 31*n*
Miles, Steven, xiv, 134*n,* 145, 150*n,* 165*n,* 176, 178, 190*n,* 196–97*n,* 205–20, 223*n,* 238*n,* 229
Mill, John Stuart, 175, 195*n*
Miller, Franklin, xv*n,* 115, 117, 133*n,* 141, 150–51*n,* 192*n,* 213, 218, 220, 223*n,* 238–39*n*
Milligan, Maureen, 237*n*
minors/legal minors, 212, 214
Misbin, Robert, 64*n,* 102*n*
Mitchell, H., 133*n*
Mogielnicki, R. Peter, 103*n*
Montanus, 18
More, Ellen, 237*n*
morphine, 34, 37
Mount, Balfour, 134*n*
Munk, William, 59–60*n*
Munson, Ronald, 64*n*
murder charges, xii

National Association of Rehabilitation Facilities Research and Information Center, 165*n*
National Hospice Organization, viii, xvi*n,* 116, 135*n*
neurological diseases, xi
Nevins, Michael, 64*n*
New Hampshire: survey of physicians, xi
New York State Task Force on Life and the Law, 142, 190–92*n*
Nielsen, Joyce, 196*n*
A Noble Death, 9
Noonan, Judge John, 212, 246
Norcross, Alastair, 103*n*
Nuland, Sherwin, 238–39*n*
Numbers, Ronald, 59*n*
nurses, 139, 147, 164
Nutton, Vivian, 29*n*

O'Connor, Justice Sandra Day, 171, 193*n*
Ogilvie, Alan, 198*n*
Oken, Donald, 62*n*
On Death and Dying, 48
opium, 34
Oregon:
    Death with Dignity Act, xii, 57, 207, 213–20, 231–32, 236
    survey of physicians, xi
Orentlicher, David, xv*n*
Orloff, Leslye, 194*n*
Orlowski, James, 198*n*
Osler, William, 61*n*

pain, x–xi, 53, 55, 69, 89, 98, 227–28
Palko v. Connecticut, 193*n*
palliative care: as alternative to physician-assisted suicide, xiii, 111, 114–17, 126–32, 138, 142, 147- 50, 210, 218, 220, 227, 234, 236
Pappas, Demetra, xiv, 205–20, 221–22*n*
Paquette, S., 135*n*
Parkinson's disease, 224
The Patient as Person, 47
patients:
    nonphysical concerns, xi
    views toward euthanasia, xi
    views toward physician-assisted suicide, xi–xii
Paul, 10, 14
Payne, R., 133*n*
Pellegrino, Edmund, xv*n,* 64*n,* 150*n,* 199*n*
People v. Kevorkian, 189*n,* 194–95*n,* 208, 243–45
Pernick, Martin, 59–60*n,* 62*n*

Persels, J., 223*n*
persons with disabilities, viii, xiii, 83, 126, 155–64, 181–82, 187, 208, 215–16, 231
  as possibly vulnerable to physician-assisted suicide, xiii–xiv, 76–77, 83, 123, 125–26, 155–64, 181–82, 208, 212, 215–16
Peter, 15
Petty, Thomas, 62*n*
pharmacists, 139
physician-assisted suicide:
  ancient Greek practices, vii
  attitudes of general public, xi–xii, 226
  attitudes of patients, xi–xii, 225
  attitudes of physicians, x–xii
  concept, viii, 208
  different from abating life-sustaining treatment, ix, 77–80
  factor of autonomy, xiii, 55, 72–77, 82, 89–91, 96, 101, 110, 119, 158, 161–64, 208–16
  factor of control, 101, 227, 229
  factor of gender, 167–70, 174–82, 186–88
  factor of suffering, 227
  guidelines, xiv
  legalization, xi–xii, xiv, 127–32, 143, 167–88, 205–20, 230–34
  liberty interest, 3, 170–86, 205, 224, 227, 230–34
  medical conditions, ix–x, 76, 78, 92–93, 123, 127
  morality, xiii, 70
  morally different from euthanasia, ix
  no moral difference from euthanasia, ix, 71–73, 77–80, 86–95, 169
  practice, xi, 70, 72
  public policy, xiv, 70, 205–21, 224–36
  role of enabler, viii, xiii
  role of physicians, viii, 43, 57, 84–85, 90, 100–102, 107–21, 123–25, 128–32, 136–50, 158–61, 163–64, 181, 184–88, 217, 224, 228–29
  safeguards, xiv, 69–71, 80–83, 97–100, 143
  surveys of physicians' opinions, x–xii
physicians:
  attitudes toward physician-assisted suicide, x
  in the Netherlands, 80–82, 118, 127,
147, 168, 184, 211, 226
  role in assisted suicide, 57, 84–85, 90, 100–102, 107–21, 123–25, 136–50, 158–61, 163–64, 181, 184, 188, 217, 224, 228–29
  surveys of opinion, x–xii, 226
  trustworthiness, xii
Pijnenborg, Loes, 135*n*, 198*n*
Pilate, 18
Pius XII, Pope, 47, 63*n*
Planned Parenthood v. Casey, 170–77, 181, 186, 192*n*, 216
Plato, 6
"A Plea for Beneficent Euthanasia," 54
Portenoy, R., 134*n*
Posner, Richard, 238*n*
Potts, S., 198*n*
Povelones, Arthur, 238*n*
Powell, John, 189*n*
Powell, R., 166*n*
President's Commission for the Study of Ethical Problems in Medicine, 50, 63*n*, 132*n*, 155, 164–65*n*, 222*n*
Proactive Responses to the Euthanasia/Assisted Suicide Debate, 116, 133*n*
process of dying, 121–25

quadriplegia, 76, 155–58
quality of life, 53, 228
Quasten, J., 30*n*
Quill, Timothy, vii, xii, xv*n*, 56, 66*n*, 120, 127, 133*n*, 134*n*, 150–51*n*, 165*n*, 191*n*, 206, 208–10, 218, 237–38*n*, 253
Quill v. Koppell, 221*n*, 253
Quill v. Vaaco, xvi*n*, 169, 174, 189*n*, 192*n*, 194*n*, 206, 238*n*, 253–55
Quimby, Isaac, 41
Quinlan, Karen, 49–50

Rachels, James, 103*n*
Raffin, T., xv*n*, 132*n*
Rakowski, Eric, 198*n*
Ramsey, Paul, 47–50, 63–65*n*
refusal of medical care, 47–51
Rehnquist, Justice William, 3, 171, 183
Reich, Warren, 58*n*
Reinhardt, Judge Stephen, 246
Reinhardt, Uwe, 201*n*
Reiser, Stanley, xv*n*, 58*n*, 63*n*
Rhode Island: survey of physicians, xi
right to die, 211

Rist, J., 29*n*
Rivlin, David, 155–63
Roberts, Dorothy, 200*n*
Robertson, T. T., 41
Rodriguez, Sue, ix
Rodriguez v. British Columbia, xvi*n*, 192*n*
Roe v. Wade, 3, 5, 182, 190*n*, 198*n*
Rogers, Carl, 123
Rosenberg, Louis, 40, 60–61*n*
Ross, Judith, 133*n*
Rothstein, Judge Barbara, 119
Rothstein, William, 58–59*n*
Rousseau, Jean-Jacques, 6
Ruark, J., 132*n*
rule of double effect, 206
Rutman, D., 222*n*
Ryan, C., 223*n*
Rynearson, Edward, 47, 63*n*

Samson, 24
sanctity of life, 6, 53, 183, 209, 236
The Sanctity of Life and the Criminal Law, 7
Saum, Lewis, 59*n*
Saunders, Cicely, 132, 134*n*
Scalia, Justice Antonin, 193–94*n,* 196*n,* 238*n*
Schloendorff v. Society of New York Hospital, 110, 164*n*
Schmitt, F., 222*n*
Schneider, A., 59*n*
Schneiderman, Lawrence, 190*n*
Scott, Richard, 56
Seaver, Anna, 135*n*
Sedler, Robert, 189*n,* 192*n,* 198*n*
Seid, J., 151*n,* 222*n*
Seidlitz, Larry, xvi*n*
Shapiro, Joseph, 165*n*
Shavelson, Lonnie, 237*n*
Shaw, Don, 65*n*
Sheldon, Tony, 198*n*
Sherwin, Susan, 189*n,* 196*n*
Shih, Willard, 190*n*
Siegler, Mark, 64*n*
Sigerist, Henry, 31*n*
Silberfeld, M., 222*n*
Simons, Marlise, 191*n*
Slome, L., xvi*n*
Smith, Emily, 58*n*
Smith, Nathan, 34
Society for Health and Human Values, viii,

xvi*n,* 165*n,* 238*n*
Solomon, A., 237*n*
Souter, Justice David, 171, 193*n*
Sperry, Willard, 40, 42–43, 60–62*n*
Spielman, Bethany, 165*n*
Spitz, René, 135*n*
St. John-Stevas, Norman, 209, 222*n*
Staquet, M., 63*n*
State v. McAfee, 165n
Steinbock, Bonnie, 103*n*
Steinfels, Peter, 63*n,* 200*n*
Stellings, Brande, 200*n*
Stevens, Justice John Paul, 171, 196*n*
Stevens, Rosemary, 62*n*
Steverns, C., 222*n*
Stoddard, Samuel, 135*n*
Stone, T. Howard, 66*n,* 238*n*
Strauss, Anselm, 44, 62*n*
suffering, x–xi, 22, 26, 38, 56, 69, 75–76, 83, 89, 98–100, 227–28
suicide:
 ancient Jewish attitudes, 6
 attitudes of Pythagoreans, 27
 decriminalization, 210–11
 definition, viii
 Durkheim's definition, 8–11
 early Stoic attitudes, 16
 factor of chastity, 20, 24
 factor of control, 101, 119
 factor of gender, 168, 174
 factor of individual well-being, xiii, 89–91, 101
 factor of self-determination, xiii, 72–77, 82, 89, 101, 110, 119, 158, 161–64
 in ancient Rome, 4
 in classical Greece, 4
 in early Christianity, 7–26
 in the Bible, 6, 10, 20
 legalization, 3, 210
 methods, viii
 societal consequences, 71, 80–83, 97–100
Sullivan, Joseph, 61*n*
Sunstein, Cass, 190*n*
Sutton, Marily, 65*n*
Swift, Jonathan, 52
Szalay, Ulrike, xvi*n*

Tabor, James, 9, 29–31*n*
Tate, P., 222*n*
Temkin, C. Lillian, 28*n*

Temkin, Owsei, 28–29*n*
Teno, J., 151*n*
terminal illness, 26, 47
terminal sedation, 117
Tertullian, 16, 30*n*
Tessler, S., 164*n*
Tilton, Margaret, 165*n*
Tolle, Susan, 150*n*
Tooley, Michael, 103*n*
Torrey, E., 64*n*
Townsend, P., 150*n*
Tribe, Laurence, 190*n*
Truog, Robert, 133*n*
Tsarouhas, Antonios, 194*n*
Tucker, Kathryn, 189*n*, 192*n*

U.S. Bureau of the Census, 197*n*
U.S. Constitution. *See* Fourth Amendment;
    U.S. Supreme Court
U.S. Court of Appeals, Second Circuit, xii,
    xiv, 167, 169, 206–208, 214, 230–33
U.S. Court of Appeals, Ninth Circuit, xii,
    xiv, 137, 167, 169, 183, 205, 212, 214,
    230–33, 246–52
U.S. District Court of Oregon, xii
U.S. Supreme Court, xii, 137, 167, 171,
    181, 207, 231–34. *See also individual
    justices by name*

Valdes, Francisco, 200*n*
Van Delden, J., 135*n*
Van der Maas, P. J., 81, 135*n*, 191*n*
van Hooff, Anton, 29*n*, 31*n*
Vance, Richard, 151*n*
Vanderpool, Harold, xiii, 33–67, 58–59*n*,
    60*n*, 63*n*, 113, 133*n*
Veatch, Robert, 49, 62–64*n*
Visser, Henk, 198*n*
Voluntary Euthanasia Legislation Society
    (Britain), 40

Waldron, Jeremy, 103*n*
Walters, LeRoy, 64*n*
Wanzer, Sidney, xv*n*, 102*n*, 132–33*n*, 191*n*

Ward, B., 222*n*
Warren, John, 60*n*
Washington:
    referendum on PAS, viii
    survey of physicians, x–xi
Washington v. Glucksberg, 189*n*, 238*n*
Waterhouse, D., 151*n*, 222*n*
Wear, Andrew, 29*n*
Weir, Jerry, xiv
Weir, Robert, xvi*n*, 65*n*, 191*n*, 238*n*
Weisbard, J., 64*n*
Welter, Barbara, 197*n*
Wennberg, Robert, 39, 61*n*
West, Robin, 194*n*
White, Margot, 199*n*
Whitehead, Alfred North, 236, 239*n*
Whiteneck, Gale, 165*n*
Wilber, Ken, 134*n*
Wilcox, Sandra, 65*n*
Williams, Glanville, 7, 29*n*, 65*n*
Williams, Robert, 65*n*
Williams, Samuel, 40
Williams, Sidney, 38
Williams, Terry, 134*n*
Williamson, William, 61*n*, 63*n*
Wilson, Jerry, 58*n*, 61*n*
Wilson, Susan, 65*n*
Winslade, William, xiv, 66*n*, 224–37, 237–
    38*n*
Wolbarst, Abraham, 61*n*
Wolf, Susan, xiv, 66*n*, 167–88, 189*n*, 190*n*,
    192*n*, 196–200*nn*
Wolhandler, Steven, 190*n*
women, xiii
    as possibly vulnerable to physician-
    assisted suicide, xiii–xiv, 167–88
Wood, Robert, 65*n*, 151*n*
Worcester, Alfred, 40, 46, 61*n*

Young, E., xv*n*
Young, James, 59*n*

Zembaty, Jane, 64*n*
Zoloth-Dorfman, Laurie, 128, 135*n*